Kathy Ogden

Laboratory Tests for the Assessment of Nutritional Status

Authors

H. E. Sauberlich, Ph.D.

J. H. Skala, Ph.D.

Department of Nutrition
Letterman Army Institute
of Research
Presidio of San Francisco, California

R. P. Dowdy, Ph.D.

Department of Human Nutrition
Foods and Food Systems Management
University of Missouri
Columbia, Missouri

CRC PRESS, INC.
Boca Raton, Florida 33431

Copyright © 1974 CRC Press, Inc.
First Published 1974

Second Printing, 1976
Third Printing, 1976
Fourth Printing, 1977
Fifth Printing, 1979

ISBN 0-8493-0121-1
Former ISBN 0-87819-123-2

Library of Congress Catalog Card No. 74-77908
Printed in the United States

This book originally appeared as Volume 4 Issue 3 of *CRC Critical Reviews in Clinical Laboratory Sciences,* a quarterly journal published by CRC Press, Inc. We would like to acknowledge the editorial assistance received by the journal's editors, Dr. John W. King, Cleveland Clinic Foundation, and Dr. Willard R. Faulkner, Vanderbilt University Medical Center. The referee for this article was Dr. Arnold E. Schaefer, Pan American Health Organization, WHO, Washington.

THE AUTHORS

H. E. Sauberlich is Chief of the Department of Nutrition, Letterman Army Institute of Research, Presidio of San Francisco, California. He received his B.A. from Lawrence University, and his M.S. and Ph.D. from the University of Wisconsin.

R. P. Dowdy is Chairman of the Department of Human Nutrition, Foods and Food Systems Management, University of Missouri, Columbia, Missouri. He received his B.S. and M.S. from West Virginia University, and his Ph.D. from North Carolina University.

J. H. Skala is Chief of the Analytical Services Division, Letterman Army Institute of Research, Presidio of San Francisco, California. He received his B.S. from Beloit College, and his M.S. and Ph.D. from the University of Minnesota.

PREFACE

Twenty years ago on February 25 and 26, 1954, a symposium was held in Chicago, Illinois, on *Methods for Evaluation of Nutritional Adequacy and Status*. The symposium was sponsored by the Quartermaster Food and Container Institute for the Armed Forces Quartermaster Research and Development Command and the Medical Nutrition Laboratory (subsequently known as the U.S. Army Medical Research and Nutrition Laboratory). The meeting was held under the guidance of the Committee on Foods of the National Academy of Sciences-National Research Council, Washington, D.C.

The publication summarizing this symposium represented the first major effort directed towards evaluating methods then available for the assessment of nutritional status of individuals or population groups. The merits of existing methods were evaluated and needs for additional techniques emphasized. Subsequently a manual for conducting nutrition surveys evolved from the efforts of the Interdepartmental Committee on Nutrition For National Defense. A "provisional edition" was issued in January 1956 and a second edition published in 1963. This manual was a guide for the nutritional assessment of populations in over 30 countries. Consequently, the biochemical methods and interpretive guides outlined in the manual received extensive application and evaluation.

Nevertheless, during the past ten years, many new or improved techniques have become available for use in the assessment of nutritional status of individuals or population groups. The ICNND nutrition surveys, the White House Conference on Nutrition held in 1969, and the Ten-State Nutrition Survey have provided an impetus for increased nutritional awareness and the need for improved laboratory tests for the evaluation of nutritional status. Consequently, it appeared timely for a review and summary of the laboratory methods currently available and to provide a recognition of their usefulness and limitations in evaluating nutritional status. Hopefully this monograph will serve as a stimulus for the further improvement of the means to assess nutritional status and in the appropriate guidelines for the interpretation of nutritional data. Unfortunately, the scope of this article did not permit a critical review of the individual biochemical methodologies available or a presentation of detailed procedures. Literature citations will provide guidance for the selection of precise methods by the reader. Additional references to articles appearing or overlooked after the completion of the manuscript have been added as an appendix.

We are gratefully indebted to Mrs. Mary Ann Zdunczyk who labored long hours in the typing and revisions of the manuscript. Our thanks are expressed to Mrs. Yvonne M. Rhodes for her tireless efforts in obtaining original articles and assistance in the translation of foreign reports. We wish to express our gratitude to Mr. Carl E. Gordon for his assistance in the preparation of the figures used in this manuscript.

February, 1974
Denver, Colorado

Howerde E. Sauberlich
Richard P. Dowdy
James H. Skala

TABLE OF CONTENTS

LABORATORY TESTS FOR THE ASSESSMENT OF NUTRITIONAL STATUS

Authors: **Howerde E. Sauberlich**
Richard P. Dowdy
James H. Skala
U. S. Army Medical Research and Nutrition Laboratory
Fitzsimons Army Medical Center
Denver, Colorado

Referee: Arnold E. Schaefer
Pan American Health Organization, W.H.O.
Washington, D.C.

I. INTRODUCTION

During the past 10 years, considerable progress has been made in the development of new or modified biochemical methods which have been useful in the evaluation of the nutritional status of individual subjects or of population groups. Moreover, the past decade has provided opportunities for experience and assessment of the available biochemical laboratory techniques through the Interdepartmental Committee on Nutrition for National Defense (ICNND) nutrition surveys of over 30 countries, the nutrition surveys of U.S. military and civilian populations, and certain other nutrition surveys. These surveys have also provided an evaluation of the interpretation standards employed in the appraisal of nutritional status. In the more recent nutrition surveys, newer techniques have been receiving increased attention as well as consideration to additional nutrients. Nutrition surveys are seldom conducted without the inclusion of some form of biochemical assessment, be it only hemoglobin or hematocrit measurements.

For the most part, biochemical measurements represent the most objective assessment of the nutritional status of an individual, frequently providing pre- or subclinical information. For the clinical case, additional biochemical laboratory tests are often available that are not practical for use in field studies or nutrition surveys. Depending upon the measurement employed, information may be obtained as to an individual's present or recent and sometimes long-range nutritional status. In many instances, nutrient intakes are reflected in their level present in blood or urine. These levels can, at least in part, be defined or related to inadequate, low, adequate, or high dietary intakes of the nutrient. Such measurements may not necessarily evaluate accurately a subclinical or marginal deficiency state but are of prognostic value. However, for many nutrients, blood or urine levels of a certain critical level, if continued without increased dietary intakes and concomitant blood or urinary increases, would lead to metabolic abnormalities. Functional biochemical measurements, such as those associated with an abnormal metabolite formation or impaired enzyme function, would detect these metabolic abnormalities and provide early indications of subclinical deficiency states.

For many nutrients, various biochemical laboratory techniques have been investigated, developed, and employed in assessing nutritional status. The majority of these techniques fall into the following categories: (a) measurement of the nutrient level in the blood, (b) measurement of the urinary excretion rate of the nutrient, (c) measurement of urinary metabolites of the nutrient, (d) measurement in blood or urine of abnormal metabolic products resulting from deficient or submarginal intakes of the nutrient, (e) measurement of changes in blood components or enzyme activities that can be related to intakes of the nutrient, and (f) load, saturation, and isotopic tests.

In order to determine nutritional status on a large scale, an important consideration is a knowledge of the type of sample available for assay. The sample should truly and accurately reflect the dietary history of the individual being surveyed, yet it must be easily obtainable. Thus, in the human population one is limited, for the most part, to urine and blood samples. Recently, hair and nails have been suggested as perhaps being appropriate biopsy samples for determining nutritional status with respect to particular nutrients, and these will be discussed briefly later. Generally then, one is restricted to measuring the concentration of a particular nutrient which is either excreted in the urine or circulating in the vascular system. Blood samples do permit the investigator a slightly greater latitude than urine since the former can be partitioned into whole blood, serum, plasma, and/or red blood cells.

Concerning the feasibility of using urine as a nutritional status assay sample, one must consider sample size. Does one attempt to collect a 24-hr sample, which is extremely difficult in a free-living (not confined to a metabolic ward, for example) population? Or would a first-voided morning urine specimen (which may be easily obtained) be adequate? Or, finally, would a randomly voided urine sample be acceptable? Ideally, the 24-hr urine specimen would provide the most accurate estimate of the amount of a particular element which is excreted daily by the renal route. However, Watson and Langford[1] point out two rather serious disadvantages to the 24-hr urine collection technique in general populations. First, it is both physically difficult and sometimes embarrassing for people to make such collections when they are away from home. And secondly, it is difficult to ascertain the completeness of the 24-hr collection since a portion of the specimen could have easily been missed. The other extreme (contrasted to a 24-hr specimen) would be the collection of random urine samples from the subjects being tested. Obvious problems with this type of specimen include: size of sample, physical activity and liquid consumption prior to the collection, and the time of day when the collection is made. All of these factors may markedly affect the concentration of nutrient, metabolite or element in the urine. Between the two extremes mentioned above of urine specimen collection would be an overnight, or first-voided morning specimen. This type of sample would seem to have some merit as it would tend to standardize physical activity and the liquid consumption during the collection period. The first-voided morning specimen also would be much less difficult to obtain than a 24-hr specimen.

In an effort to standardize the variations in urine volumes and the nutrient concentrations in urine specimens, many investigators report data as a ratio of the particular nutrient in the urine to urinary creatinine.[7,8] The rationale for using creatinine as a basis for reporting other constituents seems to be based upon the idea that the daily urinary excretion of creatinine is relatively constant, and this constancy permits extrapolation of a random specimen to a 24-hr basis. This assumption of constancy of creatinine excretion in the urine appears to be based, at least to a large extent, on the report of Clark et al.[2] who concluded that random urine samples could be corrected to a 24-hr basis by using the normal creatinine values. However, other work[3,9,10] has demonstrated a definite variation in the daily excretion of creatinine and also significant diurnal variations in creatinine excretion. Vestergaard and Leverett[4] reported pronounced variations in urinary creatinine excretion during short collection periods (less than 24 hr) and concluded that creatinine is not a good predictor of completeness of short-period urine collections. Accordingly, they suggested that creatinine values should not be used in ratio formation to standardize the excretion data of other urinary constituents. In a study of variability of random urine voidings, Clarke et al.[5] concluded that, in the random sample, creatinine-based ratios for urinary thiamin and riboflavin excretion may be useful for evaluating population nutrition but not for individuals. The usefulness of overnight samples has been found[1] to be of some value for estimating the excretion of certain cations (sodium, potassium, and calcium). However, these data were reported on a "per hour" basis which would be an extremely difficult parameter to ascertain in a large survey situation.

Thus, the problem of obtaining a useful and reliable standardizing index for measuring urinary constituents is not easily solved. For a more detailed discussion of the usefulness of the creatinine index, the reader is referred to the article by Pollack.[6]

This problem of urine volumes and standardization techniques is greatest, as has been noted, when one attempts to determine nutritional status on large numbers of persons under survey-type conditions. There are conditions in which these problems may not be quite as critical. For instance, if one were doing a metabolic ward study in which dietary intake and total excreta could be closely controlled, then 24-hr urine collections would be feasible and, thus, urinary excretion data would be quite meaningful. Also, concerning the creatinine basis, day-to-day fluctuations are much less than hour-to-hour variations.[4] Thus, in a controlled situation (metabolic or clinical ward, for example) in which 24-hr specimens can be obtained and daily individual creatinine variations ascertained, the use of creatinine as a comparator may well be justified.

When the usefulness of blood for assaying elemental nutritional status is considered, one is essentially limited to a measurement of the concentration of the element in either the whole blood, the plasma, the serum, or the red blood cells. While any of these measurements can be accomplished without a great deal of difficulty, one must remember that blood levels of nutrients reflect, to a large degree, recent dietary history rather than the preferred longer-term true nutritional status. However, the use of fasted subjects (blood samples obtained in the morning before breakfast) will correct some of the fluctuations of nutrients in the blood which result from recent dietary intake.

After various biochemical determinations have been performed on a sample of blood or urine obtained from a subject, what does this information mean with regard to the nutritional status of the individual? In this respect, it becomes exceedingly important that appropriate guidelines are available for the interpretation of the meaning of these measurements. Thus, a serum vitamin C level or a urinary value for riboflavin has little meaning in itself until it can be compared with standards or guidelines which have been developed from experimental or clinical experiences. Many of the guidelines that have been suggested for interpretation of biochemical nutritional data have been developed from information obtained from adult studies. Investigations to provide guides for the younger age groups have been limited. Indirect information has been derived from the blood and urine levels of nutrients observed in children of upper economic levels studied in nutrition surveys.

The means to assess the nutritional status of an individual will undoubtedly improve in the future as more biochemical functional tests become available which are based on the metabolic actions and interrelations of the individual nutrients at the cellular level. Biochemical techniques, as with clinical examinations, anthropometric measurements and dietary surveys, can be of considerable value in assessing nutritional status of a person providing their limitations as noted in the following sections are recognized.

REFERENCES

1. Watson, R. L. and Langford, H. G., Usefulness of overnight urines in population groups. Pilot studies of sodium, potassium, and calcium excretion, *Am. J. Clin. Nutr.*, 23, 290, 1970.
2. Clark, L. C., Jr., Thompson, H., Beck, E. I., and Jacobson, W., Excretion of creatine and creatinine by children, *Am. J. Dis. Child.*, 81, 774, 1951.
3. Best, W. R., Physiologic factors in urinary creatinine excretion, *Army Med. Nutr. Lab. Rept.*, No. 118, 1953.
4. Vestergaard, P. and Leverett, R., Constancy of urinary creatinine excretion, *J. Lab. Clin. Med.*, 51, 211, 1958.
5. Clarke, R. P., Cosgrove, L. D., and Morse, E. H., Vitamin to creatinine ratios. Variability in separate voidings of urine of adolescents during a 24 hour period, *Am. J. Clin. Nutr.*, 19, 335, 1966.
6. Pollack, H., Creatinine excretion as index for estimating urinary excretion of micronutrients or their metabolic end products, *Am. J. Clin. Nutr.*, 23, 865, 1970.
7. Krehl, W. A. and Hodges, R. H., The interpretation of nutrition survey data, *Am. J. Clin. Nutr.*, 17, 191, 1965.
8. Wilson, C. S. et al., A review of methods used in nutrition surveys conducted by the Interdepartmental Committee on Nutrition for National Defense (ICNND), *Am. J. Clin. Nutr.*, 15, 29, 1964.
9. Hegsted, D. M., Gershoff, S. N., Trulson, M. F., and Jolly, D. H., Variation in riboflavin excretion, *J. Nutr.*, 60, 581, 1956.
10. Plough, I. C. and Consolazio, C. F., The use of casual urine specimens in the evaluation of the excretion rates of thiamine, riboflavin and N'-methylnicotinamide, *J. Nutr.*, 69, 365, 1959.

II. VITAMINS

Vitamin A (Retinol)

Hypovitaminosis A is a major nutritional problem throughout the world, particularly in South and East Asia and in many of the developing countries.[1-8,14,39,98,116] Even in the United States and Canada, surveys have indicated that vitamin A is one of the three essential nutrients most likely to be supplied in marginal amounts in the diets of the North American population, particularly among the Mexican-American groups (Figure 1).[9-12,14,30,52,70] Vitamin A deficiency affects mainly the infants and children up to the age of 5 years, with night blindness representing an early symptom of the deficiency. Xerophthalmia resulting from a severe vitamin A deficiency may lead to total or partial blindness and is, in the regions noted, the most important cause of blindness in the young child.[1-7,14-18,21,23-25,37-40]

The functions of vitamin A, other than its participation in vision, remain obscure although increasing evidence for specific roles in maintenance of bone growth, maintenance of spermatogenesis, maintenance of subcellular membranes, and in mucopolysaccharide synthesis is being reported.[14,16,25,37-46,71-75,90,96,99,105-107,112,114] Consequently, at present there is no readily determined biochemical measurement of metabolic derangement due to a vitamin A deficiency. Physiological impairment of retinal function reflected in night blindness and impaired dark adaptation may occur in hypovitaminosis A. These changes may be measured by dark adaptometry, rod scotometry, reflectance spectrophotometry, and electroretinography.[15-22,24,44,45,64,68] However, these procedures require expensive and delicate equipment, trained personnel, and the cooperation of the patients, a requisite not readily attainable with children and infants. Hence, these tests are not practical for evaluating vitamin A nutritional status in the field and are seldom readily available for use with clinical cases of suspected vitamin A deficiency. Factors other than vitamin A insufficiency may also impair dark adaptation and night vision.[16,17]

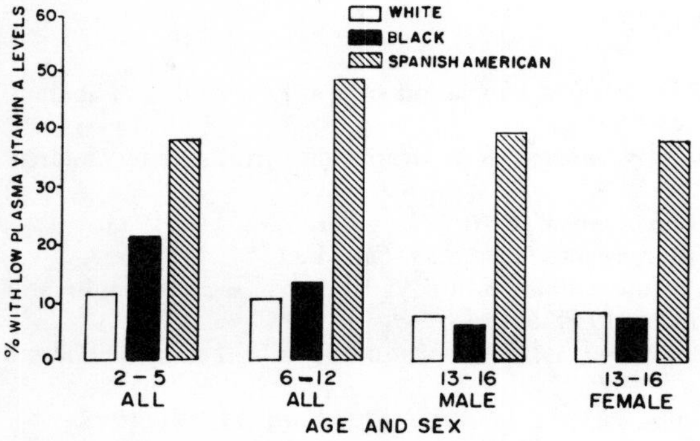

Inadequate intakes of vitamin A, either as preformed retinol or as active carotenoids, result in a tissue decrease of the vitamin.[4,6,15,39,40,99] Since the liver is a major storage organ of vitamin A in the body, the concentration of retinol and its esters in liver tissue is a direct measurement of vitamin A reserves.[4,6,10-12,15,39,40,99,100] This information can be obtained from liver biopsy specimens, but the complicated procedure is impractical for routine use in population studies; its use can be justified only in special clinical cases.

Serum measurements of vitamin A remain the only practical biochemical means of assessing the nutritive status of this nutrient.[2,9,13,23,24,27,29-31,35,39,56-64,66,67,99,117] Serum levels of vitamin A and carotene are related to the dietary intakes of these nutrients (Figure 2).[27,39,103] This relationship does not necessarily consist of a straightforward linear correlation between the serum levels and the dietary intake of vitamin A since serum levels do not necessarily reflect recent intakes of the vitamin. When large stores of retinol exist in the liver, these reserves are drawn upon when dietary intake of the vitamin is inadequate to maintain the serum vitamin A concentration at a physiologically adequate level.[39,40] However, this level will usually be considerably lower than those normally observed with adequate intakes of the vitamin.[24,27]

Prolonged low intakes of vitamin A correlate with serum vitamin A levels. Since the vitamin is stored primarily in the liver, low serum levels of vitamin A reflect not only a low intake of the nutrient but also depleted liver stores.[3,6,12,15,27,37,99,100] Serum retinol levels above 30

FIGURE 1. Percent of individuals with deficient or low vitamin A levels by ethnic group, age, and sex. (Adapted from data obtained in the Ten-State Nutrition Survey of Texas, Louisiana, Kentucky, West Virginia, and South Carolina.[9])

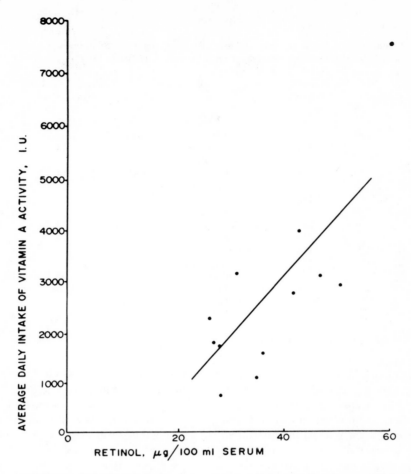

FIGURE 2. Relationship between average serum retinol levels and average daily intake of vitamin A activity in adult males in 11 countries surveyed by ICNND. (From Patwardhan.[103])

μg/100 ml of serum indicate liver stores of vitamin A, while serum levels below this value generally indicate inadequate intakes with the stores of vitamin A probably in the process of being depleted.[24,27,56] Serum vitamin A levels of 10 μg or less per 100 ml serum are indicative of depleted, or virtually so, liver reserves of the vitamin with clinical signs or symptoms of a deficiency generally evident.[6,7,24,27] Dark adaptation tests and electroretinographs readily provide such evidence (Table 1).[24,27]

Hodges and Kolder[27] in a preliminary report noted that in vitamin A depleted adult men, a daily intake of 75 μg of retinol resulted in serum retinol levels well under 10 μg/100 ml. When the intake of retinol was increased to 150 μg/day, the serum retinol level was still less than 10 μg/100 ml. At an intake of 300 μg of retinol per day, the serum retinol level was approximately 19 μg/100 ml whereas, at a daily intake of 2400 μg of retinol, the serum retinol level increased to 60 μg/100 ml. With daily intakes of 600 μg of retinol, skin lesions associated with vitamin A deficiency were corrected. These results suggest that a dose-response relationship exists between administered retinol and serum retinol levels.[27] Information as to the state of the body pool of vitamin A at each of these various intakes and serum levels of the vitamin is also needed. The FAO/WHO adopted a recommended intake of 750 μg of retinol/day for the normal adult,[23] while the NRC-NAS recommended a daily intake of 1500 μg retinol.[26] Thus, a serum retinol level of less than 20 μg/100 ml would indicate that the vitamin A intakes were considerably below the recommended allowances.

The Pan American Health Organization[8] con-

TABLE 1

Serum Retinol Levels at Time of Onset of Clinical Signs and Symptoms in Adult
Male Human Volunteers Maintained on a Vitamin A Deficient Diet*

Subject	Days on vitamin A deficient diet	Clinical signs and symptoms	Serum retinol level (μg/100 ml)
1	260	White papules (anterior and shoulders)	22
	321	Impaired dark adaptation	11
	449	Follicular hyperkeratosis (thighs and back)	11
3	185	White papules (chest, back and shoulders)	25
	282	Follicular hyperkeratosis	25
	414	Severe acne	14
	420	Impaired dark adaptation	12
8	372	Follicular hyperkeratosis (thighs)	35
	621	Impaired dark adaptation	27

*From the report of Hodges and Kolder.[27]

sidered hypovitaminosis A to be a public health problem in a population group when there existed: (a) a prevalence of less than 20 μg of retinol/100 ml plasma in 15% or more of the population, and (b) a prevalence of less than 10 μg retinol/100 ml of plasma in 5% or more of the population. Using this biochemical measurement, nutrition surveys have revealed that in Latin America, 29% of the population under 15 years of age had plasma vitamin A levels less than 20 μg/100 ml plasma; an average of 5% of the group had values less than 10 μg/100 ml plasma.

Serum β-carotene measurements provide limited information concerning vitamin A nutriture.[56,60,98] For the most part, serum concentrations of carotene reflect recent dietary intakes of the nutrient although they are not indicative of vitamin A nutritional status per se. However, a relationship between retinol and carotenoid levels in serum has been observed in population groups.[31,103] Individuals consuming only pre-formed vitamin A in their diets may have adequate vitamin A stores with little or no carotene in the serum. When low serum β-carotene levels are found in association with low serum vitamin A levels, the evidence for inadequate vitamin A nutriture is quite strong. Therefore, serum carotene values need to be interpreted with caution.[31,60] Analytical procedures employed are usually not specific for β-carotene and include in the measurement other pro-vitamin A compounds. Because of the presence of various nonconvertible yellow pigments in serum, true β-carotene values can be considerably lower than the values provided by the methods commonly used.[4,32-36,76-78,84,85]

Serum carotenoids have been reported to range from 24 to 216 μg/100 ml or greater with a mean value of about 113 to 126 μg.[30,31,56,70,78] Normally, the body would be expected to promptly convert carotene to retinol and other metabolites and effect its rapid removal from the circulation.[39,47-49,58,78,81] However, carotenemia is occasionally observed in persons with prolonged serum carotene levels over 300 μg/100 resulting in carotenoid pigments being deposited in skin of the face, hands, and feet. The condition may occur in individuals with unusual dietary habits which involve the ingestion of excessive amounts of foods high in carotene. At times, carotenemia is associated with hyperlipemia and hypercholesteremia of diabetes. Serum carotene levels increase somewhat during pregnancy.[113]

Vitamin A can be readily measured with macro- or microtechniques employing either the trifluoroacetic or antimony trichloride chromogen procedure[34,35,76,78,79] or a direct spectrophotometric method[32,33,35,76] based on the ultraviolet absorption of the vitamin. A recently developed fluorometric procedure appears promising in that the method lends itself to semiautomated instrumentation.[36,77,80,89] Samples must be handled with care and the analysis conducted with precautions in order to minimize errors that may be introduced into plasma (serum) vitamin A determinations. Fasting blood samples should be utilized whenever they can be obtained. Serum samples are preferred since the risk of encountering hemolysis is greater with plasma samples. Depending upon the method used, hemolysis may interfere in the analysis.

The mean plasma vitamin A values for normal adults range from approximately 45 to 65 μg/100 ml with higher levels noted in the older age groups (Figure 3). Males tend to have slightly higher values than females, although this difference does not appear to exist in children and the older age group.[9,29-31,56,70,78,103]

Depressed serum vitamin A levels may be encountered, unrelated to nutrition, in subjects with a febrile condition,[4,37] chronic infection,[35,91,94,101] liver diseases,[11,35,37,91,101] and sprue.[35,37,78] Children with cystic fibrosis have been observed to have below-normal levels of plasma vitamin A which are apparently due to a defect in the mobilization and transport of retinol from storage tissue rather than because of depleted tissue levels.[54,55] In contrast, women ingesting oral contraceptives have increased plasma vitamin A levels when compared to nonpregnant controls.[65]

Guidelines that have been used to evaluate serum (plasma) vitamin A levels are indicated in Table 2.[2,9,27,35,56-63,66,67,93] Serum vitamin A levels below 10 μg/100 ml indicate a deficiency in young adult men, while levels of 10 to 19 μg/100 ml indicate a low vitamin A status. Levels of 20 μg and above/100 ml of serum reflect acceptable intakes of vitamin A. Although a plasma vitamin A level of 20 μg and above/100 ml has been considered a satisfactory level,[2,9,35,67] it is interesting to note that Hodges and associates[13,27] observed clinical signs of vitamin A deficiency in subjects whose plasma retinol levels were in this "acceptable" level (Table 1). Their results would suggest that plasma retinol levels of less than 30 μg/100 ml in the adult might be considered less than an acceptable level of vitamin A. In the Sheffield study,[24] plasma vitamin A did not reach zero levels in the subjects, but changes in dark adaptation occurred when plasma vitamin A levels fell below 20 μg/100 ml. However, considerable biological variability or ability to adapt to limited vitamin A resources apparently exists with respect to this sign as Hodges and Kolder[27] failed to observe evidence of night blindness in one of their experimental subjects even though his serum vitamin A level had fallen to 9 μg/100 ml. Others have also indicated that various clinical manifestations of vitamin A deficiency do not necessarily reflect serum levels of the vitamin.[109]

The vitamin A requirement of the rapidly growing child is, on a weight basis, considered to be higher than that of the adult (50 to 18 μg/kg day vs. 12 μg/kg),[23] and this may relate to the lower mean plasma vitamin A values observed (Figure 3). For this reason, the Committee on Nutrition of the American Academy of Pediatrics considered a plasma vitamin A level of less than 30 μg/100 ml unacceptable for children (Table 2).[57] Plasma retinol levels of 30 μg/100 ml and above were considered indicative of vitamin A intakes adequate to meet the increased needs of the growing child and, as well, to permit some liver storage of the vitamin. However, the National Academy of Sciences-National Research Council[83] recommended "that, where the objective is to define populations at risk, 20 μg/100 ml plasma be used as the cutoff point for both children and adults. Any appreciable fraction of the population showing values below this level should be considered as indicative of risk." Additional efforts should be made, particularly with children, to correlate

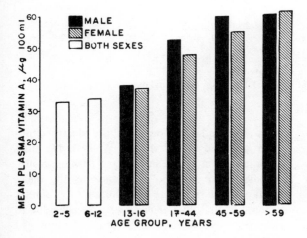

FIGURE 3. Mean plasma vitamin A levels by age and sex for white population from high income ratio states. (Adapted from the Ten-State Nutrition Survey (IV-139).[9])

TABLE 2

Guidelines Used for the Interpretation of Vitamin A Biochemical Data

Reference	Less than acceptable (at risk)		Acceptable[a] (low risk)
	Deficient (high risk)	Low (medium risk)	
	μg/100 ml	μg/100 ml	μg/100 ml
1. ICNND (35)[b]			
Plasma retinol:			
All ages	< 10	10 to 19	⩾ 20
Plasma carotene:			
All ages	–	20 to 39	⩾ 40
Pregnant women[113]			
2nd trimester	–	30 to 79	⩾ 80
3rd trimester	–	40 to 79	⩾ 80
2. Ten-state Nutrition Survey			
Plasma retinol:			
All ages	< 10	10 to 19	⩾ 20
Plasma carotene:			
16 yr and under	–	< 40	⩾ 40
17 yr and under	< 20	20 to 39	⩾ 40
3. Children's Bureau[67]			
Preschool children:			
Plasma retinol	< 10	< 20	⩾ 20
Plasma β-carotene	–	< 40	⩾ 40
4. National Nutrition Survey[57]			
Plasma retinol:			
0 to 5 months	< 10	10 to 19	⩾ 20
0.5 to 17 years	< 20	20 to 29	⩾ 30
Adults	< 10	10 to 19	⩾ 20
Plasma carotene:			
0 to 5 months	–	< 10	⩾ 10
6 to 11 months	–	< 30	⩾ 30
1 to 17 years	–	< 40	⩾ 40
Adults	< 20[c]	20 to 39	⩾ 40
Pregnant			
2nd trimester	–	30 to 79	⩾ 80
3rd trimester	–	40 to 79	⩾ 80

[a]Excessively high values may indicate abnormal clinical status or toxicity.
[b]Indicates reference cited for the guideline indicated.
[c]Very low plasma carotene levels may indicate malabsorption or unusual diet.

plasma vitamin A levels with early clinical manifestations. Kolder[83] considers dark adaptation as still probably the most sensitive and practical diagnostic test and has used the measurement successfully with children over 7 years of age. However, he did not consider it feasible to do dark adaptation tests or electroretinograms on younger children. Genest and associates[45,68] have, however, conducted electroretinography measurements in a group of children 5 to 14 years of age. In the 5 to 9-year age group, a linear relationship was found between the a-wave and the b-wave of the electroretinograph and the serum vitamin A level. No such relationship was found in the 10 to 14 age group, although there was no difference in the mean serum vitamin A level. The failure of a similar response in the older group may have been due to irreversible eye damage as a result of prolonged vitamin A deficiency occurring in earlier years. Consequently, the electroretinograph responses in the older children would have had little, if any, relationship to their serum vitamin A levels.[45]

Nevertheless, electroretinograph measurements in children are tedious and time-consuming.

Although additional means for assessing vitamin A status are presently limited, the ratio in plasma of retinol to retinol binding protein appears promising.[28,97] Vitamin A is transported in plasma by a specific retinol binding protein (RBP) which is complexed with a second protein, prealbumin (PA) to form RBP-PA.[28,39,50,82,97] Over a wide range of plasma values, there is a correlation between transport retinol binding protein and plasma vitamin A. Retinol binding protein plasma concentrations were reduced in liver disease and in hyperthyroidism. Evidence exists of a reduction of retinol binding protein in cases of kwashiorkor which may explain the lowered plasma vitamin A levels associated with this condition.[6,28,51,68,69,86-88,90,94,95,104,111] The plasma retinol binding protein is measured with the use of a radioimmunoassay which at present is too complex a determination for routine use.[97]

An impairment of both taste and smell has been reported in vitamin A deficient subjects.[27] However, measurement of these changes as a means to evaluate the nutritional status of vitamin A requires further study.

The use of isotopically labeled retinol and β-carotene has recently revealed in human studies the presence of numerous metabolites of the vitamin in the urine.[13,39,53,90,102,106,108,110,115] Whether any of these metabolites will prove useful in evaluating vitamin A nutriture remains to be seen.

Normally, little or no vitamin A is excreted in the urine. However, excessive urinary excretion of vitamin A has been reported to occur in patients with cancer, tuberculosis, chronic infections (particularly pneumonia), chronic nephritis, and urinary infections.[4,78]

The urinary excretion of the lysosmal enzymes, aryl sulfatase, and acid phosphatase, has been reported to be increased in both a deficiency of vitamin A and in acute hypervitaminosis A.[92] In studies with vitamin A deficient children, the magnitude of this increase and the variability of the excretion level appeared to indicate that this measurement would be of limited use as an index to evaluate vitamin A nutritional status.[92]

In summary, the serum retinol determination is the only practical biochemical test currently available to evaluate the vitamin A status in population groups. Serum retinol levels provide a reflection of the vitamin A intake. A low serum retinol level ($<$ 20 μg/100 ml) probably indicates both a longstanding low intake of vitamin A and a low tissue reserve of the vitamin. Serum retinol levels in the range of 20 to 30 μg/100 ml are less interpretable because of the uncertainty of the associated tissue reserves of vitamin A. Higher serum vitamin A levels can generally be considered to be associated with an appreciable tissue reserve of the vitamin. Wherever feasible, clinical cases of suspected hypovitaminosis A should be submitted to visual functional tests.

REFERENCES

1. **May, J. M.**, *Studies in Medical Geography. The Ecology of Malnutrition,* Vol. 1 – 11, Hafner Publishing Co., New York, 1961 – 1972.
2. *Nutrition Survey Reports (1957 – 1972),* Interdepartmental Committee on Nutrition for National Defense, Washington, D.C.
3. **McLaren, D. S.**, Xerophthalmia: A neglected problem, *Nutr. Rev.,* 22, 289, 1964.
4. **Moore, T.**, *Vitamin A,* Elsevier Publishing Co., Amsterdam, Netherlands, 1957.
5. **Oomen, H. A. P. C., McLaren, D. S.,** and **Escapini, H.,** A global survey on xerophthalmia. Epidemiology and public health aspects of hypovitaminosis A, *Trop. Geogr. Med.,* 16, 271, 1964.
6. **McLaren, D. S.**, *Malnutrition and the Eye,* Academic Press, Inc. New York, 1963.
7. **McLaren, D. S., Oomen, H. A. P. C.,** and **Escapini, H.,** Ocular manifestations of vitamin A deficiency in man, *Bull. W. H. O.,* 34, 357, 1966.
8. **Chopra, J. G.** and **Kevany, J.,** Hypovitaminosis A in the Americans, *Am. J. Clin. Nutr.,* 23, 231, 1970.
9. *Ten-State Nutrition Survey Reports, I-V,* Center for Disease Control, Atlanta, Georgia 30330, 1972.
10. **Hoppner, K., Phillips, W. E. J., Erdody, P., Murray, T. K.,** and **Perrin, D. E.,** Vitamin A reserves of Canadians, *Can. Med. Assoc. J.,* 101, 84, 1969.
11. **Raica, N., Scott, J., Lowry, L.,** and **Sauberlich, H. E.,** Vitamin A concentration in human tissues collected from five areas in the United States, *Am. J. Clin. Nutr.,* 25, 291, 1972.

12. **Underwood, B. A., Siegel, H., Weisell, R. C., and Dolinski, M.,** Liver stores of vitamin A in a normal population dying suddenly or rapidly from unnatural causes in New York City, *Am. J. Clin. Nutr.,* 23, 1037, 1970.

13. **Hodges, R. E. and Canham, J. E.,** Vitamin deficiencies; Studies of experimental vitamin C deficiency and experimental vitamin A deficiency in man, in *Proceedings of a Workshop on Problems of Assessment and Alleviation of Malnutrition in the United States,* Nashville, Tennessee, Jan. 13 – 14, 1970, sponsored by the Nutrition Study Section, Division of Research Grants, NIH, Washington, D.C., Pub. 916.086, 1971.

14. **Roels, O. A.,** Vitamin A physiology, *J.A.M.A.,* 214, 34, 1970.

15. **McLaren, D.,** Vitamin A and carotene. IX – B. Effects of vitamin A deficiency in man, in *The Vitamins,* Vol. I, 2nd ed., Sebrell, W. H., Jr. and Harris, R. S., Eds., Academic Press, Inc., New York, 1967, 267.

16. **Fisher, K. D., Carr, C. J., and Huber, T. E.,** A study of vision as related to dark adaptation and night vision in the soldier, August 1969 (AD693292), Life Sciences Research Office, Office of Biomedical Studies, Fed. of Am. Soc. for Exptl. Biol., Bethesda, Maryland.

17. **Carr, C. F. and Fisher, K. D.,** A Study of Individual Variability in Dark Adaptation and Night Vision in Man, December 1970 (AD722798), Life Sciences Research Office, Fed. of Am. Soc. for Exptl. Biol., Bethesda, Maryland 20014.

18. **Jayle, G. E., Ourgaud, A. G., Baisinger, L. F., and Holmes, W. J.,** *Night Vision,* Charles C Thomas, Springfield, Illinois, 1959.

19. **Carr, R. E. and Gouras, P.,** Clinical electroretinography, *J.A.M.A.,* 198, 173, 1966.

20. **Whitcomb, M. A. and Benson, W.,** Eds., Symposium on the Measurement of Visual Function, Proceedings of the Spring Meeting of 1965, Armed Forces-NRC Committee on Vision, NAS-NRC, Washington, D.C., 1968.

21. **Davson, H.,** Ed., *The Eye,* Vol. II, Academic Press, Inc., New York, 1962.

22. **Brown, K. T.,** The electroretinogram: Its components and their origins, *Vision Res.,* 8, 633, 1968.

23. Requirements of Vitamin A, Thiamine, Riboflavine and Niacin, Report of a Joint F.A.O./W.H.O. Expert Group, Rome, Italy, September 6 – 17, 1965, F.A.O. Nutrition Meetings Report Series No. 41, Rome, 1967.

24. **Hume, E. M. and Krebs, H. A.,** Vitamin A requirement of human adults: An experimental study of vitamin A deprivation in man, *United Kingdom Medical Research Council, Special Report Series* No. 264, London, 1949.

25. **Dingle, J. T. and Luch, J. A.,** Vitamin A, carotenoids, and cell structure, *Biol. Rev.,* 40, 422, 1965.

26. *Recommended Dietary Allowances,* 7th revised ed., A report of the Food and Nutrition Board, National Research Council, Publ. No. 1694, National Academy of Sciences, Washington, D.C. 20418, 1968.

27. **Hodges, R. E. and Kolder, H.,** Experimental vitamin A deficiency in human volunteers, in *Summary of Proceedings of Workshop on Biochemical and Clinical Criteria for Determining Human Vitamin A Nutriture,* Bieri, J. G., Chairman, held in Washington, D.C., January 28 – 29, 1971, Food and Nutrition Board, National Academy of Sciences-National Research Council, Washington, D.C. 20418, 1971, 10.

28. **Smith, F. R.,** Plasma retinol binding protein, in *Summary of Proceedings of Workshop on Biochemical and Clinical Criteria for Determining Human Vitamin A Nutriture,* Bieri, J. G., Chairman, held in Washington, D.C., January 28 – 29, 1971, Food and Nutrition Board, National Academy of Sciences-National Research Council, Washington, D.C. 20418, 1971, 5.

29. **DuPlessis, J. P.,** An Evaluation of Biochemical Criteria for Use in Nutrition Status Surveys, Council for Scientific and Industrial Research Report No. 261, National Nutrition Research Institute, Pretoria, South Africa, 1967, 51.

30. **Davis, T. R. A., Gershoff, S. N., and Gamble, D. F.,** Review of studies of vitamin and mineral nutrition in the United States (1950 – 1968), *J. Nutr. Educ.,* 1, 38, 1969.

31. **Leitner, Z. A., Moore, T., and Sharman, I. M.,** Vitamin A and vitamin E in human blood. I. Levels of vitamin A and carotenoids in British men and women, 1948 – 1957, *Br. J. Nutr.,* 14, 157, 1960.

32. **Bessey, O. A., Lowry, O. H., Brock, M. J., and Lopez, J. A.,** The determination of vitamin A and carotene in small quantities of blood serum, *J. Biol. Chem.,* 166, 177, 1946.

33. **McLaren, D. S., Read, W. W. C., Awdeh, Z. L., and Tchalian, M.,** Microdetermination of vitamin A and carotenoids in blood and tissue, in *Methods of Biochemical Analysis,* Vol. XV, Glick, D., Ed., John Wiley & Sons, Inc., New York, 1967, 1.

34. **Neeld, J. B., Jr. and Pearson, W. N.,** Macro- and micromethods for the determination of serum vitamin A using trifluoroacetic acid, *J. Nutr.,* 79, 454, 1963.

35. **Manual for Nutrition Surveys,** 2nd ed., Interdepartmental Committee on Nutrition for National Defense, Superintendent of Documents, U.S. Government Printing Office, Washington, D.C. 20402, 1963.

36. **Garry, P. J., Pollack, J. D., and Owen, G. M.,** Plasma vitamin A assay by fluorometry and use of a silicic acid column technique, *Clin. Chem.,* 16, 766, 1970.

37. **Goodhart, R. S.,** The vitamins. Vitamin A, in *Modern Nutrition in Health and Disease,* 4th ed., Wohl, M. G. and Goodhart, R. S., Eds., Lea & Febiger, Philadelphia, 1968, 213.

38. **Moore, T.,** The pathology of vitamin A deficiency, in *Vitamins and Hormones,* 18, 499, 1960.

39. **Wolf, G.,** International Symposium on the Metabolic Function of Vitamin A, *Am. J. Clin. Nutr.,* 22, 897, 1969.

40. **McLaren, D. S.,** Present knowledge of the role of vitamin A in health and disease, *Trans. R. Soc. Trop. Med. Hyg.,* 60, 436, 1966.

41. **Wagner, A. F. and Folkers, K.,** The vitamin A group, in *Vitamins and Coenzymes,* Interscience Publ., New York, 1964, Chap. XV, p. 280.

42. **Gloor, U. and Wiss, O.**, Fat-soluble vitamins, *Annu. Rev. Biochem.*, 33, 313, 1964.

43. **Olson, J. A.**, The metabolism of vitamin A, *Pharmacol. Rev.*, 19, 559, 1967.

44. **Dowling, J. E. and Wald, G.**, Vitamin A deficiency and night blindness, *Proc. Natl. Acad. Sci. USA*, 44, 648, 1958.

45. **Genest, A. A., Sarwono, D., and György, P.**, Vitamin A blood serum levels and electroretinogram in 5- to 14-year age group in Indonesia and Thailand, *Am. J. Clin. Nutr.*, 20, 1275, 1967.

46. **Roels, O. A.**, Present knowledge of vitamin A, *Nutr. Rev.*, 24, 129, 1966.

47. **Goodman, D. S., Huang, H. S., Kanai, M., and Shiratori, T.**, The enzymatic conversion of all-trans β-carotene into retinol, *J. Biol. Chem.*, 242, 3543, 1967.

48. **Olson, J. A. and Hayaishi, O.**, Enzymic cleavage of β-carotene into vitamin A by soluble enzymes of rat liver and intestine, *Proc. Natl. Acad. Sci. USA*, 54, 1364, 1965.

49. **Fidge, N. H. and Goodman, D. S.**, The enzymatic reduction of retinal to retinol in rat intestine, *J. Biol. Chem.*, 243, 4372, 1968.

50. **Kanai, M., Raz, A., and Goodman, D. S.**, Retinol-binding protein: The transport protein for vitamin A in human plasma, *J. Clin. Invest.*, 47, 2025, 1968.

51. **Arroyave, G., Wilson, D., Méndez, J., Béhar, M., and Scrimshaw, N. S.**, Serum and liver vitamin A and lipids in children with severe protein malnutrition, *Am. J. Clin. Nutr.*, 9, 180, 1961.

52. **Chase, H. P., Kumar, V., Dodds, J. M., Sauberlich, H. E., Hunter, R. M., Burton, R. S., and Spalding, V.**, Nutritional status of preschool Mexican-American migrant farm children, *Am. J. Dis. Child.*, 122, 316, 1971.

53. **Wallace, D. L., Baker, E. M., III, Canham, J. E., Raica, N., Jr., Sauberlich, H. E., and Hodges, R. E.**, Metabolism of vitamin A in the human, *Fed. Proc.*, 30, 584 (abstract), 1971.

54. **Underwood, B. A. and Denning, C. R.**, Correlations between plasma and liver concentrations of vitamins A and E in children with cystic fibrosis, *Bull. N. Y. Acad. Med.*, 47, 34, 1971.

55. **Underwood, B. A. and Denning, C. R.**, Blood and liver concentrations of vitamin A and E in children with cystic fibrosis of the pancreas, *Pediatr. Res.*, 6, 26, 1972.

56. **Bessey, O. A.**, Evaluation of vitamin adequacy: Blood levels, in *Methods for Evaluation of Nutritional Adequacy and Status — A Symposium*, Advisory Board on Quartermaster Research and Development, Committee on Foods, National Academy of Sciences, National Research Council, Washington, D.C., 59, 1954.

57. **O'Neal, R. M., Johnson, O. C., and Schaefer, A. E.**, Guidelines for classification and interpretation of group blood and urine data collected as part of the National Nutrition Survey, *Pediatr. Res.*, 4, 103, 1970.

58. **Pearson, W. N.**, Biochemical appraisal of the vitamin nutritional status in man, *J.A.M.A.*, 180, 49, 1962.

59. **Pearson, W. N.**, Blood and urinary vitamin levels as potential indices of body stores, *Am. J. Clin. Nutr.*, 20, 514, 1967.

60. **Pearson, W. N.**, Assessment of nutritional status: Biochemical methods, in *Nutrition: A Comprehensive Treatise*, Vol. III, Beaton, G. H. and McHenry, E. W., Eds., Academic Press, New York, 1966, 265.

61. **Jelliffe, D. B.**, *The Assessment of the Nutritional Status of the Community*, World Health Organization, Geneva, Switzerland, 1966, 88.

62. *Expert Committee on Medical Assessment of Nutritional Status*, World Health Organization Technical Report Series No. 258, World Health Organization, Geneva, Switzerland, 1963, 35.

63. **Krause, R. F.**, Laboratory aids in the diagnosis of malnutrition, in *Modern Nutrition in Health and Disease*, 4th ed., Wohl, M. G. and Goodhart, R. S., Eds., Lea and Febiger, Philadelphia, 1968, Chap. 18A, p. 519.

64. **Rodriguez, M. S. and Irwin, M. I.**, A conspectus of research on vitamin A requirements of man, *J. Nutr.*, 102, 909, 1972.

65. **Gal, I., Parkinson, C., and Craft, I.**, Effect of oral contraceptives on human plasma vitamin A levels, *Br. Med. J.*, 2, 436, 1971.

66. **Pearson, W. N.**, Biochemical appraisal of nutritional status in man, *Am. J. Clin. Nutr.*, 11, 462, 1962.

67. *Suggested Guidelines for Evaluation of the Nutritional Status of Pre-School Children*, U.S. Department of Health, Education and Welfare, Social and Rehabilitation Service, Children's Bureau, Washington, D.C. (Document No. 1967-0-275-984), 1967.

68. **György, P.**, Protein-calorie and vitamin A malnutrition in Southeast Asia, *Fed. Proc.*, 27(3), 949, 1968.

69. **Roels, O. A., Djaeni, S., Trout, M. E., Lauw, T. G., Heath, A., Poey, S. H., Tarwotjo, M. S., and Suhadi, B.**, The effect of protein and fat supplements on vitamin A-deficient Indonesian children, *Am. J. Clin. Nutr.*, 12, 380, 1963.

70. **Phillips, W. E. J., Murray, T. K., and Campbell, J. S.**, Serum vitamin A and carotenoids of Canadians, *Can. Med. Assoc. J.*, 102, 1085, 1970.

71. **Fell, H. B.**, The direct action of vitamin A on skeletal tissue in vitro, in *The Fat-soluble Vitamins*, De Luca, H. F. and Suttie, J. W., Eds., University of Wisconsin Press, Madison, 1970, 187.

72. **Wolf, G. and De Luca, L.**, Recent studies on some metabolic functions of vitamin A, in *The Fat-soluble Vitamins*, De Luca, H. F. and Suttie, J. W., Eds., University of Wisconsin Press, Madison, 1970, 257.

73. **Thompson, J. N.**, The role of vitamin A in reproduction, in *The Fat-soluble Vitamins*, De Luca, H. F. and Suttie, J. W., Eds., University of Wisconsin Press, Madison, 1970, 267.

74. **Roels, O. A.**, Vitamins A and carotene VIII, Biochemical systems, in *The Vitamins*, Vol. I, Sebrell, W. H., Jr. and Harris, R. S., Eds., Academic Press, Inc., New York, 1967, 167.

75. **Dam, H. and Søndergaard, E.,** Fat-soluble vitamins. I. Vitamin A, in *Nutrition: A Comprehensive Treatise,* Vol. II, Beaton, G. H. and McHenry, E. W., Eds., Academic Press, Inc., New York, 1964, 2.

76. **Roels, O. A. and Mahadevam, S.,** Vitamin A, in *The Vitamins,* Vol. VI, György, P. and Pearson, W. N., Eds., Academic Press, Inc., New York, 1967, 139.

77. **Thompson, J. N., Erdody, P., Brien, R., and Murry, T. K.,** Fluorometric determination of vitamin A in human blood and liver, *Biochem. Med.,* 5, 67, 1971.

78. **Roels, O. A. and Trout, M.,** Vitamin A and carotene, in *Standard Methods of Clinical Chemistry,* Vol. 7, Cooper, G. C. and King, J. S., Jr., Eds., Academic Press, Inc., New York, 1972, 215.

79. **Linhares, E. D. R.,** Microdetermination of plasma or serum vitamin A and carotene, *Microchem. J.,* 16, 467, 1971.

80. **Selvaraj, R. J. and Susheela, T. P.,** Estimation of serum vitamin A by a microfluorometric procedure, *Clin. Chim. Acta,* 27, 165, 1970.

81. **Olson, J. A. and Lakshmanan, M. R.,** Enzymatic transformation of vitamin A, with particular emphasis on carotenoid cleavage, in *The Fat-soluble Vitamins,* De Luca, H. F. and Suttie, J. W., Eds., University of Wisconsin Press, Madison, 1970, 213.

82. **Goodman, D. S.,** Retinol transport in human plasma, in *The Fat-soluble Vitamins,* De Luca, H. F. and Suttie, J. W., Eds., University of Wisconsin Press, Madison, 1970, 203.

83. **Bieri, J. G.,** Summary of Proceedings of a Workshop on Biochemical and Clinical Criteria for Determining Human Vitamin A Nutriture, held in Washington D.C., January 28 – 29, 1971, National Academy of Sciences – National Research Council, Washington, D.C.

84. **Awdeh, Z. L.,** The separation of vitamin A from carotenoids in microsamples of serum, *Anal. Biochem.,* 10, 156, 1965.

85. **Strobecker, R. and Henning, H. M.,** *Vitamin Assay-tested Methods,* Chemical Rubber Co., Cleveland, 1966, 33.

86. **Chandra, H., Venkatachalam, C., Belavady, B. V., Reddy, P., and Gopalan, C.,** Some observations on vitamin A deficiency in Indian children, *Indian J. Child Health,* 9, 589, 1960.

87. **McLaren, D., Shirajian, E., Tchalian, M., and Khoury, G.,** Xerophthalmia in Jordan, *Am. J. Clin. Nutr.,* 17, 117, 1965.

88. **Pereira, S., Begum, A., and Dumm, M.,** Vitamin A deficiency in kwashiorkor, *Am. J. Clin. Nutr.,* 19, 182, 1966.

89. **Glover, J., Moxley, L., and Muhilal,** Fluorimetric method for assay of retinol in human plasma, *Summaria,* IX International Congress of Nutrition, Mexico City, September 3 – 9, 1972, 60.

90. **Adhikari, H. R., Vakil, U. K., and Sreenivasan, A.,** Some aspects of vitamin A metabolism, *J. Sci. Ind. Res.,* 29, 364, 1970.

91. **Ralli, E. P., Papper, E., Paley, K., and Bauman, E.,** Vitamin A and carotene content of human liver in normal and in diseased subjects, *Arch. Intern. Med.,* 68, 102, 1941.

92. *Annual Report: Period 1, October 1969 to 30, September 1970,* National Institute of Nutrition, Hyderabad-7, India, 1970, 45.

93. **Varela, R. M., Teixeira, S. G., and Batista, M.,** Hypovitaminosis A in the sugarcane zone of southern Pernambuco State, Northeast Brazil, *Am. J. Clin. Nutr.,* 25, 800, 1972.

94. **McLaren, D. S.,** Prevention of xerophthalmia, in *Pre-school Child Malnutrition: Primary Deterrent to Human Progress,* National Academy of Sciences – National Research Council Publ. No. 1282, Washington, D.C., 1966, 96.

95. **Arroyave, G., Wilson, D., Couteras, C., and Béhar, M.,** Alterations in serum concentration of vitamin A associated with the hypoproteinemia of severe protein malnutrition, *J. Pediatr.,* 62, 920, 1965.

96. **Rietz, P.,** On the biological role and metabolism of vitamin A., *Acta Vit. et Enzym.,* 25, 123, 1971.

97. **Muto, Y., Smith, J. E., Milch, P. O., and Goodman, D. S.,** Regulation of retinol-binding protein metabolism by vitamin A status in the rat, *J. Biol. Chem.,* 247, 2542, 1972.

98. **Guzman, M. A., Arroyave, G., and Scrimshaw, N. S.,** Serum ascorbic acid, riboflavin, carotene, vitamin A, vitamin E and alkaline phosphatase values in Central American school children, *Am. J. Clin. Nutr.,* 9, 164, 1961.

99. **Masek, J.,** Recommended nutrient allowances, *World Rev. Nutr. Diet.,* 3, 149, 1962.

100. **Popper, H.,** Distribution of vitamin A in tissue as visualized by fluorescence microscopy, *Physiol. Rev.,* 24, 205, 1944.

101. **Popper, H., Steigmann, F., Dubin, A., Dyniewicz, H. A., and Hesser, F. P.,** Significance of vitamin A alcohol and ester partitioning under normal and pathologic circumstances, *Proc. Soc. Exp. Biol. Med.,* 68, 676, 1948.

102. **Wallace, D. L., Baker, E. M., Canham, J. E., Raica, N., Sauberlich, H. E., Teplick, R. S., and Hodges, R. E.,** Vitamin A depletion in the human male adult, *Fed. Proc.,* 31, 672 (abstract) 1972.

103. **Patwardhan, V. N.,** Hypovitaminosis A and epidemiology of xerophthalmia, *Am. J. Clin. Nutr.,* 22, 1106, 1969.

104. **Arroyave, G.,** Interrelations between protein and vitamin A and metabolism, *Am. J. Clin. Nutr.,* 22, 1119, 1969.

105. **Wasserman, R. H. and Corradino, R. A.,** Metabolic role of vitamin A and D, *Ann. Rev. Biochem.,* 40, 501, 1971.

106. **Sundaresan, P. R.,** Recent advances in the metabolism of vitamin A, *J. Sci. Ind. Res.,* 1972 (in press).

107. **De Luca, L. and Wolf, G.,** Mechanism of action of vitamin A in differentiation of mucus-secreting epithelia, *J. Agric. Food Chem.,* 20, 474, 1972.

108. **Sundaresan, P. R. and Sundaresan, G. M.,** Metabolism of retinol in the rat, *Fed. Proc.,* 31, 671 (abstract), 1972.

109. **Oomen, H. A. D. C.,** An outline of xerophthalmia, *Int. Rev. Trop. Med.,* 1, 132, 1961.

110. **Goodman, D. S., Huang, H. S., and Shiratori, T.,** Tissue distribution and metabolism of newly absorbed vitamin A in the rat, *J. Lipid Res.,* 6, 390, 1965.

111. **Mahadevan, S., Malathi, P., and Ganguly, J.,** Influence of protein absorption and metabolism of vitamin A, *World Rev. Nutr. Diet.,* 5, 210, 1965.

112. **Owen, E. C.,** Some aspects of the metabolism of vitamin A and carotene, *World Rev. Nutr. Diet.,* 5, 132, 1965.

113. **Darby, W. J. et al.,** The Vanderbilt cooperative study of maternal and infant nutrition. IV. Dietary, laboratory and physical findings in 2,129 delivered pregnancies, *J. Nutr.,* 51, 565, 1953.

114. **Mack, J. P., Lui, N. S. T., Roels, O. A. and Anderson, O. R.,** The occurrence of vitamin A in biological membranes, *Biochim. Biophys. Acta,* 288, 203, 1972.

115. **Sundaresan, P. R.,** General comments on the assessment of retinol status, *Proceedings of III Western Hemisphere Nutrition Congress,* Futura Publishing Co., Inc., Mt. Kisco, N.Y. 10549, 1972, 80.

116. **Rueda-Williamson, R.,** Vitamin A malnutrition in Latin America and the Caribbean, *Proceedings of III Western Hemisphere Nutrition Congress,* Futura Publishing Co., Inc., Mt. Kisco, N.Y. 10549, 1972, 56.

117. **Kelsay, J. L.,** A compendium of nutritional status studies and dietary evaluation studies conducted in the United States, 1957 − 1967, *J. Nutr.,* Suppl. 1, Part II, 99, 123, 1969.

Vitamin C (Ascorbic Acid)

Although ascorbic acid has long been known to prevent scurvy,[1-9] the precise biochemical functions of vitamin C have remained obscure. Ascorbic acid has been proposed to be involved in biochemical systems such as oxidation and reduction reactions, tyrosine metabolism, collagen formation and hydroxylation reactions, wound healing, steroid synthesis, and iron utilization.[1-3,7-9,33,39-42,45] More recently with the discovery of ascorbate-2-sulfate occurring in tissues and urine of man and other species,[10-16] a role for ascorbic acid in sulfation has been proposed.[10,12,16] Because of the limited knowledge concerning the metabolic functions of ascorbic acid, fully satisfactory and reliable biochemical procedures to identify a state of vitamin C deficiency or to assess vitamin C nutritional status have not been developed. Without the availability of a functional biochemical procedure that relates to vitamin C status, information concerning inadequacies in this nutrient has been derived mainly from measuring levels of ascorbic acid in serum, blood, leucocytes, and urine.[17-40,43-45,51-55,62,97-103,121]

Recognizing the limitations of the procedure, the biochemical evaluation of vitamin C status in man has been conducted usually through the determination of serum or plasma ascorbate levels. Within a relatively limited range, serum (plasma) levels of ascorbic acid show a linear relationship with the intake of vitamin C. This relationship has been considered in a number of reviews.[7,17,18,20-22,31-40] Thus, with a deprivation of vitamin C, the concentration of plasma ascorbic acid decreases rapidly[4,5,21-24] while, with a given intake of the vitamin, the plasma ascorbic acid

concentration will plateau at a given level (Table 3 and Figure 4). The maximum plasma ascorbic acid level appears to be at about 1.4 mg/100 ml at which point renal clearance of the vitamin rises abruptly.[46] However, higher plasma ascorbic acid concentrations can be attained temporarily following the ingestion of a large dose of the vitamin.

Although low plasma levels of ascorbic acid do not necessarily indicate scurvy, clinical cases of scurvy invariably have low or no serum ascorbic acid. However, continued low levels of plasma ascorbic acid of less than 0.10 mg/100 ml would probably eventually lead to signs of scurvy.[21,23] Hodges et al.[21,22] recently conducted a study with adults receiving controlled intakes of ascorbic acid and with their body pools of ascorbic acid labeled with isotopic ascorbic acid. It was observed in these studies that plasma or serum and whole blood levels of vitamin C fell rapidly with a diet free of ascorbic acid (Figure 4).[21,22] Plasma ascorbic acid fell to levels lower than those of whole blood (Table 4). Whole blood ascorbic acid fell to a stabilized low level as shown by ^{14}C-labeling, at which point body reserves of ascorbic acid continued to be depleted until signs of scurvy appeared. Ascorbic acid disappeared from the urine early in depletion.

The first signs of scurvy appeared when the plasma ascorbic acid levels ranged from 0.13 to 0.24 mg/100 ml, and the pool size had been depleted to a range of 96 to 490 mg from an average initial pool of 1,500 mg (Table 4).[21-24] There was also a definite relationship between whole blood ascorbic acid values and the body reserves of the vitamin with signs of scurvy appearing when the whole blood ascorbate level

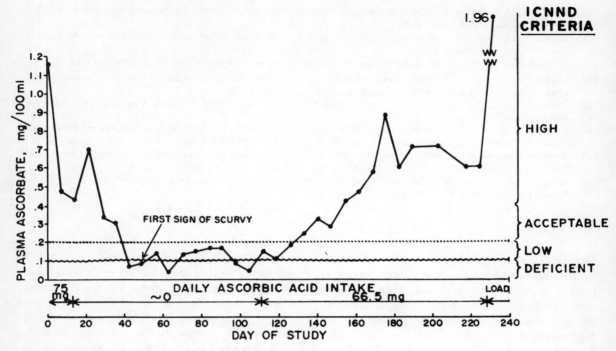

FIGURE 4. The influence of ascorbic acid intake on the plasma ascorbic acid level of adult men studied under controlled conditions. Note that during deficiency many of the plasma ascorbate values fell within the low range of acceptable as classified by ICNND. (From Hodges et al.[21])

TABLE 3

Relationship of Vitamin C Intake in Adults to Vitamin C Level in Serum and White Blood Cells

Vitamin C intake (mg/day)	Serum vitamin C (mg/100 ml)	White blood cell vitamin C (mg/100 ml)	Reference
< 7	0.20	11.5	(122)
8	0.18	11.9	(39, 43)
< 10	< 0.10	–	(18)
10 to 29	< 0.20	–	(18)
23	0.20	12.9	(39, 43)
25	0.29	12.2	(52)
32	0.48	–	(44)
33	0.47	19.5	(55)
57	0.72	–	(44)
58	0.74	26.7	(55)
75	0.84	21.3	(52)
78	0.79	24.2	(39, 43)
82	0.93	–	(44)
83	1.47	34.5	(55)
107	1.05	–	(44)
133	1.69	34.5	(55)

14

TABLE 4

Relationship of Tissue Levels of Vitamin C to Onset of Signs of Scurvy*

Signs of scurvy	Incidence in subjects	Day of depletion	Plasma ascorbic acid, mg/100 ml	Whole blood ascorbic acid mg/100 ml	Ascorbic acid body pool size mg
Petechiae	4/5	29 to 66	0.13 to 0.24	0.32 to 0.40	96 to 490
Ecchymoses	4/5	36 to 103	0.06 to 0.30	0.27 to 0.73	19 to 438
Coiled hair	2/5	42 to 74	0.14 to 0.17	0.33 to 0.50	94 to 166
Gum changes	4/5	43 to 84	0.09 to 0.16	0.30 to 0.50	63 to 360
Hyperkeratosis	5/5	45 to 100	0.00 to 0.16	0.29 to 0.47	64 to 342
Congested follicles	5/5	49 to 90	0.00 to 0.16	0.20 to 0.40	32 to 324
Sicca syndrome	5/5	58 to 123	0.06 to 0.18	0.30 to 0.42	24 to 138
Dyspnea	2/5	63 to 90	0.16 to 0.16	0.34 to 0.37	34 to 78
Arthralgia	4/5	67 to 96	0.04 to 0.16	0.30 to 0.50	45 to 217
Joint effusions	3/5	68 to 103	0.07 to 0.16	0.20 to 0.34	39 to 110
Neuropathy	1/5	71	0.15	0.37	80
Marked edema	1/5	101	0.15	0.47	67

*Adapted from reports of Hodges et al.[20-24]

fell below 0.3 mg/100 ml.[21,22] Serum (or plasma) levels of ascorbic acid may not always fully reflect vitamin C intakes or the state of the body reserves of the vitamin; nevertheless, low serum levels of ascorbic acid (below 0.3 mg/100 ml) do indicate low or inadequate intakes of the vitamin with only partial reserves present. For maximum saturated body reserves or pools of ascorbic acid, high intakes of vitamin C are required (>100 mg) and will be reflected in serum levels in excess of 1.0 mg/100 ml. Serum ascorbic acid levels are reduced in chronic inflammatory diseases[116] and in acute and chronic infections such as tuberculosis and rheumatic fever.[102] Vitamin C levels are reported to be lower in the plasma of cigarette smokers.[105-107,120] The ingestion of oral contraceptives by women has also been reported to reduce the concentration of plasma and leucocyte ascorbic acid.[108,124] Plasma and leucocyte vitamin C concentrations of men have been observed to be lower than those of women[107,111,112] and may be related to ovarian hormone activity.[109,110] The nutritional significance of these effects remains largely obscure.

The guidelines for evaluating serum vitamin C data by the Interdepartmental Committee on Nutrition for National Defense (ICNND)[47,48] and other groups[49,50] are indicated in Table 5. The ICNND has considered serum ascorbic acid levels of less than 0.10 mg/100 ml "deficient" and levels from 0.10 to 0.19 mg/100 ml as "low," while values of 0.20 mg/100 ml and above are "accept-able." The results from the studies of Hodges et al. (Table 4)[20-22] indicated that signs of scurvy may be encountered in subjects with serum ascorbic acid levels above 0.20 mg/100 ml, levels considered acceptable by ICNND (Table 5). In addition, body pools of ascorbic acid were also markedly depleted when these serum levels were observed. The results of these studies would suggest that the ICNND guidelines may need revision with an acceptable ascorbic acid serum level considered to be 0.30 mg/100 ml and above (Table 5).[56]

Whole blood ascorbic acid levels are probably a less sensitive indicator of vitamin C nutriture than serum levels of the vitamin. This is because the ascorbic acid levels in erythrocytes never fall to the low levels encountered in serum or plasma.[20-22] A similar observation was noted by Du Plessis,[38] who also studied the relationship of blood and serum ascorbic acid levels in children (Figure 5). No well-established classifications are available relating blood vitamin C values to the nutritional status of this vitamin in a population, although a tentative guide has been indicated in Table 5. However, for the low ranges, blood vitamin C levels are from 0.2 to 0.4 mg/100 ml higher than the serum levels.[20-22,38] As noted above, when the blood ascorbic acid has fallen to a level of 0.3 mg/100 ml or less, the body pool of the vitamin has been severely depleted and clinical signs of scurvy may be observed (Table 4).[20-22]

Leucocyte ascorbate concentrations are more

TABLE 5

Guidelines for the Interpretation of Vitamin C Biochemical Data (for all age groups)

| | Less than acceptable (at risk) | | |
| | Deficient (high risk) | Low (medium risk) | Acceptable (low risk) |
Measurement			
1. Serum ascorbic acid (mg/100 ml)			
(a) ICNND[47-50]	< 0.10	0.10 to 0.19	≥ 0.20
(b) Suggested revision[20-24,30]	< 0.20	0.20 to 0.29	≥ 0.30
2. White blood cell ascorbic acid (mg/100 ml)[4,7,18,39,43,44,46,52,55,98,122]	0 to 7	8 to 15	> 15
3. Whole blood ascorbic acid* (mg/100 ml)[20-22,38]	< 0.30	0.30 to 0.49	≥ 0.50

*Classification may not be valid for subjects with marked anemia.

closely related to tissue stores of the vitamin than serum levels.[4,5,43,44,98-101,121,122] Serum ascorbate levels tend to reflect, in general, recent dietary intakes of vitamin C. However, under controlled intakes of vitamin C, there is a relationship of serum ascorbate levels to the levels in the leucocytes (Table 3).

With vitamin C deprivation, serum ascorbate levels fall rather rapidly, while leucocyte ascorbate levels fall more slowly and most pronounced in association with the onset of signs of scurvy.[4,5,43] With adequate intakes of vitamin C, leucocytes will contain 12 to 35 mg of ascorbic acid/100 g of cells (Tables 3 and 5).[4,5,43,44,54,55,92,98-100,121,122,124] In clinical cases of scurvy, these levels may fall to zero.

Unfortunately, the determination of ascorbic acid in white blood cells is technically difficult and requires relatively large blood samples and is therefore not practical for routine use in nutrition surveys. For clinical cases of vitamin C deficiency, measurement of ascorbate levels in white blood cells can be a useful diagnostic procedure. However, adequate laboratory facilities must be available as improper handling of the leucocytes will cause a loss of ascorbic acid resulting in falsely low values.

Since urinary excretion of ascorbic acid falls off rapidly during a depletion of this vitamin,[21-24,122] attempts have been made to relate the ascorbic acid/creatinine ratio of random fasting urine specimens to ascorbic acid intake.[40,51,58] For this purpose, 24-hr urine collections have also been used.[46,122] Guides for the interpretation of urinary vitamin C levels in terms of nutritional status have not been established. The average 24-hr excretion of ascorbic acid by the normal well-nourished adult has been reported to range from 8 to 27 mg,[46,52,61,72] but data on this aspect are limited and unreliable in view of more recent knowledge of vitamin C metabolism and analytical methodology. Du Plessis observed in children a urinary excretion of vitamin C from 35 to 54 mg/gm of creatinine (Figure 5).[38]

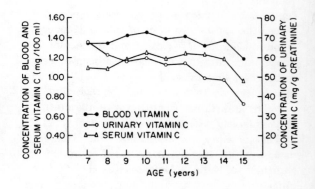

FIGURE 5. The relationship between age and the mean blood, serum, and urinary vitamin C values in Pretoria, South African children of ages 7 to 15 years. (From DuPlessis.[38])

Ritchey[103] noted the average urinary excretion of vitamin C in preadolescent children was 27.9 to 32.1 mg/day on daily intakes of ascorbic acid of 65.3 to 67.6 mg/day. Since urinary levels of ascorbic acid are probably prone to reflect immediate dietary intakes and are subject to analytical problems, measurements of urinary ascorbic acid levels are seldom undertaken. Nevertheless, in the scorbutic patient, the urinary excretion of vitamin C would be expected to be essentially nil and, hence, could provide supportive diagnostic information. In the vitamin C-depleted subjects studied by Baker et al.,[23,24] urinary loss of ascorbic acid did not occur until the body pool of the vitamin had been repleted to nearly normal levels. However, in a nutrition survey conducted in South Africa,[38] serum, blood, and urinary vitamin C levels were determined on each subject studied. It was concluded that "the blood and serum vitamin C levels are considered to give a satisfactory indication of vitamin C status in population groups, while the determination of urinary vitamin C exretion in such surveys may in fact be superfluous."[38] However, Du Plessis[38] did note that sex appeared to have no influence on the urinary excretion of vitamin C. Age did influence the urinary excretion of vitamin C when expressed on a per gram of creatinine basis (Figure 5). This would indicate that, for children of various ages, an age-adjusted sliding scale interpretive guide would be required to evaluate urinary vitamin C excretion data.

Although urinary ascorbic acid excretion rapidly declines to undetectable levels in vitamin C depletion, metabolites of ascorbic acid continue to be excreted.[21-24] The metabolites include oxalic acid,[24,59,60] ascorbate-2-sulfate[12] and, possibly, derivatives of L-threose or L-threonic acid.[57] Of these metabolites, ascorbate-2-sulfate appears to be an interesting compound for further study as an index of vitamin C status. The adult human male has been reported to excrete 30 to 60 mg of ascorbate-2-sulfate daily.[95] This level of excretion falls with the onset of scurvy.[95] With development of a simple and reliable quantitative method to measure ascorbate-2-sulfate in urine, a new approach to evaluating vitamin C nutritional status may be forthcoming.[96,119]

Ascorbic acid saturation tests are probably of little use in nutrition surveys but can be informative in individual cases where it is desired to establish tissue ascorbic acid deficit. Although a number of saturation or loading tests have been proposed,[17,31,43,51,58,61-64,72,73] the procedure of Lowry et al.[43,51] has been most commonly used. Subjects are administered 0.50 to 2.0 g of ascorbic acid in divided doses daily for 4 consecutive days. At the end of this period, the amount of ascorbic acid retained is determined with allowances being made for metabolic destruction of the vitamin. Sixty to eighty percent of the test dose will be recovered in the urine of subjects with normal ascorbic acid tissue saturation. In the tolerance test of Dutra de Oliveira,[63] vitamin C is administered orally (15 mg ascorbic acid/kg body weight) and the ascorbic acid level in the serum determined 3 hr later. The serum concentration of ascorbic acid will not increase above 0.25 mg/100 ml in patients with scurvy. Hence, this test may be of conclusive value in excluding scurvy as a diagnosis and of considerable usefulness in sustaining the diagnosis of scurvy. Although the various procedures provide some indication of the tissue depletion of vitamin C, the results must be interpreted with caution.[63] However, none of the saturation tests advocated can be considered practical for use in nutrition surveys.

Ascorbic acid can be measured with procedures employing either dinitrophenylhydrazine or 2,6-dichloroindophenol reagent.[47,49,74-77,80-94,101,113-115,123] Microautomated procedures enable the rapid analysis of large numbers of samples.[75,84,91,123] Fluorometric procedures are also available but do not appear to offer any significant advantages over the methods indicated and may suffer from the disadvantage of lower sensitivity.[86,93] However, in all instances, analytical procedures for measuring ascorbic acid in biological samples are beset with technical problems, and the methods used should be selected and conducted with extreme care with respect to specificity, reliability, reproducibility and sensitivity.[94] Moreover, ascorbic acid can be an exceedingly labile vitamin, and precautions must be taken to stabilize the ascorbic acid in serum and other biological samples to prevent losses prior to analysis.[94] Plasma or serum samples may be used with equal success providing hemolysis is prevented. Hemolyzed samples may give rise to elevated or lowered ascorbate values depending upon the storage conditions.

In this respect, it should be noted that the 2,4-dinitrophenylhydrazine method must be utilized with precaution. Blood, serum and urine samples must be incubated at temperatures not exceeding 37°C. Otherwise, variable amounts of ascorbate-2-sulfate, recently noted to be present in such samples, will be included to give rise to erroneous results.[118]

Additional procedures have been proposed to evaluate vitamin C nutritional status. For example, the rate of disappearance of intradermally injected solution of 2,6-dichloroindophenol has been proposed as an indicator of vitamin C tissue saturation. Although the method is not specific, some degree of correlation with vitamin C status has been observed.[65] However, the procedure has not been well standardized and, hence, has not been recommended for use in nutrition surveys or in clinical situations.

Similarly, the tyrosine load test is of uncertain value in the assessment of vitamin C status.[98,122] Vitamin C deficiency apparently is not the basic cause of the defective tyrosine metabolism that results in the excretion of tyrosyl metabolites, although supplements of ascorbic acid will reduce the excretion of the metabolites.[66,78,79,98,101]

More recently, the lingual vitamin C test has been studied as a procedure for evaluating ascorbic acid status.[67-71] The procedure is based on the reports of Giza et al.[67,68] that the vitamin C reserve of the body could be estimated by observing the time of decolorization of an aqueous solution of 2,6-dichloroindophenol by the tongue. The procedure has been utilized extensively by Cheraskin and associates[69,70] who have published over 25 reports on the subject.[70] However, King and Little[71] concluded from their studies that the procedure was not specific for ascorbic acid and would have little or no value when used to evaluate vitamin C nutritional status. Regardless of these differences in findings, the procedure requires further evaluation by additional investigators before any final recommendations can be made regarding the usefulness and validity of the test.

In summary, the measurement of serum (plasma) levels of ascorbic acid is the most commonly used and practical procedure for evaluating vitamin C nutritional status in population groups or individuals. The white blood cell levels of ascorbic acid provide information concerning the body stores of the vitamin, but the measurement is technically difficult to perform and its use is confined to clinical situations as an aid in the diagnosis of scurvy. Nevertheless, a correlation has been observed between the ascorbic acid levels in plasma or whole blood and the levels in white blood cells.[104,117] Information on the urinary levels of ascorbic acid and the use of vitamin C loading tests can be helpful in the clinical diagnosis of scurvy.

REFERENCES

1. **King, C. G.,** Present knowledge of ascorbic acid (vitamin C), *Nutr. Rev.,* 26, 33, 1968.
2. **Mapson, L. W.,** Ascorbic acid. IX. Biochemical systems, in *The Vitamins,* Vol. I, 2nd ed., Sebrell, W. H., Jr. and Harris, R. S., Eds., Academic Press, New York, 1967, 386.
3. **Goldsmith, G. A.,** Human requirements for vitamin C and its use in clinical medicine, *Ann. N.Y. Acad. Sci.,* 92, 230, 1961.
4. **Bartley, W. H., Krebs, H. A., and O'Brien, J. R. P.,** Vitamin C requirement of human adults, *Med. Res. Council Special Rept. Series,* 280, 142, 1953, H. M. Stationery Office, London.
5. **Crandon, J. H., Lund, C. C., and Dill, D. B.,** Experimental human scurvy, *N. Engl. J. Med.,* 223, 353, 1940.
6. **Chick, H.,** Early investigations of scurvy and the antiscorbutic vitamin, Lind Bicentenary Symposium, *Proc. Nutr. Soc.,* 12, 210, 1953.
7. **Crandon, J. H., Mikal, S., and Landeau, B. R.,** Ascorbic-acid deficiency in experimental and surgical subjects, Lind Bicentenary Symposium, *Proc. Nutr. Soc.,* 12, 273, 1953.
8. **Kark, R. M.,** Ascorbic acid in relation to cold, scurvy, ACTH, and surgery, Lind Bicentenary Symposium, *Proc. Nutr. Soc.,* 12, 279, 1953.
9. **Harris, L. J.,** The mode of action of vitamin C, Lind Bicentenary Symposium, *Proc. Nutr. Soc.,* 12, 128, 1953.
10. **Mumma, R. O.,** Ascorbic acid sulfate as a sulfating agent, *Biochim. Biophys. Acta.,* 165, 571, 1968.
11. **Mead, C. G. and Finamore, F. J.,** The occurrence of ascorbic acid sulfate in the brine shrimp, *Artemia Salina, Biochem.,* 8, 2652, 1969.
12. **Baker, E. M., III, Hammer, D. C., March, S. C., Tolbert, B. M., and Canham, J. E.,** Ascorbate sulfate: A urinary metabolite of ascorbic acid in man, *Science,* 173, 826, 1971.

13. **Mumma, R. O., Verlangieri, A. J., and Weber, W. W., II,** L-ascorbic acid 3-sulfate. Preparation and characterization, *Carbohyd. Res.,* 19, 127, 1971.

14. **Mumma, R. O. and Verlangieri, A. J.,** Isolation of ascorbic acid 2-sulfate from selected rat organs, *Biochim. Biophys. Acta.,* 273, 249, 1972.

15. **Mumma, R. O., McKee, E. E., Verlangieri, A. J., and Barron, G. P.,** Anti-scorbutic effect of ascorbic acid 2-sulfate in the guinea pig, *Nutr. Rep. Int.,* 6, 133, 1972.

16. **Halver, J. E., Johnson, C. L., Smith, R. R., Tolbert, B. M., and Baker, E. M.,** Vitamin C$_3$ reduces fish scurvy, *Fed. Proc.,* 31(2), 705 (abstract), 1972.

17. **Chatterjee, G. C.,** Ascorbic acid. X. Biochemical detection of deficiency, in *The Vitamins,* Vol. I, 2nd ed. Sebrell, W. H., Jr. and Harris, R. S., Eds., Academic Press, New York, 1967, 399.

18. **Pearson, W. N.,** Biochemical appraisal of the vitamin nutritional status in man, *J.A.M.A.,* 180, 49, 1962.

19. **Sauberlich, H. E.,** Problems of assessment of nutritional status: An overview of biochemical methodologies, in *Problems of Assessment and Alleviation of Malnutrition in the United States,* (proceedings of a workshop sponsored by Vanderbilt University, HSMHA and NIH held at Nashville, Tenn., January 13 – 14, 1970), Hansen, R. G. and Munro, H. N., Eds., U.S. Govt. Printing Office, Washington, D.C., Pub. No. 916.086, 1971.

20. **Hodges, R. E. and Canham, J. E.,** Vitamin deficiencies: Studies of experimental vitamin C deficiency and experimental vitamin A deficiency in man, in *Problems of Assessment and Alleviation of Malnutrition in the United States,* (proceedings of a workshop sponsored by Vanderbilt University, HSMHA and NIH held at Nashville, Tenn., January 13–14, 1970), Hansen, R. G. and Munro, H. N., Eds., U.S. Govt. Printing Office, Washington, D.C. Pub. No. 916.086, 1971.

21. **Hodges, R. E., Hood, J., Canham, J. E., Sauberlich, H. E., and Baker, E. M.,** Clinical manifestations of ascorbic acid deficiency in man, *Am. J. Clin. Nutr.,* 24, 432, 1971.

22. **Baker, E. M., Hodges, R. E., Hood, J., Sauberlich, H. E., March, S. C., and Canham, J. E.,** Metabolism of ^{14}C- and ^{3}H-labeled L-ascorbic acid in human scurvy, *Am. J. Clin. Nutr.,* 24, 444, 1971.

23. **Hodges, R. E., Baker, E. M., Hood, J., Sauberlich, H. E., and March, S. C.,** Experimental scurvy in man, *Am. J. Clin. Nutr.,* 22, 535, 1969.

24. **Baker, E. M., Hodges, R. E., Hood, J., Sauberlich, H. E., and March, S. C.,** Metabolism of ascorbic-1-^{14}C acid in experimental human scurvy, *Am. J. Clin. Nutr.,* 22, 549, 1969.

25. **Hood, J. and Hodges, R. E.,** Ocular lesions in scurvy, *Am. J. Clin. Nutr.,* 22, 559, 1969.

26. **Hood, J.,** Femoral neuropathy in scurvy, *N. Engl. J. Med.,* 261, 1292, 1969.

27. **Hood, J., Burns, C. A., and Hodges, R. E.,** Sjögren's syndrome in scurvy, *N. Engl. J. Med.,* 282, 1120, 1970.

28. **Abboud, F. M., Hood, J., Hodges, R. E., and Mayer, H. E.,** Automomic reflexes and vascular reactivity in experimental scurvy in man, *J. Clin. Invest.,* 49, 298, 1970.

29. **Jelliffe, D. B.,** The assessment of the nutritional status of the community, *W.H.O. Monogr. Ser.,* No. 53, World Health Organization, Geneva, Switzerland, 1966, 89.

30. *Suggested Guidelines for Evaluation of the Nutritional Status of Preschool Children,* U.S. Department of Health, Education and Welfare; Social and Rehabilitation Service, Children's Bureau, U.S. Govt. Printing Office No. 0-275-984, (revised), 1967.

31. **Woodruff, C. W.,** Ascorbic acid, in *Nutrition, A Comprehensive Treatise,* Vol. II, Chap. 4, Beaton, G. H. and McHenry, E. W., Eds., Academic Press, New York, 1964, 265.

32. *Expert Committee on Medical Assessment of Nutritional Status,* World Health Organization Technical Report Series No. 258, World Health Organization, Geneva, Switzerland, 1963, 37.

33. **Pearson, W. N.,** Assessment of nutritional status: Biochemical methods, in *Nutrition, A Comprehensive Treatise,* Vol. III, Beaton, G. H. and McHenry, E. W., Eds., Academic Press, New York, 1966, 275.

34. **Krehl, W. A. and Hodges, R. E.,** The interpretation of nutrition survey data, *Am. J. Clin. Nutr.,* 17, 191, 1965.

35. **Krause, R. F.,** Laboratory aids in the diagnosis of malnutrition, in *Modern Nutrition in Health and Disease,* 4th ed., Wohl, M. G. and Goodhart, R. S., Eds., Lea & Febiger, Philadelphia, 1968, 519.

36. **Pearson, W. N.,** Blood and urinary vitamin levels as potential indices of body stores, *Am. J. Clin. Nutr.,* 20, 514, 1967.

37. **Pearson, W. N.,** Biochemical appraisal of nutritional status in man, *Am. J. Clin. Nutr.,* 11, 462, 1962.

38. **Du Plessis, J. P.,** An evaluation of biochemical criteria for use in nutrition status surveys, *Council for Scientific and Industrial Research Report No. 261,* National Nutrition Research Institute, Pretoria, South Africa, 1967, 109.

39. **A Study of the Military Applicability of Research on Ascorbic Acid,** Griffith, W. H. and Morthland, F. W., Eds., Life Sciences Research Office, Federation of American Societies for Experimental Biology, Bethesda, Maryland, 1963.

40. **Burch, H. B.,** Methods for detecting and evaluating ascorbic acid deficiency in man and animals, *Ann. N.Y. Acad. Sci.,* 92, 268, 191.

41. **Catalano, P. M.,** Vitamin C, *Arch. Dermatol.,* 103, 537, 1971.

42. **Baker, E. M.,** Vitamin C requirements in stress, *Am. J. Clin. Nutr.,* 20, 583, 1967.

43. **Lowry, O. H., Bessey, O. A., Brock, M. J., and Lopez, J. A.,** The interrelationship of dietary, serum, white blood cell and total body ascorbic acid, *J. Biol. Chem.,* 166, 111, 1946.

44. **Dodds, M. J. and MacLeod, F. L.,** Blood plasma ascorbic acid levels on controlled intakes of ascorbic acid, *Science,* 106, 67, 1947.

45. **Masek, J.,** Recommended nutrient allowances, *World Rev. Nutr. Diet.,* 3, 149, 1962.
46. **Friedman, G. J., Sherry, S., and Ralli, E. P.,** The mechanism of the excretion of vitamin C by the human kidney at low and normal plasma levels of ascorbic acid, *J. Clin. Invest.,* 19, 685, 1940.
47. *Manual for Nutrition Surveys,* 2nd ed., Interdepartmental Committee on Nutrition for National Defense, Superintendent of Documents, U. S. Government Printing Office, Washington, D.C. 20402, 1963.
48. Nutrition Survey Reports (1957 — 1971), Interdepartmental Committee on Nutrition for National Defense, Washington, D.C.
49. Ten-State Nutrition Survey Reports, I — V, Center for Disease Control, Atlanta, Georgia 30330, 1972.
50. **O'Neal, R. M., Johnson, O. C., and Schaefer, A. E.,** Guidelines for classification and interpretation of group blood and urine data collected as part of the National Nutrition Survey, *Pediatr. Res.,* 4, 103, 1970.
51. **Lowry, O. H.,** Biochemical evidence of nutritional status, *Physiol. Rev.,* 32, 431, 1952.
52. **Davey, B. L., Wu, M. L., and Storvick, C. A.,** Daily determination of plasma, serum and white cell-platelet ascorbic acid in relationship to the excretion of ascorbic acid and homogentisic acid by adults maintained on a controlled diet, *J. Nutr.,* 47, 341, 1952.
53. **Bessey, O. A. and White, R. L.,** The ascorbic acid requirements of children, *J. Nutr.,* 23, 195, 1942.
54. **Steele, B. F., Liner, R. L., Pierce, Z. H., and Williams, H. H.,** Ascorbic acid nutriture in the human. II. Content of ascorbic acid in the white cells and sera of subjects receiving controlled low intakes of the vitamin, *J. Nutr.,* 57, 361, 1955.
55. **Morse, E. H., Potgieter, M., and Walker, G. R.,** Ascorbic acid utilization by women. Response of blood serum and white blood cells to increasing levels of intake, *J. Nutr.,* 58, 291, 1956.
56. **Bessey, O. A. and Lowry, O. H.,** Nutritional assay of 1200 New York State school children. Meals for millions — New York State Joint Legislative Committee on Nutrition, 1947, 167.
57. **Tolbert, B. M., Chen, A. W., Bell, E. M., and Baker, E. M.,** Metabolism of L-ascorbic-4-³H acid in man, *Am. J. Clin. Nutr.,* 20, 250, 1967.
58. **Johnson, R. E., Henderson, C., Robinson, P. F., and Consolazio, F. C.,** Comparative merits of fasting specimens, random specimens and oral loading tests in field nutritional surveys, *J. Nutr.,* 30, 89, 1945.
59. **Hellman, L. and Burns, J. J.,** Metabolism of L-ascorbic acid-1-C¹⁴ in man, *J. Biol. Chem.,* 230, 923, 1958.
60. **Baker, E. M., Saari, J. C., and Tolbert, B. M.,** Ascorbic acid metabolism in man, *Am. J. Clin. Nutr.,* 19, 371, 1966.
61. **Johnson, R. E., Darling, R. E., Sargent, F., and Robinson, P.,** Effects of variations in dietary vitamin C on the physical well being of manual workers, *J. Nutr.,* 29, 155, 1945.
62. **Farmer, C. J.,** Some aspects of vitamin C metabolism, *Fed. Proc.,* 3, 179, 1944.
63. **Dutra de Oliveira, J. E., Pearson, W. N., and Darby, W. J.,** Clinical usefulness of the oral ascorbic acid tolerance test in scurvy, *Am. J. Clin. Nutr.,* 7, 630, 1959.
64. **Vilter, R. W.,** Ascorbic acid. XII. Effects of ascorbic acid deficiency in man, in *The Vitamins,* Vol. I. 2nd ed., Sebrell, W. H., Jr. and Harris, R. S., Eds., Academic Press, New York, 1967, 457.
65. **Cheraskin, E., Dunbar, J. B., and Flynn, F. H.,** The intradermal ascorbic acid test: Part III. A study of forty-two dental students, *J. Dent. Med.,* 13, 135, 1958.
66. **Avery, M. E., Clow, C. L., Menkes, J. H., Ramos, A., Scriver, C. R., Stern, L., and Wasserman, B. P.,** Transient tyrosinemia of the new-born: Dietary and clinical aspects, *Pediatrics,* 39, 378, 1967.
67. **Giza, T. and Weclawowiez, J.,** Perlingual method for evaluating the vitamin C content of the body: A rapid diagnostic test for vitamin C undernutrition, *J. Vit. Res.,* 30, 327, 1960.
68. **Giza, T., Weclawowiez, J., and Zaionc, J.,** The perlingual method for evaluating vitamin C: II. The relation between decolorization time and the vitamin C content of the organs, *Int. J. Vit. Res.,* 32, 121, 1962.
69. **Ringsdorf, W. M., Jr. and Cheraskin, E.,** A rapid and simple lingual ascorbic acid test, *General Practice,* 25, 106, 1962.
70. **Cheraskin, E. and Ringsdorf, W. M., Jr.,** A fortunate erratum, *J. Oral Med.,* 26, 75, 1971.
71. **King, D. R. and Little, J. W.,** Lingual ascorbic acid test, *J. Oral Med.,* 25, 107, 1970.
72. **Roderuck, C., Burrill, L., Campbell, L. J., Brakke, Einbecker, B., Childs, M. T., Leverton, R., Chaloupka, M., Jebe, E. H., and Swanson, P. P.,** Estimated dietary intake, urinary excretion and blood vitamin C in women of different ages, *J. Nutr.,* 66, 15, 1958.
73. **Mitra, M. L.,** Vitamin-C deficiency in the elderly and its manifestations, *J. Am. Geriatr. Soc.,* 18, 67, 1970.
74. **Saari, J. C., Baker, E. M., and Sauberlich, H. E.,** Thin-layer chromatographic separation of the oxidative degradation products of ascorbic acid, *Anal. Biochem.,* 18, 173, 1967.
75. **Pelletier, O. and Brassard, R.,** A new automated serum vitamin C method, Technicon International Symposium; abstract No. PH 13, New York, June 1972, 64.
76. **Saari, J. C., Baker, E. M., and Sauberlich, H. E.,** A simplified method for the isolation of urinary ascorbic acid as the 2,4-dinitrophenylosazone, *Anal. Biochem.,* 15, 537, 1966.
77. **Schaffert, R. R. and Kingsley, G. R.,** A rapid, simple method for the determination of reduced, dehydro-, and total ascorbic acid in biological material, *J. Biol. Chem.,* 212, 59, 1955.
78. **Knox, W. E. and Goswami, M. N. D.,** The mechanism of p-hydroxyphenyl-pyruvate accumulation in guinea pigs fed tyrosine, *J. Biol. Chem.,* 235, 2662, 1960.

79. **La Da, B. N. and Zannoni, V. G.,** Tyrosyluria resulting from inhibition of p-hydroxyphenyl-pyruvic acid oxidase in vitamin C-deficient guinea pigs, *J. Biol. Chem.,* 235, 2667, 1960.

80. **Roe, J. H. and Kuether, C. A.,** The determination of ascorbic acid in whole blood and urine through the 2,4-dinitrophenylhydrazine derivative of ascorbic acid, *J. Biol. Chem.,* 147, 399, 1943.

81. **Roe, J. H.,** Appraisal of methods for the determination of L-ascorbic acid, *Ann. N. Y. Acad. Sci.,* 92, 277, 1961.

82. **Bessey, O. A., Lowry, O. H., and Brock, M. J.,** The quantitative determination of ascorbic acid in small amounts of white blood cells and platelets, *J. Biol. Chem.,* 168, 197, 1947.

83. **Lowry, O. H., Bessey, O. A., and Burch, H. B.,** Effects of prolonged high dosage with ascorbic acid, *Proc. Soc. Exp. Biol. Med.,* 80, 361, 1952.

84. **Garry, P. J. and Owen, G. M.,** Automated screening technique for vitamin C assay requiring small quantities of blood, Technicon Symposium: *Automation in Analytical Chemistry,* Vol. I, 1967, 507.

85. **Gero, E. and Candido, A.,** Une technique chimique de dosage de l'acide ascorbique total par une réaction d'oxydo-réduction, *J. Int. Vitaminol.,* 39, 252, 1969.

86. **Deutsch, M. J. and Weeks, C. E.,** Microfluorometric assay for vitamin C, *J. Assoc. Offic. Agric. Chem.,* 48, 1248, 1965.

87. **Vuillemier, J.,** Analytische probleme bei der bestimmung von vitamin C im zusammenhang mit ernährungserhebungen, *Int. Z. Vitaminforsch.,* 37, 504, 1967.

88. **Pelletier, O.,** Determination of vitamin C in serum, urine and other biological materials, *J. Lab. Clin. Med.,* 72, 674, 1968.

89. **Howard, A. N. and Constable, B. J.,** The use of homocysteine in the estimation of ascorbic acid in urine, *Clin. Chim. Acta,* 13, 387, 1966.

90. **Hughes, R. E.,** Use of a cation-exchange resin in the determination of urinary ascorbic acid, *Analyst,* 89, 618, 1964.

91. **Goad, W. C., Skala, J. H., Harding, R. S., and Sauberlich, H. E.,** A semiautomated technique for the determination of vitamin C (ascorbic acid) in serum or plasma samples, *U.S. Army Medical Research and Nutrition Laboratory Report,* Denver, Colorado 80240, June 1972.

92. **Loh, H. S. and Wilson, C. W.,** An improved method for the measurement of leucocyte ascorbic acid concentrations, *Int. J. Vit. Nutr. Res.,* 41, 90, 1971.

93. **Nobile, S.,** Fluorometric determination of vitamin C in plasma, The Vitamin Laboratories, Roche Products Proprietary, Dee Why, New South Wales, Australia, personal communication.

94. **Olliver, M.,** Ascorbic acid. IV. Estimation, in *The Vitamins,* Vol I, 2nd ed., Sebrell, W. H., Jr. and Harris, R. S., Eds., Academic Press, New York, 1967, 338.

95. **Baker, E. M., Kennedy, J. E., Tolbert, B. M., and Canham, J. E.,** Excretion and pool size of ascorbate sulfate and other ascorbate derivatives in man, *Fed. Proc.,* 31, 705 (abstract), 1972.

96. **March, S. C.,** A quantitative procedure for the assay of ascorbate-3-sulfate in biological samples, *Fed. Proc.,* 31, 705 (abstract), 1972.

97. **Woodhill, J. M. and Nobile, S.,** Vitamin C (L-ascorbic acid and dehydro-L-ascorbic acid). A contribution to the Captain Cook bicentennial celebrations, *Med. J. Aust.,* 1, 1009, 1971.

98. **Crandon, J. H., Landau, B., Mikal, S., Balmanno, J., Jefferson, M., and Mahoney, N.,** Ascorbic acid economy in surgical patients as indicated by blood ascorbic acid levels, *N. Engl. J. Med.,* 258, 105, 1958.

99. **Loh, H. S.,** The relationship between dietary ascorbic acid intake and buffy coat and plasma ascorbic acid concentrations at different ages, *Int. J. Vit. Nutr. Res.,* 42, 80, 1972.

100. **Loh, H. S.,** The differences in the metabolism of ascorbic acid between the sexes at different ages, *Int. J. Vit. Nutr. Res.,* 42, 86, 1972.

101. **Denson, K. W. and Bowers, E. F.,** The determination of ascorbic acid in white blood cells, *Clin. Sci.,* 21, 157, 1961.

102. **Manchanda, S. S., Khanna, S., and Lal, H.,** Plasma ascorbic acid as an index of vitamin C nutrition, *Indian Pediatr.,* 8, 184, 1971.

103. **Ritchey, S. J.,** Metabolic patterns in preadolescent children. XV. Ascorbic acid intake, urinary excretion and serum concentration, *Am. J. Clin. Nutr.,* 17, 78, 1965.

104. **Griffiths, L. L., Brocklehurst, J. C., Scott, D. L., Marks, J., and Blackley, J.,** Thiamine and ascorbic acid levels in the elderly, *Gerontol. Clin.,* 9, 1, 1967.

105. **Pelletier, O.,** Vitamin C status of cigarette smokers and nonsmokers, *Am. J. Clin. Nutr.,* 23, 520, 1970.

106. **Bailey, D. A., Carron, A. V., Teece, R. G., and Wehner, H. J.,** Vitamin C supplementation related to physiological response to exercise in smoking and nonsmoking subjects, *Am. J. Clin. Nutr.,* 23, 905, 1970.

107. **Brook, M. and Grimshaw, J. J.,** Vitamin C concentrations of plasma and leukocytes as related to smoking habit, age, and sex of humans, *Am. J. Clin. Nutr.,* 21, 1254, 1968.

108. **Rivers, J. M. and Devine, M. M.,** Plasma ascorbic acid concentrations and oral contraceptives, *Am. J. Clin. Nutr.,* 25, 684, 1972.

109. **Dodds, M. L.,** Sex as a factor in blood levels of ascorbic acid, *J. Am. Diet. Assoc.,* 54, 32, 1969.

110. **Loh, H. S. and Wilson, C. W. M.,** Relationship of human ascorbic-acid metabolism to ovulation, *Lancet,* 1, 110, 1971.

111. **Woodhill, J. M.,** Australian dietary surveys with special reference to vitamins, *Int. J. Vit. Res.,* 40, 520, 1970.

112. **Brin, M., Dibble, M. V., Peel, A., McMullen, E., Bourquin, A., and Chen, N.,** Some preliminary findings on the nutritional status of the aged in Onondaga County, New York, *Am. J. Clin. Nutr.,* 17, 240, 1965.

113. **Mindlin, R. L. and Butler, A. M.,** The determination of ascorbic acid in plasma: A macromethod and micromethod, *J. Biol. Chem.,* 122, 673, 1938.

114. **Bessey, O. A.,** A method for the determination of small quantities of ascorbic acid and dehydroascorbic acid in turbid and colored solutions in the presence of other reducing substances, *J. Biol. Chem.,* 126, 771, 1938.

115. **Sabry, J. H. and Dodds, M. L.,** Comparative measurements of ascorbic acid and total ascorbic acid of blood plasma, *J. Nutr.,* 64, 467, 1958.

116. **Sahud, M. A. and Cohen, R. J.,** Effect of aspirin ingestion on ascorbic-acid levels in rheumatoid arthritis, *Lancet,* 1, 937, 1971.

117. **Andrews, J. and Brook, M.,** Leucocyte-vitamin-C content and clinical signs in the elderly, *Lancet,* 1, 1350, 1966.

118. **Baker, E. M., Hammer, D. C., Kennedy, J. E., and Tolbert, B. M.,** Interference by ascorbate-2-sulfate in the dinitrophenylhydrazine assay of ascorbic acid, *Anal. Biochem.,* in press.

119. **Tolbert, B. M., Bullen, W. W., III, Downing, M., and Baker, E. M.,** Ascorbate sulfohydrolase activity of an arylsulfohydrolase A preparation, *Fed. Proc.,* 32, 931 (abstract), 1973.

120. **Pelletier, O.,** Smoking and vitamin C levels in humans, *Am. J. Clin. Nutr.,* 21, 1259, 1968.

121. **Grebenkov, S. G.,** Comparative study of the vitamin C content of the blood plasma and leucocytes in humans, *Vopr. Pitan.,* 23, 40, 1964.

122. **Steele, B. F., Hsu, C. H., Pierce, Z. H., and Williams, H. H.,** Ascorbic acid nutriture in human. I. Tyrosine metabolism and blood levels of ascorbic acid during ascorbic acid depletion and repletion, *J. Nutr.,* 48, 49, 1952.

123. **Garry, P. J. and Owen, G. M.,** Automated procedure for plasma ascorbic acid using 2,6-dichlorophenol-indophenol, IX International Congress of Nutrition, Abstracts, Mexico City, 1972, 192.

124. **McLeroy, V. J. and Schendel, H. E.,** Influence of oral contraceptives on ascorbic acid concentrations in healthy, sexually mature women, *Am. J. Clin. Nutr.,* 26, 191, 1973.

Thiamin (Vitamin B_1)

Thiamin deficiency occurs most commonly among populations of the world where rice is the staple food.[44] The condition is expressed in the classical pathological condition called beriberi.[1-3, 7,22,94] However, clinical cases of thiamin deficiency may occur frequently in association with chronic alcoholism and, in many instances, may result in Wernicke's encephalopathy.[3,4,59, 78,94] Thiamin deficiency may also develop in disease states characterized by marked anorexia, vomiting or diarrhea, and in postoperative patients.[1,3,22,77]

Various biochemical procedures have been developed which have been useful for detecting thiamin deficiency or assessing thiamin nutritional status.[2,3,5,16,22,24,25,29,96] The most commonly used procedure has been the measurement of urinary levels of thiamin.[2,3,5-7,16,88,89] Thiamin is generally measured in urine with the use of the thiochrome method[5,6,9,88,89] or by microbiological assay with *Lactobacillus viridescens* as the commonly used assay organism.[6,90] Urinary thiamin levels have been used in the ICNND nutrition surveys,[5,8,31] the Ten-State Nutrition Survey,[9] and other surveys to assess thiamin nutritional status.[26,27,30,32,91] The procedure evolved as a result of findings from various investigations that established the existence of a reasonably close correlation between the development of a thiamin deficiency and the decreasing excretion of thiamin in the urine.[10-25,92] Urinary excretion of thiamin decreases proportionally with thiamin intake to a critical point after which further lowering of intake results in only minor and variable changes in urinary excretion. Tissue stores of thiamin will be depleted with intakes of the vitamin below the critical point and, if continued, will result in symptoms of a deficiency.

The thiamin requirement of adult human has generally been considered to be about 0.30 to 0.35 mg/1,000 calories.[28,33,34] Approximately 40 to 90 μg of thiamin are excreted in the urine daily on intakes of 0.30 to 0.36 mg thiamin/1,000 calories, while 100 μg and above are excreted when the intake of thiamin is increased to 0.50 mg/1,000 calories.[5,10-12,16,28,35] When the daily intake of thiamin is reduced to only about 0.2 mg/1,000 calories, urinary excretions fall to only 5 to 25 μg of thiamin per day.[1,7,10-13,16,20,21,24,25,28, 29,35,36] In cases of beriberi, 24-hr urinary excretions of 0 to 15 μg of thiamin have been reported.[1,36] As a result of these observations, measurement of the 24-hr urinary excretion of thiamin has been useful in evaluating thiamin nutriture. Under survey conditions, however, it is usually not feasible to collect 24-hr urine samples.

Consequently, as a matter of expediency, random urine samples are obtained, preferably during fasting state, and the thiamin content related to creatinine content.[5,9,25,29,36,37,49] A correlation between the urinary excretion of thiamin per gram of creatinine and thiamin intake has been observed (Figure 6).[28,31,33] Interpretive guidelines commonly used for adults are indicated in Table 6.[5,8,9,25,29,37]

Knowledge concerning urinary thiamin excretion levels in children is limited[40] with the report of Stearns et al.[38] representing the most informative study. However, these studies and the evaluations of Pearson[25,29] revealed that children have a markedly higher level of thiamin excretion when expressed on a creatinine basis than adults. This was also exemplified in the findings of the Ten-State Nutrition Survey (Figure 7).[9] In view of this age variable, Pearson developed adjusted sliding scale interpretive guides for thiamin excretion values for children of various ages (Table 6).[25,29,41] These guides have been commonly used,[37] but some revision may be in order following an evaluation of the data obtained from the Ten-State Nutrition Survey.[9] Although thiamin urinary excretion information is subject to certain errors[24,25,29,39,40,42] (see also section on riboflavin) particularly when applied to individuals, such information has been exceedingly useful when applied to population groups. When clinical patients are encountered exhibiting suspected signs or symptoms of a thiamin deficiency, thiamin excretion levels should be measured on 24-hr urine collections. Additional supportive information should be obtained through the use of thiamin retention tests and, when feasible, through erythrocyte transketolase measurements.

Retention tests of a known dose of thiamin

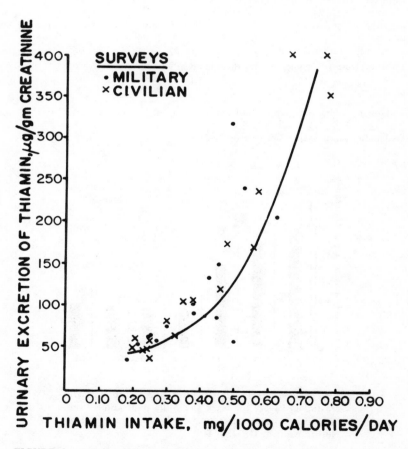

FIGURE 6.   Relationship between thiamin intake and thiamin urinary excretion in adults as observed in nutrition surveys conducted in 18 countries by ICNND.[8] (From report of a Joint FAO/WHO Expert Group.[33])

TABLE 6

Guidelines for the Interpretation of Urinary Excretion of Thiamin

| | Less than acceptable (at risk) | | |
Subjects	Deficient (high risk)	Low (medium risk)	Acceptable (low risk)
	μg/g creatinine[a]		
1 to 3 years	< 120	120 to 175	≥ 176
4 to 6 years	< 85	85 to 120	≥ 121
7 to 9 years	< 70	70 to 180	≥ 181
10 to 12 years	< 60	60 to 180	≥ 181
13 to 15 years	< 50	50 to 150	≥ 151
Adults	< 27	27 to 65	≥ 66
Pregnant			
2nd trimester	< 23	23 to 54	≥ 55
3rd trimester	< 21	21 to 49	≥ 50
	Other interpretive guidelines[b]		
Adults			
μg/24 hr	< 40	40 to 99	≥ 100
μg/6 hr	< 10	10 to 24	≥ 25
Load test (return in adults of 5 mg thiamin dose)[b]			
μg in 4 hr	< 20	20 to 79	≥ 80

[a]Adapted from the reports of O'Neal et al.[37] and others.[5,9,16,24,25,29,41,91,92]

[b]Adapted from the reports of Pearson.[5,24,29,92]

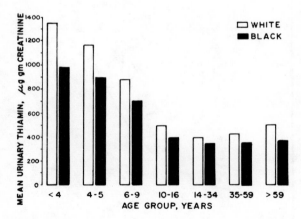

FIGURE 7. Mean urinary thiamin excretion (μg/g creatinine) by age for black and white populations from high income ratio states. (Adapted from the Ten-State Nutrition Survey (IV-226).[9])

administered orally or intramuscularly have been of value in evaluating the extent of depletion of tissue stores. Although a number of thiamin load tests have been proposed,[24,36,42,43,45] the most commonly used procedure is to administer parenterally 5 mg of thiamin and measure the urinary excretion of thiamin in the following 4-hr period. Subjects deficient in thiamin will usually excrete less than 20 μg of the dose during this period (Table 6). In nutrition surveys, the procedure has not been used extensively because of the inconvenience and extra effort required in obtaining the 4-hr urine samples following the administration of the thiamin test load. Although the test may not specifically identify clinical thiamin deficiency or indicate the severity of a deficiency, it can be useful as an indicator of low intakes and tissue deficits of the vitamin.

In recent years, erythrocyte transketolase measurements have proven to be a useful indicator of early insufficiency of thiamin prior to the appearance of clinical manifestations.[2,14,16,30,58-78,94,95] The measurement represents a functional test of thiamin adequacy and, hence, may be a more reliable indicator of thiamin insufficiency than urinary measurements of thiamin.[2,14,16,29,58,66,68] Transketolase is a thiamin-pyrophosphate-requiring enzyme which catalyzes the following two reactions in the pentose phosphate pathway:

1. Xylulose-5-phosphate + ribose-5-phosphate ⇌ sedoheptulose-7-phosphate + glyceraldehyde-3-phosphate
2. Xylulose-5-phosphate + erythrose-4-phosphate ⇌ fructose-6-phosphate + glyceraldehyde-3-phosphate

In controlled human studies, a relationship was found to exist between thiamin intake and urinary excretion of thiamin and erythrocyte transketolase activities.[2,14,28,58] Figure 8 summarizes results from a study on adults conducted at this laboratory.[28] These results support the validity of the guidelines commonly employed for interpreting thiamin nutritional status in the adult (Table 6).[5,8,9,37] The studies have also provided tentative guidelines for interpreting erythrocyte transketolase activities (Table 7).

In brief, the erythrocyte transketolase activity assay involves the incubation of hemolyzed whole blood samples in a buffered medium with an

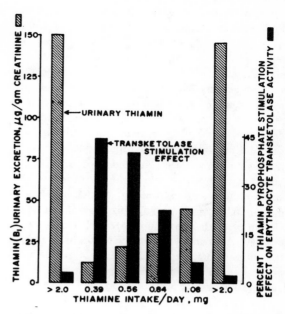

FIGURE 8. Relationship of erythrocyte transketolase activity to urinary excretion of thiamin in adult male subjects during controlled intakes of thiamin. Subjects received 3600 kcal per day.[28]

TABLE 7

Guidelines Used for Interpretation of Erythrocyte Transketolase Thiamine Pyrophosphate Stimulation Assay (all ages)*

ICNND classification[2,67]

Classification	Th PP stimulation
Acceptable (low risk)	0 to 15%
Low (medium risk)	16 to 20%
Deficient (high risk)	> 20%

Classification of Brin et al.[58,68]

Classification	T PP effect
Normal (adequate)	0 to 14%
Marginally deficient (marginal)	15 to 24%
Severely deficient (deficient)	≥ 25%

*Guidelines may require adjustment in accordance with the specific method used to measure erythrocyte transketolase activity.

excess of ribose-5-phosphate, in both the presence and the absence of excess thiamin pyrophosphate. Following an incubation period of 30 or 60 min at 37 to 43°C, the ribose-5-phosphate utilized, or sedoheptulose-7-phosphate or hexoses produced, are measured.[6,58,62,65,69] Any enhancement in enzyme activity resulting from the added thiamin pyrophosphate, expressed usually in percent, is referred to as the "ThPP stimulation" or "effect."[2,27,58,59,67] Values obtained without the addition of thiamin pyrophosphate represent the absolute enzyme activity and are dependent upon the coenzyme available in the erythrocytes. The addition of thiamin pyrophosphate permits an estimation of the amount of apoenzyme uncomplexed as well as of the maximum potential transketolase activity. A thiamin deficiency results in a reduction in the thiamin pyrophosphate available and, in some instances, may result in a reduction of the apotransketolase as well.[2,58]

Erythrocyte transketolase activity assays may be performed by manual[27,58,67] or automated procedures.[64] Both procedures have been used routinely by the authors in experimental studies, clinical situations, and in numerous nutrition surveys. Other investigators have also used erythrocyte transketolase activity measurements successfully to diagnose beriberi and evaluate thiamin nutritional status.[66-70,73,74,77,93] This is exemplified by the detailed studies of Brin.[27,58-61,72,94]

Levels of thiamin in blood and its components have also been investigated as possible indexes of thiamin nutriture.[16,29,30,46-52,96] The thiamin content of human blood and erythrocytes can be measured by fluorometric techniques or microbiological procedures.[6,53-57] Whole blood has been reported to contain about 5 to 8 $\mu g/100$ ml, although Henshaw and associates[30] found erythrocytes to contain 22.5 ± 5.88 $\mu g/100$ ml in a group of college women. White cells contain approximately 10 times more thiamin than erythrocytes. Whole blood thiamin levels less than 4.0 $\mu g/100$ ml are an indication of thiamin deficiency.[79] In deficiency, the thiamin content of erythrocytes decreased about 15 to 20%, while the mean thiamin level in whole blood in beriberi has been observed to be 3.2 $\mu g/100$ ml.[36,46] In view of the small reduction in blood thiamin in a deficiency status in addition to the technical difficulties associated with its measurement, blood thiamin levels have not proven to be a very useful index for detecting thiamin deficiency.

Additional procedures have been proposed for evaluating thiamin nutritional status.[2,3,16,29,80-82] For example, numerous metabolites of thiamin are excreted in the urine.[10,14,15,20,83-87] Although a number of the metabolites have been identified, none has proven useful thus far for evaluating thiamin nutritional status. In part, this has been due to technical difficulties encountered in developing satisfactory quantitative procedures to measure the metabolites. Additional studies may eventually reveal that the measurement of specific metabolites of thiamin will be of value as an indicator of thiamin adequacy.

Thiamin deficiency may also give rise to elevated levels of pyruvic acid in the blood,[2,3,29,80-82,94] although this effect lacks specificity and consistency.[2,29,82] The fasting levels of blood pyruvate have frequently been found to be normal in thiamin deficiency and only rise above normal following a glucose load.[2,29,80-82] Consequently, a test based on the effect of glucose and exercise on the pyruvic and lactic acid blood levels was developed and termed the "carbohydrate index."[80-82] Results are expressed in terms of the relative amounts of blood glucose, lactic acid, and pyruvic acid, 1 hr after the dose of 1.8 g of glucose/kg body weight and 5 min after completion of a standardized exercise. Unfortunately, this technique requires too much cooperation and technical ability to be useful except in experimental situations. As a result, the test has received little application, although it appears to be of value when conducted in the manner prescribed.

In summary, urinary excretion analysis for thiamin can provide information pertaining to thiamin nutriture and can be especially useful to confirm a diagnosis based on clinical symptoms. Such analyses will provide information as to thiamin intake levels, particularly with respect to the immediate intakes. Analyses of 24-hr urine collections provide more reliable information than random collections. However, the urinary thiamin analyses do not provide the desired information regarding the state of deficiency or the degree of depletion of thiamin tissue reserves. Additional information as to the physiological state with respect to thiamin can be obtained from the test-dose procedure. However, the application of the erythrocyte transketolase activity measurement as a biochemical functional test will provide more specific information. The test is convenient, feasible, specific, and sensitive.

REFERENCES

1. **Williams, R. R.,** *Toward the Conquest of Beriberi,* Harvard University Press, Cambridge, Massachusetts, 1961.
2. **Sauberlich, H. E.,** Biochemical alterations in thiamine deficiency — Their interpretation, *Am. J. Clin. Nutr.,* 20, 528, 1967.
3. **Goldsmith, G. A.,** The B vitamins: thiamine, riboflavin, niacin, in *Nutrition: A Comprehensive Treatise,* Vol. II, Beaton, G. H. and McHenry, E. W., Eds., Academic Press, New York, 1964, 109.
4. **Victor, M. and Adams, R. D.,** On the etiology of the alcoholic neurologic diseases, with special reference to the role of nutrition, *Am. J. Clin. Nutr.,* 9, 379, 1961.
5. *Manual for Nutrition Surveys,* 2nd. ed., Interdepartmental Committee on Nutrition for National Defense, Superintendent of Documents, U.S. Government Printing Office, Washington, D.C. 20402, 1963.
6. **Pearson, W. N.,** Thiamine, in *The Vitamins,* Vol. III, György, P. and Pearson, W. N., Eds., Academic Press, New York, 1967, 53.
7. **Shimazono, N. and Katasura, E.,** Eds., *Review of Japanese Literature on Beriberi and Thiamine,* Vitamin B Research Committee of Japan, Clinical Nutrition, Faculty of Medicine, Kyoto University, Kyoto, Japan, 1965.
8. *Nutrition Survey Reports (1957–1972),* Interdepartmental Committee on Nutrition for National Defense, Washington, D.C.
9. *Ten-State Nutrition Survey Reports, I – V (1972),* Center for Disease Control, Atlanta, Georgia 30330.
10. **Mickelsen, O., Caster, W. D., and Keys, A.,** A statistical evaluation of the thiamine and pyramin excretions of normal young men on controlled intakes of thiamine, *J. Biol. Chem.,* 168, 415, 1947.
11. **Mason, H. L. and Williams, R. D.,** The urinary excretion of thiamine as an index of the nutritional level: Assessment of the value of a test dose, *J. Clin. Invest.,* 21, 247, 1942.
12. **Oldham, H. C., Davis, M. V., and Roberts, L. J.,** Thiamine excretions and blood levels of young women on diets containing varying levels of the B vitamins, with some observations on niacin and pantothenic acid, *J. Nutr.,* 32, 163, 1946.
13. **Horwitt, M. K., Liebert, E., Kreisler, O., and Wittmann, P.,** Investigations of human requirements for B-complex vitamins, *National Research Council Bull. No. 116,* National Research Council, Washington, D.C., 1948.
14. **Ziporin, Z. Z., Nunes, W. T., Powell, R. C., Waring, P. P., and Sauberlich, H. E.,** Excretion of thiamine and its metabolites in the urine of young adult males receiving restricted intakes of the vitamin, *J. Nutr.,* 85, 287, 1965.
15. **Ziporin, Z. Z., Nunes, W. T., Powell, R. C., Waring, P. P., and Sauberlich, H. E.,** Thiamine requirement in the adult human as measured by urinary excretion of thiamine metabolites, *J. Nutr.,* 85, 297, 1965.
16. **Pearson, W. N.,** Blood and urinary vitamin levels as potential indices of body stores, *Am. J. Clin. Nutr.,* 20, 514, 1967.
17. **Holt, L. E., Jr. and Snyderman, S. E.,** The influence of dietary fat on thiamine loss from the body, *J. Nutr.,* 56, 495, 1955.
18. **Holt, L. E., Jr., Nemir, R. L., Snyderman, S. E., Albanese, A. A., Ketron, K. C., Guy, L. P., and Carretero, R.,** The thiamine requirement of the normal infant, *J. Nutr.,* 37, 53, 1949.
19. **Jolliffe, N., Goodhart, R., Ginnis, J., and Cline, J. K.,** The experimental production of vitamin B_1 deficiency in normal subjects. The dependence of the urinary excretion of thiamine on the dietary intake of vitamin B_1, *Am. J. Med. Sci.,* 198, 198, 1939.
20. **Pollack, H., Ellenberg, M., and Dolger, H.,** Study of the excretion of thiamine and its degradation products in humans, *J. Nutr.,* Suppl. 10, 21, 1941.
21. **Melnick, D.,** Vitamin B_1 (thiamine) requirement of man, *J. Nutr.,* 24, 139, 1942.
22. **Wuest, H. M., Furness, F. N., White, E. W., and Beckel, W. S.,** Eds., Unsolved problems of thiamine, *Ann. N.Y. Acad. Sci.,* 98, 384, 1962.
23. **Oldham, H. G.,** Thiamine requirements of women, *Ann. N.Y. Acad. Sci.,* 98, 542, 1962.
24. **Pearson, W. N.,** Biochemical appraisal of the vitamin nutritional status in man, *J.A.M.A.,* 180, 49, 1962.
25. **Pearson, W. N.,** Biochemical appraisal of nutritional status in man, *Am. J. Clin. Nutr.,* 11, 462, 1962.
26. **Thanangkul, O. and Whitaker, J. A.,** Childhood thiamine deficiency in northern Thailand, *Am. J. Clin. Nutr.,* 18, 275, 1966.
27. **Brin, M., Dibble, M. V., Peel, A., McMullen, E., Bourquin, A., and Chen, N.,** Some preliminary findings on the nutritional status of aged in Onondaga County, New York, *Am. J. Clin. Nutr.,* 17, 240, 1965.
28. **Sauberlich, H. E., Stevens, C. O., and Herman, Y. F.,** Thiamin requirement of the adult human, *Am. J. Clin. Nutr.,* 23, 671, (detailed manuscript submitted for publication), 1970.
29. **Pearson, W. N.,** Assessment of nutritional status: Biochemical methods, in *Nutrition: A Comprehensive Treatise,* Vol. III, Beaton, G. H. and McHenry, E. W., Eds., Academic Press, New York, 1966, 265.
30. **Henshaw, J. L., Noakes, G., Morris, S. O., Bennion, M., and Gubler, C. J.,** Method for evaluating thiamine adequacy in college women, *J. Am. Diet. Assoc.,* 57, 436, 1970.
31. **Plough, I. C. and Bridgefort, E. B.,** Relations of clinical and dietary findings in nutrition surveys, *Publ. Health Rep.,* 75, 699, 1960.
32. **Krehl, W. A. and Hodges, R. E.,** The interpretation of nutrition survey data, *Am. J. Clin. Nutr.,* 17, 191, 1965.

33. Requirements of vitamin A, thiamine, riboflavine and niacin, Report of a Joint FAO/WHO Expert Group, *FAO Nutrition Meeting Report Series No. 41,* Food and Agriculture Organization of the United Nations, Rome, 1967.

34. *Recommended Dietary Allowances,* 7th revised ed., Publication 1694, National Academy of Sciences, Washington D.C., 1968.

35. Elsom, K., O'Shea, J. G., Nicholson, J. T. L., and Chornock, C., Studies of the B vitamins in the human subject. V. The normal requirement for thiamine; some factors influencing its utilization and excretion, *Am. J. Med. Sci.,* 203, 569, 1942.

36. Spector, H., Peterson, M. S., and Friedemann, T. E., Eds., Methods for evaluation of nutritional adequacy and status, National Academy Science – National Research Council Publication, Washington, D.C., 1954.

37. O'Neal, R. M., Johnson, O. C., and Schaefer, A. E., Guidelines for classification and interpretation of group blood and urine data collected as part of the National Nutrition Survey, *Pediatr. Res.,* 4, 103, 1970.

38. Stearns, G., Adamson, L., McKinley, J. B., Lenner, T., and Jeans, P. C., Excretion of thiamine and riboflavin by children, *Am. J. Dis. Child.,* 95, 185, 1958.

39. Plough, I. C. and Consolazio, C. F., The use of casual urine specimens in the evaluation of the excretion rates of thiamine, riboflavin and N'-methylnicotinamide, *J. Nutr.,* 69, 365, 1959.

40. Du Plessis, J. P., An evaluation of biochemical criteria for use in nutrition status surveys, National Nutrition Research Institute, *Council for Scientific and Industrial Research Report No. 261,* Pretoria, South Africa, 1967, 65.

41. *Suggested Guidelines for Evaluation of the Nutritional Status of Preschool Children,* revised 1967, U.S. Department of Health, Education and Welfare, Social and Rehabilitation Service, Children's Bureau, Washington, D.C.

42. Johnson, R. E., Henderson, C., Robinson, P., F., and Consolazio, C. F., Comparative merits of fasting specimens, random specimens, and oral loading tests in field nutrition surveys, *J. Nutr.,* 30, 89, 1945.

43. Lossy, F. T., Goldsmith, G. A., and Sarett, H. P., A study of test dose excretion of five B complex vitamins in man, *J. Nutr.,* 45, 213, 1951.

44. May, J. M., *Studies in Medical Geography. The Ecology of Malnutrition,* Vol. 1 – 11, Hafner Publishing Co., New York, 1961 – 1972.

45. Dewhurst, W. G. and Morgan, H. G., Importance of urine volume in assessment of thiamin deficiency, *Am. J. Clin. Nutr.,* 23, 379, 1970.

46. Burch, H. B., Salcedo, J., Jr., Carrasco, E. O., Intengan, C. L., and Caldwell, A. B., Nutrition survey and tests in Bataan, Philippines, *J. Nutr.,* 42, 9, 1950.

47. Burch, H. B., Bessey, O. A., Love, R. H., and Lowry, O. H., The determination of thiamine and thiamine phosphates in small quantities of blood and blood cells, *J. Biol. Chem.,* 198, 477, 1952.

48. Dube, R. B., Johnson, E. C., Yu, H. H., and Storvick, C. A., Thiamine metabolism of women on controlled diets. 2. Daily blood thiamine values, *J. Nutr.,* 48, 307, 1952.

49. Louhi, H. A., Yu, H. H., Hawthorne, B. E., and Storvick, C. A., Thiamine metabolism of women on controlled diets. I. Daily urinary thiamine excretion and its relation to creatinine excretion, *J. Nutr.,* 48, 297, 1952.

50. Fennelly, J., Frank, O., Baker, H., and Leevy, C. M., Transketolase activity in experimental thiamine deficiency and hepatic necrosis, *Proc. Soc. Exp. Biol. Med.,* 116, 875, 1964.

51. Foltz, E. E., Barborka, C. J., and Ivy, A. C., The level of vitamin B-complex in the diet at which detectable symptoms of deficiency occur in man, *Gastroenterology,* 2, 323, 1944.

52. Burch, H. B., Salcedo, J., Jr., Carrasco, E. O., and Intengan, C., Nutrition resurvey in Bataan, Philippines, 1950, *J. Nutr.,* 46, 239, 1952.

53. Baker, H., Frank, O., Pasher, I., Ziffer, H., and Sobotka, H., Pantothenic acid, thiamine and folic acid levels at parturition, *Proc. Soc. Exp. Biol. Med.,* 103, 321, 1960.

54. Myint, T. and Houser, H. B., The determination of thiamine in small amounts of whole blood and serum by a simplified thiochrome method, *Clin. Chem.,* 11, 617, 1965.

55. Frank, O., Baker, H., and Sobotka, H., Blood- and serum-levels of water-soluble vitamins in man and animals, *Nature,* 197, 490, 1963.

56. Baker, H., Frank, O., Pasher, I., Sobotka, H., and Hunter, S., Vitamin levels in blood and serum, *Nature,* 191, 78, 1961.

57. Houser, H. B., Myint, T., and Weir, D. R., Estimation of red blood cell thiamine concentration from whole blood and serum thiamine by adjustment for hematocrit, *Am. J. Clin. Nutr.,* 20, 46, 1967.

58. Brin, M., Functional evaluation of nutritional status: Thiamine, in *Newer Methods of Nutritional Biochemistry,* Vol. III, Albanese, A. A., Ed., Academic Press, New York, 1967, 407.

59. Brin, M., Erythrocyte transketolase in early thiamine deficiency, *Ann. N.Y. Acad. Sci.,* 98, 528, 1962.

60. Brin, M., Tai, M., Ostashever, A. S., and Kalinsky, H., The effect of thiamine deficiency on the activity of erythrocyte hemolysate transketolase, *J. Nutr.,* 71, 273, 1960.

61. Brin, M., Erythrocyte as a biopsy tissue for functional evaluation of thiamine adequacy, *J.A.M.A.,* 187, 762, 1964.

62. Dreyfus, P., Clinical application of blood transketolase determinations, *N. Engl. J. Med.,* 267, 596, 1962.

63. Sauberlich, H. E., Problems of assessment of nutritional status: An overview of biochemical methodologies in *Proceedings of a Workshop on Problems of Assessment and Alleviation of Malnutrition in the United States,* Nashville, Tennessee, January 13 – 14, 1970, sponsored by the Nutrition Study Section, Division of Research Grants, Nat. Inst. of Health, Washington, D.C., Pub. 916.086.

64. **Stevens, C. O., Sauberlich, H. E., and Long, J. L.,** An automated assay for transketolase determinations, in *Automation in Analytical Chemistry,* Mediad Inc., Publishers, New York, 1968.

65. **Warnock, L. G.,** A new approach to erythrocyte transketolase measurement, *J. Nutr.,* 100, 1057, 1970.

66. **Tanphaichitr, V., Vimokesant, S. L., Dhanamitta, S., and Valyasevi, A.,** Clinical and biochemical studies of adult beriberi, *Am. J. Clin. Nutr.,* 23, 1017, 1970.

67. **Sauberlich, H. E. and Bunce, G. E.,** Interdepartmental Committee on Nutrition for National Defense, *Union of Burma Nutrition Survey Report,* U.S. Government Printing Office, Washington, D.C., May 1963, 163.

68. **Chong, Y. H. and Ho, G. S.,** Erythrocyte transketolase activity, *Am. J. Clin. Nutr.,* 23, 261, 1970.

69. **Schouten, H., Statius Van Eps, L. W., and Struyker Boudier, A. M.,** Transketolase in blood, *Clin. Chim. Acta,* 10, 474, 1964.

70. **Tripathy, K.,** Erythrocyte transketolase activity and thiamine transfer across human placenta, *Am. J. Clin. Nutr.,* 21, 739, 1968.

71. **Brubacher, G., Haenel, A., and Ritzel, G.,** Transketolaseaktivität, thiaminausscheidung und blutthiamingehalt bein menschen zur beurteilung der vitamin-B$_1$-versorgung, *Int. J. Vit. Nutr. Res.,* 42, 190, 1972.

72. **Brin, M.,** Thiamine deficiency and erythrocyte metabolism, *Am. J. Clin. Nutr.,* 12, 107, 1963.

73. **Burgener, M. and Jürgens, P. G.,** Thiamine excretion and transketolase activity in chronic alcoholism and Wernicke's encephalopathy, *Ger. Med. Mon.,* 12, 396, 1967.

74. **Akbarian, M. and Dreyfus, P. M.,** Blood transketolase activity in beriberi heart disease, *J.A.M.A.,* 203, 77, 1968.

75. **Kraut, H., Wildeman, L., and Böhm, M.,** Untersuchungen zum thiaminbedarf des menschem, *Int. J. Vit. Res.,* 36, 157, 1966.

76. **Reuter, H., Gassmann, B., and Erhardt, V.,** Beitrag zur frage des menschlichen thiaminbedarfs, *Int. J. Vit. Res.,* 37, 315, 1967.

77. **Coon, W. W. and Bizer, L. S.,** Subclinical thiamine deficiency in postoperative patients, *Surg. Gynecol. Obst.,* 121, 37, 1965.

78. **Konttinen, A., Louhija, A., and Härtel, G.,** Blood transketolase in assessment of thiamine deficiency in alcoholics, *Ann. Med. Exp. Biol. Fenn.,* 48, 172, 1970.

79. **Abe, T.,** Department of Medicine, Toho University School of Medicine, personal communication.

80. **Horwitt, M. K. and Kreisler, O.,** The determination of early thiamine-deficient states by estimation of blood lactic and pyruvic acids after glucose administration and exercise, *J. Nutr.,* 37, 411, 1949.

81. **Horwitt, M. K., Liebert, E., Kreisler, O., and Wittman, P.,** Investigations of human requirements for B-complex vitamins, *Natl. Res. Council Philipp. Bull. 116,* Washington D.C., 1948.

82. **Thompson, R. H. S.,** The value of blood pyruvate determinations in the diagnosis of thiamine deficiency, in *Thiamine Deficiency: Biochemical Lesions and Their Clinical Significance,* Wolstenholme, G. E. W., Ed., Ciba Foundation Study Group No. 28, Churchill, London, 1967.

83. **Ariaey-Nejad, M. R., Balaghi, M., Baker, E. M., and Sauberlich, H. E.,** Thiamin metabolism in man, *Am. J. Clin. Nutr.,* 23, 764, 1970.

84. **Ziporin, Z. Z., Beier, E., Holland, D. C., and Bierman, E. L.,** A method for determining the metabolites of thiamine in urine, *Anal. Biochem.,* 3, 1, 1962.

85. **White, W. W., III, Amos, W. H., Jr., and Neal, R. A.,** Isolation and identification of the pyrimidine moiety of thiamin in rat urine using gas chromatography-mass spectrometry, *J. Nutr.,* 100, 1053, 1970.

86. **Amos, W. H. and Neal, R. A.,** Gas chromatography-mass spectrometry of the trimethylsilyl derivatives of various thiamine metabolites, *Anal. Biochem.,* 36, 332, 1970.

87. **Neal, R. A.,** Vitamin deficiencies: Thiamin, in *Proceedings of a Workshop on Problems of Assessment and Alleviation of Malnutrition in the United States,* Nashville, Tennessee, January 13 – 14, 1970, sponsored by the Nutrition Study Section, Division of Research Grants, Nat. Inst. of Health, Washington, D.C., 1971, Pub. 916.086.

88. **Pelletier, O. and Madère, R.,** New automated method for measuring thiamine (vitamin B$_1$) in urine, *Clin. Chem.,* 18, 937, 1972.

89. **Leveille, G. A.,** Modified thiochrome procedure for the determination of urinary thiamin, *Am. J. Clin. Nutr.,* 25, 273, 1972.

90. *Difco Supplementary Literature,* Difco Laboratories, Detroit, 48232, May 1972, 449.

91. **Darby, W. J. et al.,** The Vanderbilt cooperative study of maternal and infant nutrition. IV. Dietary, laboratory and physical findings in 2,129 delivered pregnancies, *J. Nutr.,* 51, 565, 1953.

92. Suggested guide for interpreting dietary and biochemical data, Interdepartmental Committee on Nutrition for National Defense, *Public Health Rep.,* 75, 687, 1960.

93. **Van Reen, R., Minard, D., Consolazio, C. F., and Matoush, L. O.,** Nutrition of 96 Naval recruits during a shelter habitability study, *J. Am. Diet. Assoc.,* 42, 117, 1963.

94. **Wolstenholme, G. E. W. and O'Connor, M.,** Eds., Thiamine deficiency: Biochemical lesions and their clinical significance, *CIBA Foundation Study Group No. 28,* Little, Brown, and Co., Boston, 1967.

95. **Upjohn, D. R., Dohm, G. L., and Ziporin, Z. Z.,** An enzyme method for the assay of transketolase activity in the red blood cell, submitted for publication in *J. Nutr.,* 1973.

96. **Lamden, M. P.,** Thiamine IX. Biochemical detection of deficiency, in *The Vitamins,* Vol. V, 2nd ed., Sebrell, W. H., Jr. and Harris, R. S., Eds., Academic Press, New York, 1972, 134.
97. **Kelsay, J. L.,** A compendium of nutritional status studies and dietary evaluation studies conducted in the United States, 1957 – 1967, *J. Nutr.,* Suppl. 1, Part II, 99, 123, 1969.
98. **Davis, T. R. A., Gershoff, S. N., and Gamble, D. F.,** Review of studies of vitamin and mineral nutrition in the United States (1950 – 1968), *J. Nutr. Educ.,* 1, Suppl. I, 41, 1969.

Riboflavin

Evidence of riboflavin nutritional inadequacies has been commonly observed in nutrition surveys,[18,75,76] including those conducted by the Interdepartmental Committee on Nutrition for National Defense (ICNND)[1] and the U.S. Ten-State Nutrition Survey.[2] Clinical cases of riboflavin deficiency are also reported on occasion.[3-5] The evidence for riboflavin inadequacies has usually been based on urinary levels of riboflavin, although in some instances it has been supported by riboflavin load tests or by erythrocyte riboflavin levels.

Since considerable information is available concerning riboflavin dietary intake to urinary excretion, measurement of urinary riboflavin excretion has come into common use for evaluating the nutritional status of this nutrient.[1,2,66] Moreover, riboflavin is unique in that the body appears to metabolize little of the vitamin[66-69] and, hence, urinary excretions appear to correlate well with reserves and intakes of the vitamin.[6-15,47,48] However, in conditions of negative nitrogen balance and in fasting, deceptive and abnormally high excretion levels of riboflavin may be encountered.[6,16,17,19,24] Sleep and short periods of heavy physical work have been reported to decrease riboflavin excretion, while enforced bed rest and heat stress may increase riboflavin excretion.[17]

Correlations between dietary intakes of riboflavin and urinary excretions of the vitamin have been established through carefully controlled human studies.[9,14,73] Adult males maintained on a daily intake of 0.55 mg of riboflavin developed clinical signs of a riboflavin deficiency.[14,73] Their urinary riboflavin excretion was approximately 50 μg/day or 20 to 30 μg/g of creatinine. As their riboflavin intakes were increased, urinary riboflavin excretions slowly increased. However, at an intake of 1.3 to 1.6 mg/day, the urinary excretion of riboflavin markedly increased indicating that at this level tissue saturation was maintained (Figure 9). A similar break in the excretion curve of

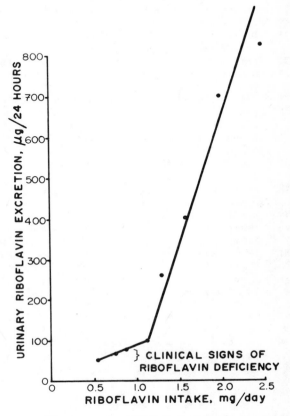

FIGURE 9.   Relationship of riboflavin intake to urinary excretion of riboflavin as observed in the studies of Horwitt et al.[14,73]

riboflavin was observed in young adult women.[8,9] From these studies, it was considered that a 24-hr urinary riboflavin excretion of less than 100 μg was indicative of a recent dietary regimen providing less than the minimum requirement of riboflavin.[14] Guidelines for interpreting urinary riboflavin excretion data have been extrapolated from these controlled studies[1,2,25,29-33] (Table 8).

Such guidelines must be used with caution when evaluating the riboflavin nutritional status of an individual.[22,23] Urinary riboflavin levels tend to reflect the recent dietary intake of riboflavin

TABLE 8

Guidelines for the Interpretation of Erythrocyte Levels and Urinary Excretion of Riboflavin

Less than acceptable (at risk)

Subjects	Deficient (high risk)	Low (medium risk)	Acceptable (low risk)
μg/g creatinine[a]			
1 to 3 years	< 150	150 to 499	⩾ 500
4 to 6 years	< 100	100 to 299	⩾ 300
7 to 9 years	< 85	85 to 269	⩾ 270
10 to 15 years	< 70	70 to 199	⩾ 200
Adults	< 27	27 to 79	⩾ 80
Pregnant, 2nd trimester	< 39	39 to 119	⩾ 120
Pregnant, 3rd trimester	< 30	30 to 89	⩾ 90

Other Interpretive Guidelines[b]

Adults:			
μg/24 hr	< 40	40 to 119	⩾ 120
μg/6 hr	< 10	10 to 29	⩾ 30

Load Test (return in adults of 5 mg riboflavin dose):[b]

μg in 4 hr	< 1000	1000 to 1399	⩾ 1400

Erythrocyte Riboflavin:[c]

μg/100 ml cells	< 10.0	10.0 to 14.9	⩾ 15.0

[a]Adapted from the reports of O'Neal et al.[31] and others.[2,25,29,32,33,36]
[b]Adapted from the reports of Pearson.[25,29,32]
[c]From ICNND guide.[25]

and, hence, are prone to considerable variation. In nutrition surveys, for practical reasons but at the expense of precision, random urine samples are collected and analyzed with the results expressed in terms of creatinine level. Expressing urinary riboflavin excretions per gram of creatinine has the advantage of tending to correct variations due to body size.[20,23] If nonfasting samples are collected, urinary riboflavin levels may be misleadingly elevated. This is exemplified by the study of Clarke et al.[74] (Figure 10). However, this effect is minimal in individuals subsisting on marginal or inadequate intakes of riboflavin whose body stores are depleted or unsaturated. Under these conditions, any riboflavin ingested would be largely retained rather than excreted. Thus, the errors associated with random samples are of reduced concern since the errors would be greatest in those individuals with adequate intakes of riboflavin.

In some studies, 2-hr urine collections have been used in place of 24-hr samples. Results, when expressed as μg of riboflavin per gram of creatinine, were not significantly different between the two sample collections.[21] In other instances, 6-hr urine collections have been used.[20,23] Although the use of 6-hr or 2-hr urine collections or random, fasting or nonfasting, samples are open to certain criticisms, their use in population groups or in surveys provides a general indication of the riboflavin nutrition status.[1,2,20-23] Nevertheless, when clinical cases of suspected riboflavin deficiency are encountered,

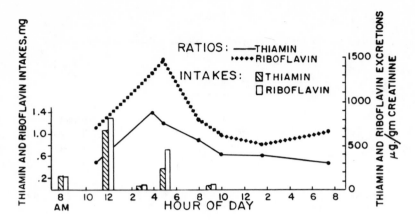

FIGURE 10. Urinary excretion of thiamin and riboflavin as influenced by intakes of these vitamins and the time of urine collection. (Adapted from Clarke et al.[74])

24-hr urine collections should be obtained if at all possible.

Riboflavin may be measured in urine with the use of fluorometric techniques[1,2,21,25,26,49] or microbiological assays.[26,27,44] The authors have used the fluorometric and microbiological procedures with equal success. Recently, automated procedures have become available for the determination of riboflavin in urine.[70,72]

Information on the relationship of riboflavin nutritional status and their urinary excretion of the vitamin is limited in infants and children.[7,15,28] But as in the case of niacin and thiamin, children excrete more riboflavin per gram of creatinine than adults[1,2,21,33,65] (Figure 11). From the limited information available, Pearson,[33] using the creatinine coefficients of Stearns et al.[34] and the mean weights obtained from the Jackson-Kelly[35] growth charts, developed a sliding-scale tentative guide for the interpretation of riboflavin excretions by children (Table 8). The guides have been commonly accepted and applied in numerous nutrition surveys.[1,2,25,31] Data from the recent Ten-State Nutrition Survey[2] (Figure 11) appear to provide support to the validity of these guidelines for children.

In clinical cases with suspected riboflavin deficiency, the use of a riboflavin load test has been suggested.[14,19,20,39,43] The procedure most commonly used consists of measuring the urinary excretion of riboflavin in the 4-hr period following the oral administration of a 5-mg test dose of the vitamin.[39] On occasion, the test has been used in

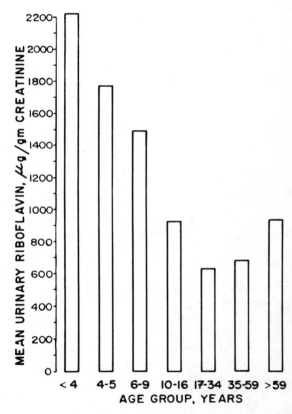

FIGURE 11. Mean urinary riboflavin levels (μg/g creatinine) by age for white population from high income ratio states. (Adapted from the Ten-State Nutrition Survey (IV-221).[2])

the ICNND nutrition surveys[1] and the results evaluated using the guides indicated in Table 8. It should be recognized that these guides are tentative and have been derived from rather limited information and, therefore, must be used with reservations. The procedure has apparently not been developed for use with children. In general, the riboflavin load test has received only limited use. Nevertheless, whenever it is used, additional supporting information should be obtained on the subject. This may be in the form of measuring nonload urinary riboflavin excretion or determining the erythrocyte glutathione reductase activity coefficient (see below).

The measurement of blood riboflavin levels has also been proposed to evaluate riboflavin nutritional status.[32,33] This approach has been largely related to the study of Bessey et al.[37] Riboflavin, flavin mononucleotide (FMN), and flavin dinucleotide (FAD) may be measured in blood, plasma, and erythrocytes with the use of a fluorometric procedure.[26,38,40] Microbiological assay procedures have not been very satisfactory for this purpose.[26] However, Baker et al.[45] have developed a protozoological assay, using *Tetrahymena pyriformis,* to measure riboflavin in blood. Under conditions of restricted riboflavin intakes, the riboflavin content of erythrocytes decreased.[38] Plasma levels of riboflavin were less affected. The erythrocyte riboflavin content was 20.2 to 27.6 $\mu g/100$ ml of cells in the supplemented subjects and 10.0 to 13.1 $\mu g/100$ ml in the deficient subjects, which showed clinical signs of ariboflavinosis.[38] Nevertheless, the analysis of riboflavin in blood or its components as a means of evaluating riboflavin adequacy appears to be of limited value. As pointed out by Horwitt[41] from the result of his experiences,[14,37] the level of riboflavin in the blood does not change until after other more easily determined parameters have been altered. As Horwitt stated,[41] "One can obtain much more information from the analysis of urine samples for riboflavin with less technical difficulty since there is only a 2-fold difference between adequacy and deficiency in blood cell riboflavin."

Other investigators have also observed that the free riboflavin level in human serum appeared to be influenced by recent dietary intakes and was too variable to serve as a useful index of riboflavin status.[21,42] The variations were not due to age or sex. In another report, the level of dietary intake of riboflavin within the range studied did not bear a significant relationship to the level of riboflavin in erythrocytes of healthy children.[46] However, infants tended to have higher levels of riboflavin in the erythrocytes than children 10 years of age and over. In a nutrition study by DuPlessis and Lange[21,65] on 7- to 15-yr-old children, total red blood cell riboflavin, serum riboflavin content, and serum FAD content proved unsatisfactory for assessing riboflavin status. However, riboflavin excretion per gram of creatinine in 2-hr urine specimens provided a reasonably good criterion of riboflavin nutrition status. In contrast, using the ICNND guidelines (Table 8), the nutritional evaluation of Central America and Panama revealed a significant proportion of the subjects studied to have "low" or "deficient" levels of riboflavin in the red cells.[71] These findings were supported by a high proportion of the subjects with "low" and "deficient" values for urinary riboflavin, by low dietary intakes of riboflavin, and by clinical evidence of riboflavin deficiency.[71]

A recently available biochemical procedure that holds promise as being the method of choice for evaluating riboflavin nutriture is the erythrocyte glutathione reductase (EGR) measurement.[50–63] Erythrocyte glutathione reductase activity represents a functional test of nutritional adequacy of riboflavin.[50,51] The enzyme catalyzes the reduction of oxidized glutathione (GSSG) in the following manner:

$$NADPH \,(NADH) + H^+ + GSSG$$

$$\rightarrow NADP^+ \,(NAD^+) + 2\,GSH$$

Erythrocyte glutathione reductase assays can be readily performed spectrophotometrically requiring only a small quantity of blood.[50–52,64] The assay results are usually expressed in terms of "activity coefficients" (AC), representing the degree of stimulation resulting from the in vitro addition of flavin adenine dinucleotide (FAD).[50–52,64] The activity coefficient may be expressed as follows:

$$AC = \frac{\text{Reduction of absorbance with added FAD/10 min.}}{\text{Reduction of absorbance without added FAD/10 min.}}$$

In normal subjects, an AC of approximately 1.00 ± 0.10 is obtained indicating little or no stimulation. With an inadequate intake of riboflavin, a marked stimulation occurs. An AC value of 1.20 and above has been considered as indicative of inadequate riboflavin nutriture.[50-52] In subjects on controlled riboflavin intakes, Tillotson and Baker[50] found the erythrocyte glutathione reductase activity coefficient measurement to be a sensitive procedure for assessing riboflavin status (Figure 12). Urinary riboflavin measurements, although useful, were a less sensitive assessment of nutritional status and reflected recent dietary riboflavin intakes. Similar observations were reported by Bamji.[53] The enzyme measurement has been applied in a number of recent nutrition surveys.[51,52,61-63,77] Subjects observed with elevated AC values responded promptly to riboflavin administration.[51,52] For the most part, subjects with elevated EGR activity coefficients had urinary excretion levels considered low or deficient.[51] Similarly, elevated activation coefficients appear to be associated with reduced levels of riboflavin in the erythrocytes.[58]

Measurement of EGR activity coefficients is a simple, reproducible, functional test of riboflavin status in the human. As noted earlier, the procedure can be readily performed involving only a small quantity of blood. The enzyme involved is

moderately stable and, hence, samples can be collected, stored and analyzed at laboratories distant from collecting locations. Although fasting blood samples are usually obtained, this does not appear to be as essential as in the case of urine specimens used for riboflavin evaluation. Thus, EGR activity coefficient measurements largely avoid the limitations associated with urinary excretion data.[22,23] Since the erythrocyte glutathione reductase activity coefficient values appear to be age and sex independent, a single guide can be used for all age groups (Table 9). An activity coefficient greater than 1.20 cannot be accepted with complete certainty at present as an absolute

TABLE 9

Tentative Guides for the Interpretation of Erythrocyte Glutathione Reductase Activity Coefficients[50-52]

	Less than acceptable (at risk)		
Subjects	Deficient (high risk)	Low (medium risk)	Acceptable (low risk)
All Ages	> 1.40	1.20 to 1.40	< 1.20

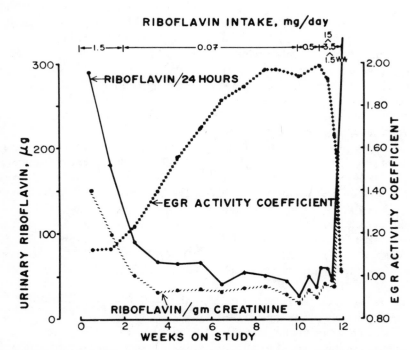

FIGURE 12.   Relationship of riboflavin intake to urinary riboflavin excretion and erythrocyte glutathione reductase activity coefficients. Mean values for six young adult males. (Adapted from Tillotson and Baker.[50])

cutoff level for evidence of inadequate riboflavin nutrition. Nevertheless, the value appears to be in keeping with information available from controlled human riboflavin deficiency studies.[50,53] Further investigations will be required to ascertain the possible influence of certain clinical diseases on the erythrocyte glutathione reductase activity coefficient.[55,57,60]

In brief, clinical cases of suspected riboflavin deficiency can be evaluated biochemically by measuring the riboflavin content of 24-hr urine collections and expressing the results in terms of μg per 24-hr and per gram of creatinine. When feasible, erythrocyte glutathione reductase activity coefficient values should also be determined.

In field surveys, erythrocyte glutathione reductase activity coefficient values should be determined in addition to the measurement of riboflavin levels on random fasting urine samples with the results related to per gram of creatinine.

REFERENCES

1. *Nutrition Survey Reports of the Interdepartmental Committee on Nutrition for National Defense,* National Institute of Health, Office of International Research, Department of Health, Education, and Welfare, Bethesda, Maryland.
2. *Reports of the Ten-State Nutrition Survey: 1968–1970,* U.S. Department of Health, Education, and Welfare, Health Services and Mental Health Administration, Center for Disease Control, Atlanta, Georgia 30333, 1972.
3. **Lai, C. S. and Ransome, G. A.,** Burning-feet syndrome. Case due to malabsorption and responding to riboflavine, *Br. Med. J.,* 2, 151, 1970.
4. **Clarke, H. C.,** The riboflavin deficiency syndrome of pregnancy, *Surg. Forum,* 22, 394, 1971.
5. **Coon, W. W.,** Riboflavin metabolism in surgical patients, *Surg. Gynecol. Obst.,* 120, 1289, 1965.
6. **Bro-Rasmussen, F.,** The riboflavin requirement of animals and man and associated metabolic functions. Part II: Relation of requirement to the metabolism of protein and energy, *Nutr. Abstr. Rev.,* 28, 369, 1958.
7. **Snyderman, S. E., Ketron, K. C., Burch, H. B., Lowry, O. H., Bessey, O. A., Guy, L. P., and Holt, L. E., Jr.,** The minimum riboflavin requirement of the infant, *J. Nutr.,* 39, 219, 1949.
8. **Brewer, W., Porter, T., Ingalls, R., and Ohlson, M. A.,** The urinary excretion of riboflavin by college women, *J. Nutr.,* 32, 583, 1946.
9. **Davis, M. V., Oldham, H. G., and Roberts, L. J.,** Riboflavin excretion of young women on diets containing varying levels of the B-vitamins, *J. Nutr.,* 32, 143, 1946.
10. **Friedemann, T. E., Ivy, A. C., Jung, F. T., Sheft, B. B., and Kinney, V. M.,** Work at high altitude. IV. Utilization of thiamin and riboflavin, *Q. Bull. Northwest Univ. Med. Sch.,* 23, 177, 1949.
11. **Friedemann, T. E., Ivy, A. C., Sheft, B. B., and Kinney, V. M.,** V. The relation between daily oral intake and excretion of thiamin and riboflavin, *Q. Bull. Northwest. Univ. Med. Sch.,* 23, 438, 1949.
12. **Oldham, H., Sheft, B. B., and Porter, T.,** Thiamine and riboflavin intakes and excretions during pregnancy, *J. Nutr.,* 41, 231, 1950.
13. **Horwitt, M. K., Hills, O. W., Harvey, C. C., Liebert, E., and Steinberg, D. L.,** Effects of dietary depletion of riboflavin, *J. Nutr.,* 39, 357, 1949.
14. **Horwitt, M. K., Harvey, C. C., Hills, O. W., and Liebert, E.,** Correlation of urinary excretion of riboflavin with dietary intake and symptoms of ariboflavinosis, *J. Nutr.,* 41, 247, 1950.
15. **Oldham, H., Johnston, F., Kleiger, D., and Hedderich-Arismendi, H.,** A study of the riboflavin and thiamine requirements of children of preschool age, *J. Nutr.,* 27, 435, 1944.
16. **Windmueller, H. G., Anderson, A. A., and Mickelsen, O.,** Elevated riboflavin levels in urine of fasting human subjects, *Am. J. Clin. Nutr.,* 15, 73, 1964.
17. **Tucker, R. G., Mickelsen, O., and Keys, A.,** The influence of sleep, work, diuresis, heat, acute starvation, thiamine intake and bed rest on human riboflavin excretion, *J. Nutr.,* 72, 251, 1960.
18. **May, J. M.,** *Studies in Medical Geography. The Ecology of Malnutrition,* Vol. 1-11, Hafner Publishing Co., New York, 1961–1972.
19. **Unglaub, W. G. and Goldsmith, G. A.,** Evaluation of vitamin adequacy: Urinary excretion tests, in *Methods for Evaluation of Nutritional Adequacy and Status – A Symposium,* Advisory Board on Quartermaster Research and Development, Committee on Foods, National Academy of Sciences, National Research Council, Washington D.C., 1954, 69.
20. **Lowry, O. H.,** Biochemical evidence of nutritional status, *Physiol. Rev.,* 32, 431, 1952.
21. **DuPlessis, J. P.,** An evaluation of biochemical criteria for use in nutrition status surveys, National Nutrition Research Institute, *Council for Scientific and Industrial Research Report No. 261,* Pretoria, S. Africa, 1967, 77.
22. **Hegsted, D. M., Gershoff, S. N., Trulson, M. F., and Jolly, D. H.,** Variation in riboflavin excretion, *J. Nutr.,* 60, 581, 1956.
23. **Plough, I. C. and Consolazio, F. C.,** The use of casual urine specimens in the evaluation of the excretion rates of thiamine, riboflavin and N'-methylnicotinamide, *J. Nutr.,* 69, 365, 1959.

24. **Pollack, H. and Bookman, J. J.,** Riboflavin excretion as a function of protein metabolism in the normal, catabolic and diabetic human being, *J. Lab. Clin. Med.,* 38, 561, 1951.

25. *Manual for Nutrition Surveys.* 2nd ed., Interdepartmental Committee on Nutrition for National Defer se. Superintendent of Documents, U.S. Government Printing Office, Washington, D.C. 20402, 1963.

26. **Pearson, W. N.,** Riboflavin, in *The Vitamins,* Vol. VII, 2nd ed., György, P. and Pearson, W. N., Eds., Academic Press, New York, 1967, 99.

27. *Difco Supplementary Literature,* Difco Laboratories, Detroit 48232, 1972, 448.

28. **Stearns, G., Adamson, L., McKinley, J. B., Lenner, T., and Jeans, P. C.,** Excretion of thiamine and riboflavin by children, *Am. J. Dis. Child.,* 95, 185, 1958.

29. **Pearson, W. N.,** Biochemical appraisal of the vitamin nutritional status in man, *J.A.M.A.,* 180, 49, 1962.

30. **Pearson, W. N.,** Blood and urinary vitamin levels as potential indices of body stores, *Am. J. Clin. Nutr.,* 20, 514, 1967.

31. **O'Neal, R. M., Johnson, O. C., and Schaefer, A. E.,** Guidelines for classification and interpretation of group blood and urine data collected as part of the National Nutrition Survey, *Pediatr. Res.,* 4, 103, 1970.

32. **Pearson, W. N.,** Assessment of nutritional status: Biochemical methods, in *Nutrition,* Vol. III, Beaton, G. H. and McHenry, E. W., Eds., Academic Press, New York, 1966, 265.

33. **Pearson, W. N.,** Biochemical appraisal of nutritional status in man, *Am. J. Clin. Nutr.,* 11, 462, 1962.

34. **Stearns, G., Newman, K. J., McKinley, J. B., and Jeans, P. C.,** The protein requirements of children from 1 to 10 years of age, *Ann. N.Y. Acad. Sci.,* 69, 857, 1958.

35. **Jackson, R. L. and Kelly, H. G.,** Growth charts for use in pediatric practice, *J. Pediatr.,* 27, 215, 1945.

36. **Darby, W. J. et al.,** The Vanderbilt cooperative study of maternal and infant nutrition. IV. Dietary, laboratory and physical findings in 2,129 delivered pregnancies, *J. Nutr.,* 51, 565, 1953.

37. **Bessey, O. A., Horwitt, M. K., and Love, R. H.,** Dietary deprivation of riboflavin and blood riboflavin levels in man, *J. Nutr.,* 58, 367, 1956.

38. **Burch, H. B., Bessey, O. A., and Lowry, O. H.,** Fluorometric measurements of riboflavin and its natural derivatives in small quantities of blood, serum and cells, *J. Biol. Chem.,* 175, 457, 1948.

39. **Lossy, F. T., Goldsmith, G. A., and Sarett, H. P.,** A study of test dose excretion of five B complex vitamins in man, *J.Nutr.,* 45, 213, 1951.

40. **Clarke, H. C.,** A photodecomposition fluorimetric method for the determination of riboflavin in whole blood, *Int. J. Vit. Res.,* 39, 182, 1969.

41. **Horwitt, M. K.,** personal communication.

42. **Suvarnakich, K., Mann, G. V., and Stare, F. J.,** Riboflavin in human serum, *J. Nutr.,* 47, 105, 1952.

43. **Arroyave, G., Valenzuela, S., and Faillace, A.,** Deficiency of riboflavine in pregnant women of the city of Guatemala, *Rev. Col. Méd. Guatemala,* 9, 7, 1958.

44. **DeRitter, E., Moore, M. E., Hirschberg, E., and Rubin, S. H.,** Critique of methods for the determination of riboflavin in urine, *J. Biol. Chem.,* 175, 883, 1948.

45. **Baker, H., Frank, O., Feingold, S., Gellene, R. A., Leevy, C. M., and Hunter, S. H.,** A riboflavin assay suitable for clinical use and nutritional surveys, *Am. J. Clin. Nutr.,* 19, 17, 1966.

46. **Beal, V. A. and VanBuskirk, J. J.,** Riboflavin in red blood cells in relation to dietary intake of children, *Am. J. Clin. Nutr.,* 8, 841, 1960.

47. **Kraut, H., Ramaswamy, S. S., and Wildemann, L.,** Riboflavin requirement and riboflavin excretion, *Int. Zeit. Vit.,* 32, 25, 1961.

48. **Morley, H. H., Edwards, M. A., Moller, I. I., Woodring, M. J., and Storvick, C. A.,** Riboflavin in the blood and urine of women on controlled intakes, *J. Nutr.,* 69, 191, 1959.

49. **Mellar, N. P. and Maass, A. R.,** A simplified automated determination of riboflavin in urine, Technicon International Symposium; Abstract No. PH 16, New York, June 1972, 64.

50. **Tillotson, J. A. and Baker, E. M.,** An enzymatic measurement of the riboflavin status in man, *Am. J. Clin. Nutr.,* 25, 425, 1972.

51. **Sauberlich, H. E., Judd, J. H., Nichoalds, G. E., Broquist, H. P., and Darby, W. J.,** Application of the erythrocyte glutathione reductase assay in evaluating riboflavin nutritional status in a high school student population, *Am. J. Clin. Nutr.,* 25, 756, 1972.

52. **Glatzle, D., Körner, W. F., Christeller, S., and Wiss, O.,** Method for the detection of a biochemical riboflavin deficiency, *Int. J. Vitam. Nutr. Res.,* 40, 166, 1970.

53. **Bamji, M. S.,** Glutathione reductase activity in red blood cells and riboflavin nutritional status in humans, *Clin. Chim. Acta,* 26, 263, 1969.

54. **Beutler, E.,** The correction of glutathione reductase deficiency by riboflavin administration, *J. Clin. Invest.,* 48, 7a, 1969.

55. **Beutler, E.,** Effect of flavin compounds on glutathione reductase activity: in vivo and in vitro studies, *J. Clin. Invest.,* 48, 1957, 1969.

56. **Beutler, E.,** Glutathione reductase: stimulation in normal subjects by riboflavin supplementation, *Science,* 165, 613, 1969.

57. **Flatz, G.,** Population study of erythrocyte glutathione reductase activity. I. Stimulation of the enzyme by flavin adenine dinucleotide and by riboflavin supplementation, *Humangenetik,* 11, 269, 1971.

58. **Glatzle, D.,** Dependency of the glutathione reductase activity on the riboflavin status, *Clinical Enzymology,* S. Karger, Basel, 1970, 2, 89.

59. **Glatzle, D., Weber, F., and Wiss, O.,** Enzymatic test for the detection of a riboflavin deficiency, *Experientia,* 24, 1122, 1968.

60. **Sharada, D. and Bamji, M. S.,** Erythroctye glutathione reductase activity and riboflavin concentration in experimental deficiency of some water soluble vitamins, *Int. J. Vitam. Nutr. Res.,* 42, 43, 1972.

61. **Thurnham, D. I., Migasena, P., and Pavapootanon, N.,** The ultramicro red-cell glutathione reductase assay for riboflavin status: Its use in field studies in Thailand, *Microchim. Acta (Wien),* 5, 988, 1970.

62. **Thurnham, D. I., Migasena, P., Vudhivai, N., and Supawan, V.,** A longitudinal study on dietary and social influences on riboflavin status in pre-school children in Northeast Thailand, *South-East Asian J. Trop. Med. Publ. Health,* 2, 552, 1971.

63. **Buzina, R., Jusić, M., Brodarec, A., Milanović, N., Brubacher, G., Viulleumier, J. P., and Wiss, O.,** The assessment of dietary vitamin intake of 24 Istrian farmers: II. Comparison between the dietary intake and biochemical status of ascorbic acid, vitamin A, thiamine, riboflavin and niacin, *Int. J. Vitam. Nutr. Res.,* 41, 289, 1971.

64. **Tillotson, J. A. and Sauberlich, H. E.,** Effect of riboflavin depletion and repletion on the erythrocyte glutathione reductase in the rat, *J. Nutr.,* 101, 1459, 1971.

65. **DuPlessis, J. P. and De Lange, D. J.,** Biochemical evaluation of the nutrition status of urban school children of 12−15 years − riboflavin status, *S. Afr. Med. J.,* 40, 518, 1966.

66. **Horwitt, M. K.,** Nutritional requirements of man, with special reference to riboflavin, *Am. J. Clin. Nutr.,* 18, 458, 1966.

67. **Rivlin, R. S.,** Riboflavin metabolism, *N. Engl. J. Med.,* 283, 463, 1970.

68. **McCormick, D. B.,** The fate of riboflavin in the mammal, *Nutr. Rev.,* 30, 75, 1972.

69. **McCormick, D. B.,** Vitamin deficiencies: The fate of riboflavin, in *Problems of Assessment and Alleviation of Malnutrition in the United States* (proceedings of a workshop sponsored by Vanderbilt University, HSMHA and NIH, held at Nashville, Tennessee, Jan. 13−14, 1970), Hansen, R. G. and Munro, H. N., Eds., U.S. Govt. Printing Office, Pub. #916.086, Washington, D.C., 1971.

70. **Pelletier, O. and Madère, R.,** Automated determination of riboflavin (vitamin B_2) in urine, Research Laboratories, Food and Drug Directorate, Department of National Health and Welfare, Ottawa, Canada, personal communication.

71. *Nutritional Evaluation of the Population of Central America and Panama: 1965−1967,* Report of the Institute of Nutrition of Central America and Panama and of the Nutrition Program, Center for Disease Control, U.S. Department of Health, Education, and Welfare Publication No. (HSM) 72−8120, 1972.

72. **Mellor, N. P. and Maass, A. R.** (Smith, Kline & French Laboratories, Philadelphia), A simplified automated determination of riboflavin in urine, *Technicon International Congress on Advances in Automated Analysis, 12−14 June, 1972;* Abstracts, New York, 64.

73. **Horwitt, M. K.,** Riboflavin XII. Requirements and factors influencing them, in *The Vitamins,* Vol. V, 2nd ed., Sebrell, W. H., Jr. and Harris, R. S., Eds., Academic Press, New York, 1972, 88.

74. **Clarke, R. P., Cosgrove, L. DeG., and Morse, E. H.,** Vitamin to creatinine ratios. Variability in separate voidings of urine of adolescents during a 24 hour period, *Am. J. Clin. Nutr.,* 19, 335, 1966.

75. **Kelsay, J. L.,** A compendium of nutritional status studies and dietary evaluation studies conducted in the United States, 1957−1967, *J. Nutr.,* Suppl. 1, Part II, 99, 123, 1969.

76. **Davis, T. R. A., Gershoff, S. N., and Gamble, D. F.,** Review of studies of vitamin and mineral nutrition in the United States (1950−1968), *J. Nutr. Educ.,* Suppl. I, 1, 41, 1969.

77. **Canham, J. E.,** Nutrition surveys of military populations, personal communication.

Vitamin B_6

Vitamin B_6 was delineated by György in 1934 as a distinct entity which prevented skin lesions in the rat.[1,2] During the intervening years, this vitamin has been demonstrated to serve as the coenzyme, pyridoxal-5-phosphate, for well over 60 different enzyme systems.[3-5] Although the majority of these enzymes, functions are associated with amino acid and protein metabolism, functions related to the metabolism of carbohydrates and fats have been observed.[3-5]

Because of the widespread distribution of vitamin B_6 among foods, serious outbreaks of vitamin B_6 deficiency have not been observed throughout the world. Nevertheless, greater attention has been paid in recent years to the vitamin B_6 nutriture of the human because of its (a) ease of depletion to produce deficiency symptoms, (b) participation in numerous metabolic functions, (c) association with brain metabolism and development, (d) apparent increased needs with pregnancy, (e) marked losses in food processing, and (f) antagonisms by certain drugs and hormones.[3-9,58] As a consequence, various biochemical procedures have been developed and used in the evaluation of vitamin B_6 nutritional status.[3,5,6,8-16,58] Biochemical techniques currently employed in the assessment of the vitamin B_6 nutritional status in the human were recently reviewed.[17]

Tryptophan Load Test

Following the observation that vitamin B_6-deficient rats[18] and dogs[19] excreted increased amounts of xanthurenic acid, Greenberg et al.[20] demonstrated that a dietary restriction of vitamin B_6 in man also resulted in an increased excretion of xanthurenic acid following a loading with tryptophan. Subsequently, other urinary metabolites of tryptophan, including 3-hydroxykynurenine, kynurenine, and kynurenic acid were observed to increase in vitamin B_6 deficiency following a tryptophan load (Figure 13).[3,6,11,21] A test load of 2 or 5 g of L-tryptophan results in little or no increase in the metabolite excretion in individuals receiving adequate levels of vitamin B_6.[9,11,12,17,22-24,107] As a result of these observations, the tryptophan load test has been a very useful procedure for detecting or in evaluating vitamin B_6 deficiency, particularly in clinical cases and in controlled research studies.[3,6,9,10, 17,21,22,25,26,36,70,103,104,107,108,110,160]

Usually, either a 2-g or a 5-g L-tryptophan oral load is employed in studies with adults. In some instances, L-tryptophan at a level of 50 or 100 mg/kg of body weight has been used.[70] The larger load dose of tryptophan may be important in detecting and evaluating very early stages of vitamin B_6 insufficiency.[12] Other investigators, however, have considered the 2-g load adequate.[13,104,106,107] For tests with children and infants, the administration of L-tryptophan at a level of 100 of mg/kg body weight has been used satisfactorily.[16,70]

Under survey or field conditions, it is usually not feasible to obtain 24-hr urine collections. As an alternative, although a less satisfactory procedure, subjects are given the test load of tryptophan and the urine collected for the following 6-hr period.[9,27,28] In not all instances, however, would the presence of a vitamin B_6 insufficiency be detected. In experimentally induced vitamin B_6 deficiency, some subjects were observed to excrete the majority of the tryptophan metabolites during the following 18-hr period rather than during the initial 6-hr period. Nevertheless, adult subjects with an appreciable degree of vitamin B_6 depletion will usually excrete significantly abnormal levels of xanthurenic acid during the first 6 hr after a 5-g L-tryptophan load. For an adult, xanthurenic acid values in excess of 25 mg for the 6-hr collections are an indication of vitamin B_6 insufficiency.[17,28]

Protein intake, exercise, lean body mass, individual variations, amount of tryptophan used in the loading test, as well as other factors may

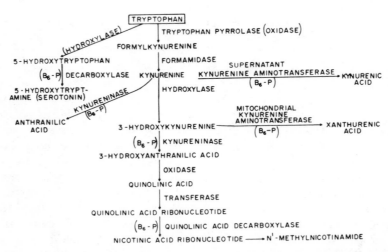

FIGURE 13.   Metabolic pathways of tryptophan in the human with reactions involving pyridoxal phosphate (B_6-P) indicated.

influence the level of tryptophan metabolites excreted in the urine of the subject deficient or marginally deficient in vitamin B_6[9],[29-32] but, in the subject adequately nourished in vitamin B_6, these factors appear to be without effect. Women ingesting oral contraceptives may excrete in the urine increased amounts of tryptophan metabolites following a tryptophan load.[2],[4-6],[9],[17],[26],[33-45],[58] The abnormal excretions of tryptophan metabolites are reduced to normal or near normal levels with the administration of relatively large doses of pyridoxine.[2],[9],[26],[33],[36] Pregnant women may also excrete abnormal amounts of kynurenine, xanthurenic acid and 3-hyrdoxykynurenine.[5],[36],[46-48],[58],[70]

Of the tryptophan metabolites excreted in the urine, xanthurenic acid is the easiest to measure.[11],[16],[21],[70] The use of the more sophisticated methods required for the determination of the other metabolites of tryptophan after loading is to be advocated, but the technical difficulties and increased laboratory equipment and personnel requirements would normally preclude the routine use of these procedures under population survey conditions or with the occasional clinical case.[21],[24] Moreover, whether the measurement of other metabolites of tryptophan would furnish any added information concerning vitamin B_6 nutritional status remains uncertain. Xanthurenic acid and other tryptophan metabolites can be measured in urine with the use of various manual or automated procedures.[16],[21-24],[28],[44],[45],[49-57],[59],[60],[70],[103-105],[116]

Urinary Excretion of Vitamin B_6

When population groups or large numbers of subjects are involved, the tryptophan load test is not a practical means for evaluating vitamin B_6 nutritional status. In recent years, a number of studies have been conducted to ascertain the usefulness of measuring urinary levels of vitamin B_6 for this purpose.[9],[10-12],[14],[17],[22],[61-64],[109] The vitamin appears in the urine mainly as pyridoxal and, to a lesser amount, as pyridoxamine, although quantities of pyridoxine and the phosphorylated forms may be present.[63],[65] In controlled studies with adult subjects, the urinary excretion of free vitamin B_6 correlated closely with the level of intake of the vitamin (Figures 14 and 15).[12],[17],[22],[63],[64] With an intake of 1.5 mg/day of pyridoxine, a level that marginally meets the requirement of the adult male or

female,[5],[9-12],[23],[24],[64],[66] a urinary excretion of 35 to 55 μg/day is usually observed (20 μg vitamin B_6/g creatinine (Figures 14 and 15). This level of vitamin B_6 intake usually prevents the excretion of abnormal levels of tryptophan metabolites following a 5-g L-tryptophan load.[9-12],[17] The results of several studies with adult subjects on known intakes of vitamin B_6 have suggested that urinary excretions of less than 20 μg/g creatinine are indicative of marginal or inadequate dietary

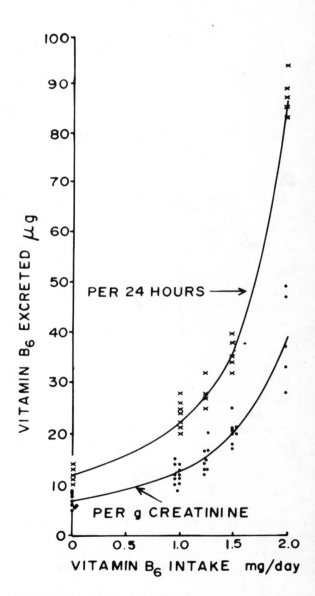

FIGURE 14. Relationship of vitamin B_6 intake to the level of urinary excretion of free vitamin B_6 in the adult human.

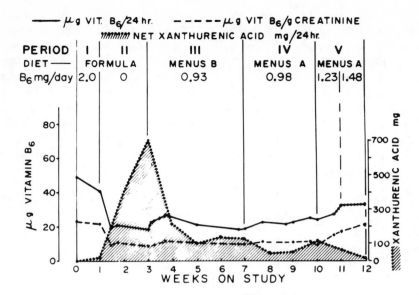

FIGURE 15. Relationship of vitamin B_6 intake in young adults to urinary excretion of free vitamin B_6 and to xanthurenic acid excretion following a 5-g L-tryptophan load.

intakes of vitamin B_6.[17] Although the vitamin B_6 requirement of the human is related to the level of protein ingested, dietary protein appears to have little effect on the urinary excretion of vitamin B_6.[9,12,22,63] The urinary level of vitamin B_6 may be of limited value per se as an indication of the severity of a vitamin B_6 deficiency in an individual; it is useful as a reflection of the subject's recent dietary intakes of vitamin B_6.

In nutrition surveys, as well as with most clinical cases, precise 24-hr urine collections are difficult to obtain. As an alternative, random fasting urine collections have been commonly employed and the urinary excretions of nutrients, expressed in terms of per gram of creatinine, used as an index of intake of nutrients.[67,68,116] In the case of vitamin B_6, random morning urine samples, preferably fasting, were found to be reasonably indicative of the total 24-hr excretion.[9,27,28] When the mean vitamin B_6 excretion per gram of creatinine is evaluated in terms of age groups, an age-excretion difference is observed similar to that observed for thiamin and riboflavin. This is exemplified by the unpublished data from the Ten-State Nutrition Survey (Figure 16).[68] Utilizing these data along with information obtained from controlled adult vitamin B_6 excretion studies and employing the creatinine excretion information of Stearns and associates,[69] a

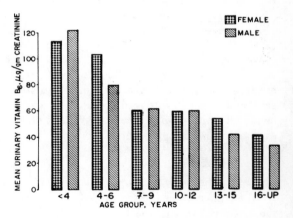

FIGURE 16. Mean urinary free vitamin B_6 levels (μg/g creatinine) by age and sex. (Adapted from unpublished data obtained during the Ten-State Nutrition Survey.[68])

tentative interpretive guide can be established for various age groups (Table 10).[17] For the occasional subject receiving vitamin B_6 antagonists, such as isoniazid, penicillamine, or cycloserine, urinary measurements for vitamin B_6 would probably not be valid.[4,6,7,9,58] The ingestion of oral contraceptives does not appear to influence the urinary excretion of vitamin B_6.[43]

Vitamin B_6 or the various individual forms of the vitamin may be measured in urine by various procedures.[5,16,71-97] However, microbiological

TABLE 10

A Tentative Guide for the Interpretation of Urinary Levels of Vitamin B_6 for Various Age Groups[a,b]

μg/g creatinine

Age group (years)	Unacceptable level	Acceptable level
1 to 3	< 90	≥ 90
4 to 6	< 75	≥ 75
7 to 9	< 50	≥ 50
10 to 12	< 40	≥ 40
13 to 15	< 30	≥ 30
Adults	< 20	≥ 20

[a]Based on *Saccharomyces uvarum* assay of unhydrolyzed urine.
[b]Adapted from Figures 14-16 and reports of Sauberlich et al.[17,109]

assays have been most commonly employed using *Saccharomyces uvarum* ATCC No. 9080 (formerly known as *Saccharomyces carlsbergenis* ATCC No. 9080)[92] as the test organism.[16,75,91,93,96] Pyridoxine, pyridoxal and pyridoxamine are essentially equally active on a molar basis for this yeast,[16,96] although strains of the organism have been reported to respond to pyridoxamine to a lesser extent.[75,87] Less commonly, the protozoan *Tetrahymena pyriformis*[62,75,90] and other microorganisms have been utilized in the assays.[16,75,87-93,96] Unfortunately, facilities to conduct microbiological assays are often not available in clinical laboratories.

Urinary Excretion of 4-Pyridoxic Acid

The major urinary metabolite of all forms of vitamin B_6 is 4-pyridoxic acid. Between 20 to 50% of the ingested vitamin B_6 is reported to be converted to 4-pyridoxic acid in the adult with the remainder excreted as the various forms of vitamin B_6 along with a number of unidentified metabolities.[63,65,98] Recently, 4-pyridoxic acid 5′-phosphate was reported to account for as much as 20% of the vitamin B_6 metabolites present in urine.[99] Theoretically, 4-pyridoxic acid levels in the urine should reflect the dietary intake of vitamin B_6. Some evidence for such a relationship has been observed in human experimental studies in which the intake of vitamin B_6 was controlled.[11,14,63,64,100-102,160] With a marked vitamin B_6 deficiency, no 4-pyridoxic acid was detected in the

urine.[11,14] The percent of vitamin B_6 converted to 4-pyridoxic acid has been reported to vary considerably according to age. Adult males converted 40 to 50% of the ingested vitamin B_6 to 4-pyridoxic acid,[14,63,65,98,111] while young adult females converted 22 to 35%[64] and preadolescent girls converted only 2.5 to 6%.[112]

The methods for measuring 4-pyridoxic acid in urine are rather tedious and involved and, hence, have seldom been used to evaluate vitamin B_6 nutritional status.[16,113,114] The potential interference of 4-pyridoxic acid 5′-phosphate in the analytical methods requires further evaluation[99] since, depending upon the treatment of the samples, variable amounts of this recently recognized metabolite may be measured as 4-pyridoxic acid. Moreover, in none of the human investigations was the influence of graded intakes of vitamin B_6 on urinary 4-pyridoxic acid excretion extensively studied. Therefore, the relationship of dietary vitamin B_6 intake to the level of urinary excretion of 4-pyridoxic acid has not been assuredly established.[17] Until the usefulness of the measurement has been reasonably established, urinary 4-pyridoxic acid analyses cannot be recommended as an index for evaluating vitamin B_6 nutriture in clinical cases. Moreover, 4-pyridoxic acid measurements as with urinary levels of vitamin B_6, furnish information primarily as to the immediate dietary intake of vitamin B_6 and probably do not indicate with certainty the body reserves of the vitamin.

Provisional guidelines for evaluating 4-pyridoxic acid excretion data can be arrived by tentatively accepting a conversion of 40% of the daily ingested vitamin B_6 to 4-pyridoxic acid.[17] Thus, the adult male would excrete 0.8 mg of 4-pyridoxic acid when ingesting the recommended daily intake of 2.0 mg of vitamin B_6 (Table 11). Information is not available as to whether or not random urine samples could be employed with the 4-pyridoxic acid levels related to creatinine excretion.

Blood Transaminase Activities

Transaminase measurements represent a biochemical functional test which possesses the possibility of providing information regarding the state of deficiency or degree of depletion of vitamin B_6 reserves. Controlled human vitamin B_6 depletion studies have demonstrated that glutamate-oxaloacetate transaminase (GOT) and glutamate-pyruvate transaminase (GPT) activities fall in erythro-

TABLE 11

Tentative Guidelines for Evaluating Vitamin B_6 Nutritional Status in the Adult Human[a]

Biochemical measurement[b]	Vitamin B_6 status	
	Marginal or inadequate	Acceptable
Tryptophan load test (net increase in excretion)		
Xanthurenic acid, mg/day	> 50	< 25
3-OH-kynurenine, mg/day	> 50	< 25
Kynurenine, mg/day	> 50	< 10
Quinolinic acid, μmol/day	> 50	< 25
Urinary measurements		
Vitamin B_6, μg/g creatinine[c]	< 20	$\geqslant$ 20
4-pyridoxic acid, mg/day	< 0.5	$\geqslant$ 0.8
Blood measurements		
EGPT index[d]	< 1.25	$\leqslant$ 1.25
EGOT index[d]	< 1.5	$\leqslant$ 1.5
Plasma vitamin B_6, ng/ml[e]	< 25	$\geqslant$ 50

[a]Adapted from Sauberlich et al.[17]
[b]As analytical procedures are improved and standardized, guidelines will undoubtedly require revision.
[c]Based on *Saccharomyces uvarum* assay of unhydrolyzed urine.
[d]The index will depend upon the methods used and the level of pyridoxal phosphate added in the in vitro stimulation assay.
[e]Adapted from the report of Baker et al.[90,115,143]

cytes, leukocytes and serum.[9,11,12,14,16,25,29,64,117-119] Serum (plasma) contains considerably less transaminase activities than do the erythrocytes.[129] Moreover, serum transaminase activities observed in normal individuals show a wide range. As a consequence, serum or plasma GPT and GOT activity measurements appear to be of limited use for assessing vitamin B_6 nutriture.[9,12,14,16,119]

The measurement of these enzymes in erythrocytes appears to be of value for detecting and evaluating human deficiencies of vitamin B_6.[26,43,64,120-124,160,161] Erythrocyte transaminase activities provide a much closer reflection of vitamin B_6 status than serum transaminase activities.[118,119] The GPT activity of whole blood and erythrocytes (EPGT) is only one tenth or less that of the EGOT activity.[16,24,118-120,161] Nevertheless, both enzyme activities decline with inadequate intakes of vitamin B_6, and both are accompanied by increases in the percentage stimulation produced by in vitro supplied pyridoxal phosphate.[25,29,117-119] The measurement of the stimulation of EGOT and EGPT activities induced by the in vitro addition of pyridoxal phosphate to the assay reaction appears to provide a reasonably satisfactory indication of

vitamin B_6 status. However, the in vitro addition of pyridoxal phosphate, usually in amounts of 50 or 100 μg per reaction vessel, stimulates transaminase activities significantly in erythrocytes obtained from normal subjects.[17,25,29,64,118,119,121-124,161] Considerable individual variation exists with normal individuals as to the erythrocyte transaminase activities either with or without the addition of pyridoxal phosphate. The amount of stimulation varies somewhat according to the method used, but generally, with normal erythrocytes, the EGOT activity is seldom stimulated more than 50% or the EGPT more than 25%.[17,25,29,118,119,123,124,138] Erythrocyte transaminase levels have been reported to be influenced by a concomitant riboflavin deficiency.[122,153]

In order to overcome some of the differences in methods of measurement and in erythrocyte transaminase activities between normal healthy individuals, the use of an erythrocyte transaminase index has been suggested:[17]

$$\text{EGOT index} = \frac{\text{EGOT} + \text{pyridoxal PO}_4}{\text{EGOT} (-\text{pyridoxal PO}_4)}$$

$$\text{EGPT index} = \frac{\text{EGPT} + \text{pyridoxal PO}_4}{\text{EGPT} (-\text{pyridoxal PO}_4)}$$

Based on the reports of several studies on erythrocyte transaminase activities,[17,25,29,118,119,123,124] normal subjects would probably have an EGOT index of less than 1.5 and an EGPT index of less than 1.25 (Table 11).[17] Nevertheless, additional studies with normal individuals and with known vitamin B_6 deficient subjects are needed before the validity and usefulness of such indexes can be established. The GOT and GPT activities have been measured in erythrocytes by various methods.[16,25,64,118-138] Unfortunately, the procedures used represent modifications of methods designed for measuring serum transaminases. The most commonly used colorimetric methods are based on the procedure of Reitman and Frankel,[129] and the generally used spectrophotometric methods are modifications of the procedures of Karmen[130] or Wroblewski and La Due.[136] A comparative study was conducted by Giusti et al.[127] on some of the procedures used for the determination of serum GOT and GPT. The enzymes appear to be stable for at least several weeks in samples held in a low-temperature freezer (-40 to -70°C).[139,140] For nutrition surveys or with large group studies, the present erythrocyte transaminase assay methods leave much to be desired.[17] The development of reliable, rapid and standardized methods would encourage their employment and would thereby assist in evaluating the usefulness of erythrocyte transaminase measurements in assessing vitamin B_6 nutritional status.

Blood Levels of Vitamin B_6

The vitamin B_6 levels in plasma, erythrocytes, and whole blood fall rapidly during vitamin B_6 depletion and rise following supplementation with a reflection of intake.[14,63,64] Consequently, a number of attempts have been made to utilize the levels of vitamin B_6 in plasma, whole blood or leukocytes as an indication of vitamin B_6 nurture.[9,16,17,48,61,62,64,76,90,93,95,100,115,138,141-145] Normal adult subjects have been observed to have plasma (serum) levels of vitamin B_6 in excess of 50 ng/ml whereas, in subjects with biochemical evidences of a vitamin B_6 deficiency, the levels fell below 25 ng/ml.[17,90,143] Plasma has been reported to contain approximately three times more vitamin B_6 than the erythrocytes (13 to 31 ng/ml cells),[62,90,142-144,146-148] although others have reported high levels of the vitamin in erythrocytes (336 ng/ml cells).[64] The

only nutrition survey in which a significant number of serum samples were analyzed for vitamin B_6 levels was the study of Baker et al.[115] A mean vitamin B_6 serum level of 36 ng/ml was observed in a group of New York City school children, ages 10 to 13 years. Baker et al.[62,90] have reported vitamin B_6 levels for whole blood, red cells and plasma in normal subjects as 37 ± 6, 20 ± 3 and 59 ± 13 ng/ml, respectively.

Pyridoxal phosphate levels have also been measured in serum, employing various analytical procedures.[14,16,71,75,80-83,85,88,94,95,138,141] A considerable range of values has been reported (0 to 35 ng/ml serum), reflecting in part the poor sensitivity of some of the methods employed.[16] Serum pyridoxal phosphate levels have been reported to fall with increasing age[88,145,150] and in pregnancy.[48,149,151] Recently, improvements have been reported in the procedures used for measuring pyridoxal phosphate in serum and other biological materials.[71,80-83,88] In the experiences of the reviewers, modifications of the procedures of Haskell and Snell[80] and of Chabner and Livingston[81] appear to be the most promising methods possessing the sensitivity necessary to reliably measure the low levels of pyridoxal phosphate present in plasma and erythrocytes.

In general, measurements of plasma or blood levels of vitamin B_6 appear to hold promise as an index for evaluating the status of this vitamin in human population groups. The technical difficulties associated with the analytical procedures have, however, discouraged their use. Until the methods have been simplified and standardized and appropriate guidelines developed, widespread acceptance and application cannot be expected.

Other Measurements That May Reflect Vitamin B_6 Status

During a vitamin B_6 deficiency, a number of additional biochemical changes have been observed that have suggested the possibility of other techniques for evaluating the nutritional status of this vitamin.[17] Of these techniques, the methionine load test appears to be worthy of further investigation.[154] In vitamin B_6-depleted adult men, methionine loading induced a marked excretion of cystathionine which was prevented with vitamin B_6 supplementation.[154] The methionine load test consists of administering 3 g of L-methionine orally, collecting the postload urine for 24 hr and analyzing the urine samples for cystathionine and cysteine sulfinic acid. The methionine load test was employed recently in a group of pregnant women with signs of a pyridoxine deficiency and in a group of normal nonpregnant women.[155] The pregnant women were observed to excrete large amounts of cystathionine following the methionine load test, and the ratio of cystathionine:cysteine sulfinic acid was elevated. Therapy with pyridoxine corrected these biochemical abnormalities.[155] The increases in urinary excretion of taurine and sulfate after a loading dose of methionine or cystine in vitamin B_6-deficient subjects were not sufficient to serve as a means of assessing vitamin B_6 nutriture.[17,156]

The urinary excretion of quinolinic acid, a precursor of nicotinic acid, is markedly increased in vitamin B_6-deficient subjects following a tryptophan load.[157] Although this observation deserves further evaluation, the measurement of quinolinic acid excretion levels does not appear to offer any advantages over measurements for xanthurenic acid, kynurenine or 3-hydroxykynurenine as a means of assessing vitamin B_6 status. Changes in plasma and urinary levels of free amino acids may occur in pyridoxine deficiency.[12,64,152,158,159] None of these changes appears suitable as the basis for a satisfactory technique to detect a vitamin B_6 deficiency. Other measurements, such as blood urea nitrogen levels after an alanine load test and urinary levels of oxalic acid or o-phosphory-

lethanolamine, do not appear to be sufficiently dependable, sensitive, or specific to serve as indices for evaluating vitamin B_6 nutriture.[17]

Summary

The biochemical techniques described can furnish information as to the dietary supply of vitamin B_6 provided the body through reflections in urine excretion rates and in blood levels of the vitamin. For the most part, such measurements would not distinguish between a dietary deficiency and abnormal states such as poor absorption, dependency syndromes, abnormal utilization, or drug interactions. Nevertheless, such measurements can aid in indicating the possibility of a vitamin B_6 deficiency. More specific indications of an inadequacy of vitamin B_6 intake or reduced tissue reserves can be obtained with biochemical tests that reveal metabolic changes such as the tryptophan load or blood transaminase activity measurements. Although the tryptophan load test is relatively easy to perform in clinical cases and has been widely used to evaluate vitamin B_6 deficiency, the results of the test need to be interpreted with care in view of the interrelated metabolic and hormonal factors involved in tryptophan metabolism.[6,26,58] As a consequence, additional biochemical indices should be employed whenever feasible to assess vitamin B_6 nutritional status. For this purpose, measurements of urinary levels of vitamin B_6 and erythrocyte transaminase activities appear the most useful.

REFERENCES

1. **György, P.,** The history of vitamin B_6, *Vitam. Horm.,* 22, 361, 1964.
2. **György, P.,** Developments leading to the metabolic role of vitamin B_6, *Am. J. Clin. Nutr.,* 24, 1250, 1971.
3. **Sauberlich, H. E.,** Vitamin B_6 group. IX. Biochemical systems and biochemical detection of deficiency, in *The Vitamins,* Vol. II, 2nd ed., Sebrell, W. H., Jr. and Harris, R. S. Eds., Academic Press, New York, 1968, chap. 3, p. 44.
4. **Sauberlich, H. E.,** Recent advances in the knowledge of vitamin function and metabolism: Pyridoxine, Symposia Proceedings IX International Congress of Nutrition, Mexico City, S. Karger, Basle, 1972, in press.
5. **Sauberlich, H. E. and Canham, J. E.,** Vitamin B_6, in *Modern Nutrition in Health and Disease,* Goodhart, R. S. and Shils, M. E., Eds., Lea and Febiger, Philadelphia, 1973.
6. **Kelsall, M. A.,** Ed., Vitamin B_6 in metabolism of the nervous system, *Ann. N.Y. Acad. Sci.,* 166, 1, 1969.
7. **Sauberlich, H. E.,** Vitamin B_6 group. VIII. Active compounds and antagonists, in *The Vitamins,* Vol. II, 2nd ed., Sebrell, W. H., Jr. and Harris, R. S., Eds., Academic Press, New York, 1968, 33.
8. International Symposium on Vitamin B_6, *Vitam. Horm.,* 22, 399, 1964.
9. **Sauberlich, H. E., Canham, J. E., Baker, E. M., Raica, N., Jr., and Herman, Y. F.,** Human vitamin B_6 nutriture, *J. Sci. Ind. Res.,* 29(8), 528, 1970.
10. **Sauberlich, H. E.,** Human requirements for vitamin B_6, *Vitam. Horm.,* 22, 807, 1964.
11. **Linkswiler, H.,** Biochemical and physiological changes in vitamin B_6 deficiency, *Am. J. Clin. Nutr.,* 20, 547, 1967.

12. **Canham, J. E., Baker, E. M., Harding, R. S., Sauberlich, H. E., and Plough, I. C.,** Dietary protein – its relationship to vitamin B_6 requirement and function, *Ann. N.Y. Acad. Sci.,* 166, 16, 1969.

13. **Coon, W. W. and Nagler, E.,** The tryptophan load as a test for pyridoxine deficiency in hospitalized patients, *Ann. N.Y. Acad. Sci.,* 166, 30, 1969.

14. **Baysal, A., Johnson, B. A., and Linkswiler, H.,** Vitamin B_6 depletion in man: blood vitamin B_6, plasma pyridoxal-phosphate, serum cholesterol, serum transaminases and urinary vitamin B_6 and 4-pyridoxic acid, *J. Nutr.,* 89, 19, 1966.

15. **György, P.,** Vitamin B_6 group. XI. Vitamin B_6 deficiency effects in man, in *The Vitamins,* Vol. II, 2nd ed., Sebrell, W. H., Jr. and Harris, R. S., Eds., Academic Press, New York, 1968, 90.

16. **Sauberlich, H. E.,** Vitamin B_6, in *The Vitamins,* Vol. VII, 2nd ed., György, P. and Pearson, W. N., Eds., Academic Press, New York, 1967, 169.

17. **Sauberlich, H. E., Canham, J. E., Baker, E. M., Raica, N., Jr., and Herman, Y. F.,** Biochemical assessment of the nutritional status of vitamin B_6 in the human, *Am. J. Clin. Nutr.,* 25, 629, 1972.

18. **Lepkovsky, S. and Nielson, E.,** A green pigment-producing compound in urine of pyridoxine-deficient rats, *J. Biol. Chem.,* 144, 135, 1942.

19. **Fouts, P. J. and Lepkovsky, S.,** A green pigment-producing compound in urine of pyridoxine-deficient dogs, *Proc. Soc. Exp. Biol. Med.,* 50, 221, 1942.

20. **Greenberg, L. D., Bohr, D. F., McGrath, H., and Rinehart, J. F.,** Xanthurenic acid excretion in the human subject on a pyridoxine-deficient diet, *Arch. Biochem.,* 21, 237, 1949.

21. **Price, J. M., Brown, R. R., and Yess, N.,** Testing the functional capacity of the tryptophan-niacin pathway in man by analysis of urinary metabolites, *Adv. Metab. Disord.,* 2, 159, 1965.

22. **Baker, E. M., Canham, J. E., Nunes, W. T., Sauberlich, H. E., and McDowell, M. E.,** Vitamin B_6 requirement for adult men, *Am. J. Clin. Nutr.,* 15, 59, 1964.

23. **Miller, L. T. and Linkswiler, H.,** Effect of protein intake on the development of abnormal tryptophan metabolism by men during vitamin B_6 depletion, *J. Nutr.,* 93, 53, 1967.

24. **Yess, N., Price, J. M., Brown, R. R., Swan, P. B., and Linkswiler, H.,** Vitamin B_6 depletion in man: urinary excretion of tryptophan metabolites, *J. Nutr.,* 84, 229, 1964.

25. **Cinnamon, A. D. and Beaton, J. R.,** Biochemical assessment of vitamin B_6 status in man, *Am. J. Clin. Nutr.,* 23, 696, 1970.

26. **Brown, R. R., Miller, O. N., Coursin, D. B., and Rose, D. P.** (organizing committee), Biochemistry and pathology of tryptophan metabolism and its regulation by amino acids, vitamin B_6 and steroid hormones, *Am. J. Clin. Nutr.,* 24, 653, 1971.

27. **Canham, J. E., Baker, E. M., Sauberlich, H. E., Raica, N., Jr., and Nunes, W. T.,** Human requirements and various aspects of vitamin B_6 metabolism: fractional urinary excretion of tryptophan metabolites, creatinine and vitamin B_6 status, *U.S. Army Med. Res. Nutr. Lab. Ann. Prog. Rep.,* 151, 1963.

28. **Interdepartmental Committee on Nutrition for National Defense,** *Union of Burma Nutritional Survey, October-December 1961,* Washington, D.C., U.S. Govt. Printing Office, 1963.

29. **Canham, J. E., Baker, E. M., Raica, N., Jr., and Sauberlich, H. E.,** Vitamin B_6 requirement of adult men, *Proc. Seventh Intern. Congr. Nutr., Hamburg,* Vol. 5, Pergamon Press, Elmsford, New York, 1966, 558.

30. **Rapoport, M. I. and Beisel, W. R.,** Circadian periodicity of tryptophan metabolism, *J. Clin. Invest.,* 47, 934, 1968.

31. **Vinyard, E., Joven, C. B., Swendseid, M. E., and Drenick, E. J.,** Vitamin B_6 nutriture studied in obese subjects during 8 weeks of starvation, *Am. J. Clin. Nutr.,* 20, 317, 1967.

32. **Drenick, E. J., Vinyard, E., and Swendseid, M. E.,** Vitamin B_6 requirements in starving obese males, *Am. J. Clin. Nutr.,* 22, 10, 1969.

33. **Rose, D. P.,** The influence of oestrogens on tryptophan metabolism in man, *Clin. Sci.,* 31, 265, 1966.

34. **Rose, D. P.,** Excretion of xanthurenic acid in the urine of women taking progestogen-oestrogen preparations, *Nature,* 210, 196, 1966.

35. **Baker, E. M., Sauberlich, H. E., and Canham, J. E.,** The effects of short-term ingestion of contraceptive steroids on tryptophan metabolism in female subjects, *U.S. Army Med. Res. Nutr. Lab. Ann. Prog. Rep.,* 239, 1968.

36. **Brown, R. R., Rose, D. P., Price, J. M., and Wolf, H.,** Tryptophan metabolism as affected by anovulatory agents, *Ann. N.Y. Acad. Sci.,* 166, 44, 1969.

37. **Price, J. M., Brown, R. R., and Thornton, M. J.,** Tryptophan metabolism of women using steroid hormones for ovulation control, *Am. J. Clin. Nutr.,* 18, 312, 1966 (abstract).

38. **Price, J. M., Thornton, M. J., and Mueller, L. M.,** Tryptophan metabolism in women using steroid hormones for ovulation control, *Am. J. Clin. Nutr.,* 20, 452, 1967.

39. **Baumblatt, M. J. and Winston, F.,** Pyridoxine and the pill, *Lancet,* 1, 832, 1970.

40. **Luhby, A. L., Davis, P., Murphy, M., Gordon, M., Brin, M., and Spiegel, H.,** Pyridoxine and oral contraceptives, *Lancet,* 2, 1083, 1970.

41. **Theuer, R. C.,** Effect of oral contraceptive agents on vitamin and mineral needs: A review, *J. Reprod. Med.,* 8, 13, 1972.

42. **Moursi, G. E., Abdel-Daim, M. H., Kelada, N. L., Abdel-Tawab, G. A., and Girgis, L. H.,** The influence of sex, age, synthetic oestrogens, progestogens and oral contraceptives on the excretion of urinary tryptophan metabolites, *Bull. W.H.O., 43, 651, 1970.*

43. **Aly, H. E., Donald, E. A., and Simpson, M. H. W.,** Oral contraceptives and vitamin B_6 metabolism, *Am. J. Clin. Nutr., 24, 297, 1971.*

44. **Price, S. A., Rose, D. P., and Toseland, P. A.,** Effects of dietary vitamin B_6 deficiency and oral contraceptives on the spontaneous urinary excretion of 3-hydroxyanthranilic acid, *Am. J. Clin. Nutr., 25, 494, 1972.*

45. **Toseland, P. A. and Price, S.,** Tryptophan and oral contraceptives, *Br. Med. J., 1, 777, 1969.*

46. **Brown, R. R., Thornton, M. J., and Price, J. M.,** The effect of vitamin supplementation on the urinary excretion of tryptophan metabolites by pregnant women, *J. Clin. Invest., 40, 617, 1961.*

47. **Wachstein, M.,** Evidence for a relative vitamin B_6 deficiency in pregnancy and some disease states, *Vitam. Horm., 22, 705, 1964.*

48. **Hamfelt, A. and Hahn, L.,** Pyridoxal phosphate concentration in plasma and tryptophan load test during pregnancy, *Clin. Chim. Acta., 25, 91, 1969.*

49. **Arend, R. A., Leklem, J. E., and Brown, R. R.,** Direct and steam distillation autoanalyzer methods for assay of diazotizable aromatic amine metabolites of tryptophan in urine and in serum, *Biochem. Med., 4, 457, 1970.*

50. **Wolf, H., Price, J. M., Brown, R. R., and Madsen, P. O.,** Studies on tryptophan metabolism in male subjects treated with progestational agents, *Scand. J. Clin. Lab. Invest., 25, 237, 1970.*

51. **Brown, R. R. and Price, J. M.,** Quantitative studies on metabolites of tryptophan in the urine of the dog, cat, rat and man, *J. Biol. Chem., 219, 985, 1956.*

52. **Brown, R. R.,** The isolation and determination of urinary hydroxykynurenine, *J. Biol. Chem., 227, 649, 1957.*

53. **Satoh, K. and Price, J. M.,** Fluorometric determination of kynurenic acid and xanthurenic acid in human urine, *J. Biol. Chem., 230, 781, 1958.*

54. **Watanabe, M., Watanabe, Y., and Okada, M.,** A new fluorimetric method for the determination of 3-hydroxykynurenine, *Clin. Chim. Acta, 27, 461, 1970.*

55. **Nowak, H. and Körner, W. F.,** Automatic determination of xanthurenic acid, *Anal. Biochem., 17, 154, 1966.*

56. **Atkins, R., Wilson, L., and Horton, J.,** Automated fluorometric analysis of urine xanthurenic and kynurenic acid, *Technicon Q., 4(1), 20, 1972.*

57. **Wallace, M. J., Vaillant, H. W., and Salhanick, H. A.,** Method for quantitative measurement of xanthurenic acid in urine, *Clin. Chem., 17, 505, 1971.*

58. **Brown, R. R.,** Normal and pathological conditions which may alter the human requirement for vitamin B_6, *J. Agric. Food Chem., 20, 498, 1972.*

59. **Toseland, P. A., Michelin, M. J., and Price, S. A.,** The determination of 3-hydroxyanthranilic acid in human urine by thin-layer electrophoresis and fluorimetry, *Clin. Chim. Acta, 37, 477, 1972.*

60. **Watanabe, M. and Hayashi, K.,** A fluorometric method for 3-hydroxyanthranilic acid in human urine, *Clin. Chim. Acta, 37, 417, 1972.*

61. **Baker, H. and Frank, O.,** Vitamin status in metabolic upsets, *World Rev. Nutr. and Diet., 9, 124, 1968.*

62. **Baker, H., Frank, O., Ning, M., Gellene, R. A., Hutner, S. H., and Leevy, C. M.,** A protozoological method for detecting clinical vitamin B_6 deficiency, *Am. J. Clin. Nutr., 18, 123, 1966.*

63. **Kelsay, J., Baysal, A., and Linkswiler, H.,** Effect of vitamin B_6 depletion on the pyridoxal, pyridoxamine and pyridoxine content of the blood and urine of men, *J. Nutr., 94, 490, 1968.*

64. **Donald, E. A., McBean, L. D., Simpson, M. H. W., Sun, M. F., and Aly, H. E.,** Vitamin B_6 requirement of young adult women, *Am. J. Clin. Nutr., 24, 1028, 1971.*

65. **Tillotson, J. A., Sauberlich, H. E., Baker, E. M., and Canham, J. E.,** Use of carbon-14 labeled vitamins in human nutrition studies: pyridoxine, *Proc. Seventh Int. Congr. Nutr., 5, 554, 1966.*

66. *Recommended Dietary Allowances.* 7th revised ed., A report of the Food and Nutrition Board, National Research Council, Publication No. 1694, National Academy of Sciences, Washington, D.C. 20418, 1968.

67. *Manual for Nutrition Surveys.* 2nd ed., Interdepartmental Committee on Nutrition for National Defense, Superintendent of Documents, U. S. Government Printing Office, Washington, D.C. 20402, 1963.

68. Ten-State Nutrition Survey Reports, I–V, 1972, Center for Disease Control, Atlanta, Georgia 30330.

69. **Stearn, G., Newman, K. J., McKinley, J. B., and Jeans, P. C.,** The protein requirements of children from one to ten years of age, *Ann. N. Y. Acad. Sci., 69, 857, 1958.*

70. **Musajo, L. and Benassi, C. A.,** Aspects of disorders of the kynurenine pathway of tryptophan metabolism in man, *Adv. Clin. Chem., 7, 63, 1964.*

71. **Okuda, K., Fujii, S., and Wada, M.,** Microassay of pyridoxal phosphate using tryptophan-^{14}C with tryptophanase, in *Methods in Enzymology,* Vol. 18A, McCormick, D. B. and Wright, L. D., Eds., Academic Press, New York, 1970, 505.

72. **Polansky, M. M. and Murphy, E. W.,** Vitamin B_6 components in fruits and nuts, *J. Am. Diet. Assoc., 48, 109, 1966.*

73. **Toepfer, E. W. and Lehmann, J.,** Procedure for chromatographic separation and microbiological assay of pyridoxine, pyridoxal and pyridoxamine in food extracts, *J. Assoc. Off. Agric. Chem., 44, 426, 1961.*

74. **Toepfer, E. W., Polansky, M. M., Richardson, L. R., and Wilkes, S.,** Comparison of vitamin B_6 values of selected food samples by bioassay and microbiological assay, *J. Agric. Food. Chem., 11, 523, 1963.*

75. Storvick, C. A., Benson, E. M., Edwards, M. A., and Woodring, M. J., Chemical and microbiological determination of vitamin B_6, in *Methods of Biochemical Analysis*, Vol. XII, Glick, D., Ed., Interscience Publishers, New York, 1964, 183.

76. Donald, E. A. and Ferguson, R. F., A micro method for determination of pyridoxal phosphate in leukocytes and liver, *Anal. Biochem.*, 7, 335, 1964.

77. Ahrens, H. and Korytnyk, W., Pyridoxine chemistry. XXI. Thin-layer chromatography and thin-layer electrophoresis of compounds in the vitamin B_6 group, *Anal. Biochem.*, 30, 413, 1969.

78. Korytnyk, W., Fricke, G., and Paul, B., Pyridoxine chemistry. XII. Gas chromatography of compounds in the vitamin B_6 group, *Anal. Biochem.*, 17, 66, 1966.

79. Prosser, A. R., Sheppard, A. J., and Libby, D. A., Gas-liquid chromatography of vitamin B_6 (pyridoxal, pyridoxol, and pyridoxamine) and its application to pharmaceuticals containing pyridoxol, *J. Assoc. Off. Agric. Chem.*, 50, 1348, 1967.

80. Haskell, B. E. and Snell, E. E., An improved apotryptophanase assay for pyridoxal phosphate, *Anal. Biochem.*, 45, 567, 1972.

81. Chabner, B. and Livingston, D., A simple enzymic assay for pyridoxal phosphate, *Anal. Biochem.*, 34, 413, 1970.

82. Sundaresan, P. R. and Coursin, D. B., Microassay of pyridoxal phosphate using L-tyrosine-1-^{14}C and tyrosine apodecarboxylase, in *Methods in Enzymology*, Vol. 18A, McCormick, D. B. and Wright, L. D., Eds., Academic Press, New York, 1970, 509.

83. Evangelopoulos, A. E., Karni-Katsadimas, I., and Kalogerakos, T. G., Simultaneous determination of pyridoxal-P and pyridoxamine-P by an enzyme-substrate complex of aspartate transaminase, *Enzymologia*, 40, 37, 1971.

84. Smith, M. A. and Dietrich, L. S., Preparative thin-layer chromatography for the separation of the various forms of vitamin B_6 in tissues. Vitamin B_6 content of chick embryo liver during the midperiod of development, *Biochim. Biophys. Acta*, 230, 262, 1971.

85. Takanashi, S. and Tamura, Z., Preliminary studies for fluorometric determination of pyridoxal and of its 5'-phosphate, *J. Vitaminol.*, 16, 129, 1970.

86. Colombini, C. E. and McCoy, E. E., Rapid thin-layer electrophoretic separation and estimation of all vitamin B_6 compounds and of some 5-hydroxyindoles, *Anal. Biochem.*, 34, 451, 1970.

87. Barton-Wright, E. C., The microbiological assay of the vitamin B_6 complex (pyridoxine, pyridoxal and pyridoxamine) with *Kloeckera brevis*, *Analyst*, 96, 314, 1971.

88. Anderson, B. B., Peart, M. B., and Fulford-Jones, C. E., The measurement of serum pyridoxal by a microbiological assay using *Lactobacillus casei*, *J. Clin. Pathol.*, 23, 233, 1970.

89. Benson, E. M., Edwards, M. A., Peters, J. M., and Storvick, C. A., Vitamin B_6-amino acid-peptide interrelationship in *Streptococcus faecium* φ51, *Int. J. Vit. Res.*, 40, 184, 1970.

90. Baker, H. and Frank, O., Vitamin B_6, in *Clinical Vitaminology*, Interscience Publishers, New York, 1968, 66.

91. *Difco Supplementary Literature*, Difco Laboratories, Detroit, Michigan 48232, May, 1972, 448.

92. The American Type Culture Collection, 12301 Parklawn Drive, Rockville, Maryland 20852.

93. Storvick, C. A. and Peters, J. M., Methods for the determination of vitamin B_6 in biological materials, *Vitam. Horm.*, 22, 833, 1964.

94. Maruyama, H. and Coursin, D. B., Enzymic assay of pyridoxal phosphate using tyrosine apodecarboxylase and tyrosine-1-^{14}C, *Anal. Biochem.*, 26, 420, 1968.

95. Hamfelt, A., Enzymatic determination of pyridoxal phosphate in plasma by decarboxylation of L-tyrosine-^{14}C(U) and a comparison with the tryptophan load test, *Scand. J. Clin. Lab. Invest.*, 20, 1, 1967.

96. Haskell, B. E. and Snell, E. E., Microbiological determination of the vitamin B_6 group, in *Methods in Enzymology*, Vol. 18A, McCormick, D. B. and Wright, L. D., Eds., Academic Press, New York, 1970, 512.

97. Brin, M., A simplified Toepfer-Lehmann assay for the three vitamin B_6 vitamers, in *Methods in Enzymology*, Vol. 18A, McCormick, D. B. and Wright, L. D., Eds., Academic Press, New York, 1970, 519.

98. Johansson, S., Lindstedt, S., Register, U., and Wadstrom, L., Studies on the metabolism of labeled pyridoxine in man, *Am. J. Clin. Nutr.*, 18, 185, 1966.

99. Contractor, S. F. and Shane, B., 4-pyridoxic acid 5'-phosphate: A metabolite of pyridoxal in the rat, *Biochem. Biophys. Res. Commun.*, 39, 1175, 1970.

100. Gailani, S. D., Holland, J. F., Nussbaum, A., and Olson, K. B., Clinical and biochemical studies of pyridoxine deficiency in patients with neoplastic diseases, *Cancer*, 21, 975, 1968.

101. Snyderman, S. E., Holt. L. E., Jr., Carretero, R., and Jacobs, K., Pyridoxine deficiency in the human infant, *Am. J. Clin. Nutr.*, 1, 200, 1953.

102. Ziegler, E., Reinken, L., and Berger, H., Die Ausscheidung von Pyridoxinsäure beim Neugeborenen und ihre Beeinflussung durch Pyridoxinbelastung, *Int. Z. Vitaminforsch.*, 39, 192, 1969.

103. Wolf, H., Brown, R. R., Price, J. M., and Madsen, P. O., Studies on tryptophan metabolism in male subjects treated with female sex hormones, *J. Clin. Endocrinol Metab.*, 31, 397, 1970.

104. Coon, W. W., The tryptophan load and pyridoxine deficiency, *Am. J. Clin. Pathol.*, 46, 345, 1966.

105. Tompsett, S. L., The determination in urine of some metabolites of tryptophan – kynurenine, anthranilic acid and 3-hydroxy-anthranilic acid – and reference to the presence of *o*-aminophenol in urine, *Clin. Chim. Acta*, 4, 411, 1959.

106. Coursin, D. B., Recommendations for standardization of the tryptophan load test, *Am. J. Clin. Nutr.*, 14, 56, 1964.

107. Wolf, H. and Brown, R. R., The effect of tryptophan load and vitamin B_6 supplementation on urinary excretion of tryptophan metabolites in human male subjects, *Clin. Sci.*, 41, 237, 1971.

108. Gibbs, D. A. and Watts, R. W. E., The action of pyridoxine in primary hyperoxaluria, *Clin. Sci.*, 38, 277, 1970.

109. Sauberlich, H. E., Goad, W., Herman, Y. F., Milan, F., and Jamison, P., Biochemical assessment of the nutritional status of the Eskimos of Wainwright, Alaska, *Am. J. Clin. Nutr.*, 25, 437, 1972.

110. Faber, S. R., Feitler, W. W., Bleiler, R. E., Ohlson, M. A., and Hodges, R. E., The effects of an induced pyridoxine and pantothenic acid deficiency on excretions of oxalic and xanthurenic acids in the urine, *Am. J. Clin. Nutr.*, 12, 406, 1963.

111. McCoy, E. E. and England, J., Excretion of 4-pyridoxic acid during deoxypyridoxine and pyridoxine administration to mongoloid and non-mongoloid subjects, *J. Nutr.*, 96, 525, 1968.

112. Ritchey, S. J. and Feeley, R. M., The excretion patterns of vitamin B_6 and B_{12} in preadolescent girls, *J. Nutr.*, 89, 411, 1966.

113. Woodring, M. J., Fisher, D. H., and Storvick, C. A., A microprocedure for the determination of 4-pyridoxic acid in urine, *Clin. Chem.*, 10, 479, 1964.

114. Reddy, S. K., Reynolds, M. S., and Price, J. M., The determination of 4-pyridoxic acid in human urine, *J. Biol. Chem.*, 233, 691, 1958.

115. Baker, H., Frank, O., Feingold, S., Christakis, G., and Ziffer, H., Vitamins, total cholesterol, and triglycerides in 642 New York City school children, *Am. J. Clin. Nutr.*, 20, 850, 1967.

116. *Manual for Nutrition Surveys*, 1st ed., Interdepartmental Committee on Nutrition for National Defense, Superintendent of Documents, U.S. Government Printing Office, Washington, D.C. 20402, 1957.

117. Canham, J. E., Sauberlich, H. E., Baker, E. M., and Raica, N., Jr., Human studies in vitamin B_6 metabolism, *U.S. Army Med. Res. Nutr. Lab. Ann. Prog. Rep.*, 1965, 119.

118. Cheney, M., Sabry, Z. I., and Beaton, G. H., Erythrocyte glutamic-pyruvic transaminase activity in man, *Am. J. Clin. Nutr.*, 16, 337, 1965.

119. Raica, N., Jr. and Sauberlich, H. E., Blood cell transaminase activity in human vitamin B_6 deficiency, *Am. J. Clin. Nutr.*, 15, 67, 1964.

120. Jacobs, A., Cavill, I. A. J., and Hughes, J. N. P., Erythrocyte transaminase activity. Effect of age, sex, and vitamin B_6 supplementation, *Am. J. Clin. Nutr.*, 21, 502, 1968.

121. Brubacher, G., Ritzel, G., and Schlettwein-Gsell, D., Über die Versorgung eines ausgewählten Kollektivs von Studenten mit einigen Nährstoffen durch die tägliche Nahrung. II. Blutchemische Vitamenanalysen, *Int. Z. Vitaminforsch.*, 40, 199, 1970.

122. Krishnaswamy, K., Erythrocyte transaminase activity in human vitamin B_6 deficiency, *Int. J. Vitam. Nutr., Res.*, 41, 240, 1971.

123. Woodring, M. J. and Storvick, C. A., Effect of pyridoxine supplementation on glutamic-pyruvic transaminase and in vitro stimulation in erythrocytes of normal women, *Am. J. Clin. Nutr.*, 23, 1385, 1970.

124. Doberenz, A. R., Van Miller, J. P., Green, J. R., and Beaton, J. R., Vitamin B_6 depletion in women using oral contraceptives as determined by erythrocyte glutamic-pyruvic transaminase activities, *Proc. Soc. Exp. Biol. Med.*, 137, 1100, 1971.

125. Babson, A. L., Shapiro, P. O., Williams, P. A. R., and Phillips, G. E., The use of a diazonium salt for the determination of glutamic-oxalacetic transaminase in serum, *Clin. Chim. Acta*, 7, 199, 1962.

126. Babson, A. L. and Phillips, G. E., An improved colorimetric transaminase assay, *Clin. Chem.*, 11, 533, 1965.

127. Giusti, G., Ruggiero, G., and Cacciatore, L., A comparative study of some spectrophotometric and colorimetric procedures for the determination of serum glutamic-oxaloacetic and glutamic-pyruvic transaminase in hepatic diseases, *Enzymol. Biol. Clin.*, 10, 17, 1969.

128. Karmen, A., Wróblewski, F., and LaDue, J. S., Transaminase activity in human blood, *J. Clin. Invest.*, 34, 126, 1955.

129. Reitman, S. and Frankel, S., A colorimetric method for the determination of serum glutamic oxalacetic and glutamic pyruvic transaminases, *Am. J. Clin. Pathol.*, 28, 56, 1957.

130. Karmen, A., A note on the spectrophotometric assay of glutamic oxaloacetic transaminase in human blood serum, *J. Clin. Invest.*, 34, 131, 1955.

131. Heddle, J. G., McHenry, F. W., and Beaton, G. H., Penicillamine and vitamin B_6 interrelationship in the rat, *Can. J. Biochem. Physiol.*, 41, 1215, 1963.

132. Tonhazy, N. E., White, N. G., and Umbreit, W. W., A rapid method for the estimation of the glutamic-aspartic transaminase in tissues and its application to radiation sickness, *Arch. Biochem.*, 28, 36, 1950.

133. Cabaud, P., Leeper, R., and Wróblewski, F., Colorimetric measurement of serum glutamic oxaloacetic transaminase, *Am. J. Clin. Pathol.*, 26, 1101, 1956.

134. Salvatore, F., Bocchini, V., and Cimmino, P., Methods for the determination of some transaminase activities in biological fluids, *Enzymologia*, 22, 357, 1961.

135. Umbreit, W. W., Rahway, N. J., Kingsley, G. R., Schaffert, A. B., and Siplet, H., A colorimetric method for transaminase in serum or plasma, *J. Lab. Clin. Med.*, 49, 454, 1957.

136. Wróblewski, F. and LaDue, J. S., Serum glutamic pyruvic transaminase in cardiac and hepatic disease, *Proc. Soc. Exp. Biol. Med.,* 91, 569, 1956.

137. Wróblewski, F. and Cabaud, P., Colorimetric measurement of serum glutamic pyruvic transaminase, *Am. J. Clin. Pathol.,* 27, 235, 1957.

138. Hamfelt, A., Pyridoxal phosphate concentration and aminotransferase activity in human blood cells, *Clin. Chim. Acta,* 16, 19, 1967.

139. Mosley, J. W. and Goodwin, R. F., Stability of serum glutamic pyruvic transaminase activity on storage, *Am. J. Clin. Pathol.,* 44, 591, 1965.

140. Fleshood, H. L. and Sauberlich, H. E., U.S. Army Medical Research and Nutrition Laboratory, Denver, Colorado 80240, unpublished data.

141. Coburn, S. P. and Seidenberg, M., Leukocyte pyridoxal phosphate and alkaline phosphatase in Down's syndrome and other retardates, *Am. J. Clin. Nutr.,* 22, 1197, 1969.

142. Leevy, C. M., Baker, H., Ten Hove, W., Frank, O., and Cherrick, G. R., B-complex vitamins in liver disease of the alcoholic, *Am. J. Clin. Nutr.,* 16, 339, 1965.

143. Leevy, C. M., Cardi, L., Frank, O., Gellene, R., and Baker, H., Incidence and significance of hypovitaminemia in a randomly selected municipal hospital population, *Am. J. Clin. Nutr.,* 17, 259, 1965.

144. Ning, M., Baker, H., and Leevy, C. M., Effect of protein intake on the development of abnormal tryptophan metabolism by men during vitamin B_6 depletion, *Proc. Soc. Exp. Biol. Med.,* 121, 27, 1966.

145. Hamfelt, A., Age variation of vitamin B_6 metabolism, *Clin. Chim. Acta,* 10, 48, 1964.

146. Baker, H., Frank, O., Thomson, A. D., and Feingold, S., Vitamin distribution in red blood cells, plasma, and other body fluids, *Am. J. Clin. Nutr.,* 22, 1469, 1969.

147. Baker, H., Frank, O., and Pasher, I., Vitamin levels in blood and serum, *Nature,* 191, 78, 1961.

148. Frank, O., Baker, H., and Sobotka, H., Blood and serum levels of water-soluble vitamins in man and animals, *Nature,* 197, 490, 1963.

149. Contractor, S. F. and Shane, B., Blood and urine levels of vitamin B_6 in the mother and fetus before and after loading of the mother with vitamin B_6, *Am. J. Obstet. Gynecol.,* 107, 635, 1970.

150. György, P., Philadelphia General Hospital, Philadelphia, personal communication, 1972.

151. Hamfelt, A. and Tuvemo, T., Pyridoxal phosphate and folic acid concentration in blood and erythrocyte aspartate aminotransferase activity during pregnancy, *Clin. Chim. Acta,* 41, 287, 1972.

152. Park, Y. K. and Linkswiler, H., Effect of vitamin B_6 depletion in adult man on the plasma concentration and the urinary excretion of free amino acids, *J. Nutr.,* 101, 185, 1971.

153. Krishnaswamy, K., Erythrocyte glutamic oxaloacetic transaminase activity in patients with oral lesions, *Int. J. Vitam. Nutr. Res.,* 41, 247, 1971.

154. Park, Y. K. and Linkswiler, H., Effect of vitamin B_6 depletion in adult man on the excretion of cystathionine and other methionine metabolites, *J. Nutr.,* 100, 110, 1970.

155. Krishnaswamy, K., Methionine load test in pyridoxine deficiency, *Int. J. Vitam. Nutr. Res.,* 42, 468, 1972.

156. Swan, P., Wentworth, J., and Linkswiler, H., Vitamin B_6 depletion in man: Urinary taurine and sulfate excretion and nitrogen balance, *J. Nutr.,* 84, 220, 1964.

157. Kelsay, J., Miller, L. T., and Linkswiler, H., Effect of protein intake on the excretion of quinolinic acid and niacin metabolites by men during vitamin B_6 depletion, *J. Nutr.,* 94, 27, 1968.

158. Harding, R. S., Sauberlich, H. E., and Canham, J. E., The free amino acids in the plasma and urine of human subjects on a vitamin B_6-deficient diet, in *Automation in Analytical Chemistry — Technicon Symposia,* Skeggs, L. T., Jr., Ed., Mediad, New York, 1965, 643.

159. Merrow, S. B., Babcock, M. J., Radke, F. H., and Rasmussen, A. T., Effects of vitamin B_6 on amino acids and their metabolites in the rat and man, *Vt. Agric. Exp. Stn. Bull.,* No. 647, Burlington, Vermont, 1966.

160. Rose, D. P., Strong, R., Adams, P. W., and Harding, P. E., Experimental vitamin B_6 deficiency and the effect of oestrogen-containing oral contraceptives on tryptophan metabolism and vitamin B_6 requirements, *Clin. Sci.,* 42, 465, 1972.

161. Rose, D. P., Strong, R., Folkard, J., and Adams, P. W., Erythrocyte aminotransferase activities in women using oral contraceptives and the effect of vitamin B_6 supplementation, *Am. J. Clin. Nutr.,* 26, 48, 1973.

Folacin (Folic Acid, Pteroylmonoglutamic Acid, Folate)

Folic acid nutriture has received increased interest in recent years. The prevalence of folate deficiency throughout the world is uncertain, but recent studies would suggest that the incidence and importance of folate deficiency has been underestimated.[1,3,12,13,19,151] Megaloblastic anemia resulting from folate deficiency may be observed in 2.5 to 5.0% of pregnant women in the developed countries with a considerably higher incidence noted in pregnant women of the developing countries.[1-6,12,19,136] In many of the developing countries and to a lesser extent in the developed countries, folate deficiency may also occur in men, nonpregnant women and children.[1,2,12,143] Although a folate deficiency occurs most commonly from inadequate dietary intakes of the vitamin, a deficiency may result from impaired absorption, metabolic derangements and excessive demands by tissues of the body.[8,9,12,13,15,18-22,125,136,140,141,144,149]

The chemistry of folic acid is rather complex, owing to its presence in nature in various forms, and to its serving as a coenzyme in numerous metabolic reactions. Hence, terms such as "folacin," "folate," and "folacin activity" are used to express folic acid or folacin activity of the various forms of the vitamin which serve to support growth and hematopoiesis in animals and man and support growth of microorganisms. These aspects of folic acid have been the subject of a number of extensive review articles.[7-22,64,125,142]

The earliest hematological sign of a folate deficiency is an increase in the hypersegmentation of the nuclei of the neutrophilic polymorphonuclear leucocytes (Figure 17).[12,13,18,23-28] With the onset of megaloblastic anemia the neutrophils, instead of having a normal average lobe number of approximately 3.2, will be observed to have an increase in the percentage of cells with five or more nuclear lobes.[12,13,23-28] However, this sign of folate deficiency must be assessed with care in pregnant women in whom a tendency to hyposegmentation occurs.[12,13,28,29,137] Following the changes in the neutrophils, the next hematologic alteration that may be noted in folacin deficiency is a gradual appearance of macroovalocytosis, with a gradual increase in the mean corpuscular volume.[12,13]

Megaloblastic bone marrow changes also occur with dietary folate deprivation.[12,13,19] Usually the severity of the bone marrow changes will relate directly with the degree of anemia present. However, the morphological changes in the peripheral blood usually occur before the appearance of an overtly megaloblastic bone marrow,[23,25] although the data to support this view are limited.[12]

It should be noted that the histological findings indicated above are identical for the megaloblastic anemias caused by either a deficiency in folic acid or vitamin B_{12}. Hence, morphological changes alone cannot be used to distinguish between these two vitamin deficiencies. For this purpose, a number of biochemical measurements are available to provide information concerning the nutritional status of folacin in the individual subject.[7-13,15,17-20,23,140,144] Such procedures include the assay of folate levels in serum, whole blood, red cells, leucocytes, or liver biopsy specimens, the use of folacin loading tests, and measurement of urinary excretion of formiminoglutamic acid (FIGLU), urocanic acid or aminoimidazolecarboxamide.

Of the procedures indicated, measurement of serum folic acid levels is most commonly performed. In a controlled folacin deficiency study conducted by Herbert,[13,23-25] serum folacin levels fell rapidly to below-normal levels well before the appearance of hematological changes (Figure 17). Unfortunately, the number of sub-

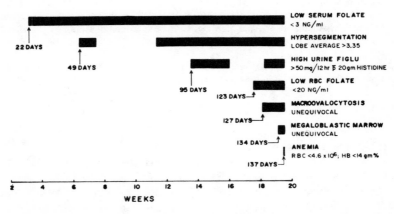

FIGURE 17. Hematologic and biochemical sequence of events in experimentally induced dietary folate deficiency in a healthy 35-year-old, 77-kg male. (From Herbert.[13,25])

jects studied on controlled intakes of folacin has been very limited.[9,12,18,20,30-32] However, from these studies and from comparisons between normal subjects and patients considered to have a folacin deficiency, it has been considered that serum folate determinations provide an easy, sensitive and early assessment of folate deficiency.[9,13,15,19,20,24,29,33,36,41,45,46,140]

Serum folate levels are probably a poor indicator of the degree of folate deficiency.[12,15,24] Low serum folate levels may not necessarily be associated with megaloblastic anemia or any abnormal biochemical changes.[12,20,23,24] Such low serum levels may be a reflection of only recent low dietary intakes of the vitamin and provide little information concerning tissue reserves. However, continued low serum folacin levels would eventually be accompanied by signs of megaloblastic anemia and megaloblastic bone marrow changes.[25] Megaloblastic anemia is a manifestation of a rather advanced deficiency of the vitamin.[9,12,25] Almost invariably, megaloblastic anemia caused by a folate deficiency is accompanied by low serum folate levels.[12,13,15,24,34-36] Only seldom is a low serum folate level found in patients with a vitamin B_{12} deficiency.[12] Thus, a low serum folate level in association with megaloblastic anemia provides strong evidence that the anemia is due to a folate deficiency rather than to a vitamin B_{12} deficiency. On the other hand, borderline or normal serum levels of folacin could be encountered in patients with megaloblastic anemia but in whom the anemia could be in the process of correction due to a recent increased dietary intake of folacin. Serum folate levels appear to be a less dependable index of the presence or likely development of megaloblastic changes in pregnant women than in nonpregnant subjects,[12,136] although a good correlation between serum and erythrocyte folate levels and neutrophil lobe indices has been reported.[137] However, serum folate levels usually fall significantly during pregnancy, although bone marrow morphology changes and megaloblastic anemia may not occur.[12,38,119,124,126,136,137,151] The fall in serum folate levels is probably in response to the marked increased demands for the vitamin during the third trimester of pregnancy, but the folate deficiency may not be of sufficient duration to produce hematological changes. Such changes could occur in patients who went into

pregnancy with inadequate reserves of folic acid.[38,85,124,126] In patients with a primary vitamin B_{12} deficiency, elevated serum levels of folacin may be encountered.[26,39]

The assay of folate levels in whole blood and red blood cells has come into increased use in recent years.[12,15,24,31,41,42,130,136,137,141] The red cell folate level has been regarded as a more accurate and less variable quantitative index than serum folate as to the severity of folacin deficiency in patients.[12,23,24] The red blood cell folate levels reflect the body folacin status at the time the red cells were formed. However, the procedure is more involved in that both serum and whole blood folate levels must be measured and the folate level in the red cells calculated on the basis of the hematocrit value.[12,23,24,40] It should be noted that red blood cell folate measurements do not distinguish between megaloblastic anemia due to vitamin B_{12} deficiency and that due to a folacin deficiency (Figure 18). In patients with a primary vitamin B_{12} deficiency, folate levels in the serum may be elevated while low levels may be encountered in the red cells.[12,13,20,24,26,29,36,39,143] However, a low folate value for both serum and red blood cells is strong evidence that a folacin deficiency exists which is probably accompanied by bone marrow morphology and/or hematological changes (Figure 19).[24,36] In patients free of a vitamin B_{12} deficiency, a good correlation has been observed between red blood cell folate level and severity of folate deficiency as assessed by hematological and bone marrow morphology changes.[24,136,140] Red cell folate measurements have also proven to be a useful biochemical test for evaluating folacin nutritional status in pregnancy.[12,28,29,43,136,137]

In evaluating folate levels in serum and red blood cells, it must be recognized that the period of folate deficiency which must pass before the red blood cell folate levels decrease is much longer than that causing a decrease in the serum level of folacin (Figure 17).[13,25] Guidelines that have been used in evaluating serum and red blood cell folacin data are indicated in Table 12. Such guidelines can be regarded only as tentative and must be considered in terms of the microbiological assay procedures employed to measure serum and red blood cell folate levels. Fasting serum folate levels less than 3.0 ng (mμg)/ml have been considered "deficient" and levels from 3.0 to 5.9

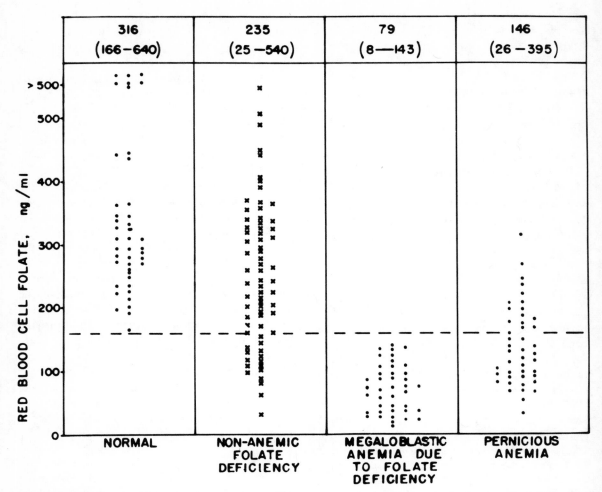

FIGURE 18. The mean, range and distribution of red blood cell folate levels of healthy control subjects, nonanemic patients with subnormal serum folate levels, patients with megaloblastic anemia due to folate deficiency, and patients with pernicious anemia. (From Hoffbrand, Newcombe, and Mollin.[24])

ng/ml as "low," while values of 6.0 ng/ml and above as "acceptable."[44] Hoffbrand et al.[24] observed that patients with serum folate levels less than 3.0 ng/ml almost always had megaloblastic anemia or obvious morphological changes of folate deficiency (Figures 18 and 19). However, these subjects had subnormal levels of red blood cell folate. In patients with borderline serum folate levels (3.0 to 5.9 ng/ml), hematological changes varied widely as did the red blood cell folate levels. Others have also considered serum folacin levels of 3.0 ng/ml or less as evidence of a folate deficiency.[12,13,25,29,39,47,72,86,140]

Red blood cell folacin levels less than 140 ng/ml of cells have been considered "deficient"

and levels from 140 to 159 ng/ml as "low," while values of 160 ng/ml and above as "acceptable" (Table 12, Figures 18 and 19).[24,29,44] Age and sex of the subjects appear to have little influence on the folate levels.[40]

Leucocytes also contain relatively high levels of folacin. Leucocytes from normal subjects have been reported to contain 60 to 123 ng of folacin/ml of packed cells with a mean value of 92 ng/ml.[48] Values as high as 262 to 1,028 ng/ml cells have also been reported.[141] The leucocyte folacin levels correlated well with red cell folate values but less so with serum folate values.[48,52] The procedure did not distinguish between patients with pernicious anemia and those

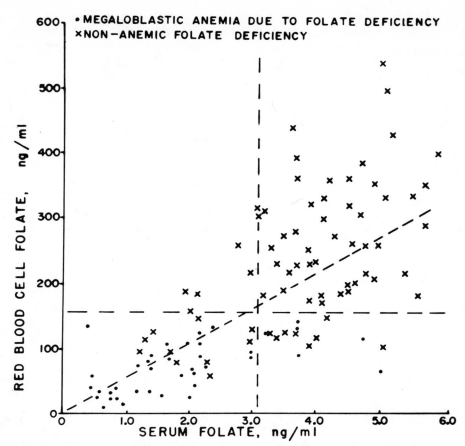

FIGURE 19. The relation of red blood cell folate levels to serum folate levels in human patients. The horizontal dotted line represents the lower limit of the normal red blood cell level and the vertical dotted line, the upper limit of the range of serum folate levels usually found in severe folate deficiency. (From Hoffbrand, Newcombe, and Mollin.[24])

TABLE 12

Guidelines for the Interpretation of Serum and Red Blood Cell Folacin Levels[a,b]

	Less than acceptable (at risk)		
Determination	Deficient (high risk)	Low (medium risk)	Acceptable (low risk)
	ng (mµg)/ml	ng (mµg)/ml	ng (mµg)/ml
Serum folacin (all ages)	< 3.0	3.0 to 5.9	≥ 6.0
Red blood cell folacin (all ages)	< 140	140 to 159	≥ 160

[a]Adapted from the reports of O'Neal et al.,[44] WHO report[2] and others.[12,13,24,25,29,72,86,145]

[b]Guidelines should be regarded as tentative and must be considered in terms of the microbiological assay procedure employed. Values based on the use of *Lactobacillus casei* as the test organism.

deficient in folacin.[48] Hence, considering the technical difficulties involved, the method provides no apparent advantage over the measurement of folacin in serum and red blood cells.

The liver contains a significant reserve store of folacin in the body (5 to 10 ng/g wet liver). Several investigators have made measurements on the folacin levels in human liver biopsy specimens in an attempt to detect and assess folate deficiency.[49-51] Liver levels of folacin correlated reasonably well with serum folate values and formiminoglutamate excretion. Although liver biopsy measurements are neither practical nor usually feasible, the studies cited provide an indication that serum folate levels do provide a reflection of tissue folacin stores.[13,51]

Normally, only small amounts of folacin are excreted in the urine,[53-58] representing about 1% of the dietary folate intake.[56] The amounts excreted are increased after injected or oral test doses of folic acid.[56,59-65] Measurements of urinary levels of folacin, with or without folic acid test doses, have not been of value for evaluating folacin nutritional status but have been useful in detecting folacin malabsorption states.[12,15,53-65] Radioactively labeled folic acid has also been used in the test for folacin absorption.[66-68,134]

The rate of plasma clearance of an intravenous test dose of folic acid has also been investigated as an index of folacin deficiency.[69-71,135] Folic acid is administered intravenously at a level of 15 μg/kg of body weight and the plasma level of folacin assayed after 3, 15, 30, and 60 min. In folacin deficiency, the administered folic acid is rapidly cleared from the plasma. An oral folic acid tolerance test has also been developed.[72] However, since the procedure does not clearly distinguish between folate and vitamin B_{12} deficiencies, it has not been widely used.

Microbiological assay procedures are used almost entirely to measure folacin levels in serum, red blood cells, urine, and other biological samples,[7,8,10-12,14-17,20,24,33,40,45,64,73-89,142,146] although isotopic assay procedures have been recently described.[132,147,148,150,153] The organisms most commonly used have been *Lactobacillus casei* (ATCC 7469), *Streptococcus faecalis* (ATCC 8043), and *Pediococcus cerevisiae* (ATCC 8081). For evaluating folacin nutritional status in the human, *L. casei* is the organism of choice since it responds to the major folic acid analogs present in serum. The main folates in serum are the

N^5-methylfolates which support growth of *L. casei* but not *S. faecalis* or *P. cerevisiae*.[17,45] A majority of the folate activity in red blood cells is as conjugated forms which must be deconjugated prior to assay.[24,40,78,80,88] A number of procedures have been outlined in detail using *L. casei* for assaying folacin levels in serum[10,33,40,45,74-81,142] and red blood cells.[24,40,78,80,142] Several automated procedures are also available.[79,80] Microbiological assays for folacin must be conducted with extreme care to avoid erroneously low or high values.[40,73,82,83] Fasting samples should be employed to avoid the effects of immediate dietary intakes of folacin. Due to the high levels of folacin in the erythrocytes, hemolyzed samples will result in erroneously high serum values. Another potential source of error is the presence of antibiotics or other growth-inhibiting materials in serum or blood samples.[89] Blood samples properly handled and preserved with ascorbic acid to protect the labile folates can be held frozen for several months without any appreciable loss in folacin activity.[24,40,45,75] The addition of ascorbate to serum or plasma samples before freezing is unnecessary if the folate analyses are to be performed within 6 months after collection.[26,40] Moreover, if the same serum samples are to be analyzed for vitamin B_{12}, the addition of ascorbic acid would partially destroy this vitamin.[26]

Several indirect tests for evaluating folacin status are based on the increased urinary excretion formiminoglutamic acid (FIGLU) and of its immediate precursor, urocanic acid, that occurs in the folacin-deficient subject.[12,13,15,20,136,137] These compounds arise from histidine metabolism which is normally converted to glutamic acid through the participation of formiminotransferase and tetrahydrofolic acid.[15] In folacin deficiency, the conversion is inhibited and the amounts of FIGLU and urocanic acid in the urine are increased.[12,15,34] The excretion of these compounds can be greatly increased in the folacin-deficient subject by administering an oral load of 2 to 15 g of L-histidine.[12,15,34,90-93,124,136,137]

The excretion of FIGLU or of FIGLU-plus-urocanic acid has been a useful index of folate deficiency, particularly in research studies. For nutrition surveys, the procedure is impractical. The abnormal excretion of the metabolites appears to correlate better with red cell folate than with serum folate.[24,48] However, the measurement of urocanic acid in addition to FIGLU after a histidine load may provide no advantage over measuring only FIGLU.[91,92] Unfortunately, the FIGLU and urocanate excretion test is not entirely specific. Patients with pernicious anemia often have a positive test[13,24,26,94,95] and, hence, the test does not distinguish between the anemia of vitamin B_{12} deficiency and the anemia of folacin deficiency. Similarly, abnormal amounts of FIGLU and urocanic acid may be excreted by subjects suffering from liver damage, protein malnutrition, and congenital formiminotransferase deficiency.[12,15,91,96-98] A number of methods are available for measuring FIGLU and urocanic acid.[15,95,98,99,131]

Depending upon the analytical procedure employed, normal adult subjects excrete 0 to 15 μg of FIGLU/ml of urine. After a histidine load (0.12 g/lb of body weight), normal adults excreted 10 to 50 μg of FIGLU/ml of urine or approximately 5 to 20 mg in the post 8-hr urine collection. Folacin-deficient adult subjects may excrete five to ten times these levels following a histidine load.

Additional procedures have been proposed for evaluating folacin nutritional status, but none have received wide acceptance. For example, amino-imidazolecarboxamide (AIC) is excreted in elevated amounts in subjects with pernicious anemia or deficient in folacin,[100-104,133] and the excretion can be enhanced in patients with the use of an AIC load.[102] Since the procedure does not appear to distinguish between a folate deficiency and pernicious anemia, the technique offers no advantage over the previous methods described and thus has not received general use. An increase in urinary formate has been observed in children with leukemia who had received folacin antagonist therapy.[105] However, the measurement of this metabolite has apparently not been studied further as a possible diagnostic test for folacin deficiency. The measurement of expired $^{14}CO_2$ following a tracer dose of ^{14}C-histidine (C-2 of the imidazole ring) has also been proposed as a test for folacin deficiency.[15,106] Since this carbon atom of histidine requires folacin for its conversion to CO_2, less $^{14}CO_2$ would appear in the expired air in a given time in a folate-deficient subject. In addition to the radiation hazard, the procedure appears to have the same limitations as the FIGLU test.[13,23] Elevated plasma lactate dehydrogenase values have been related to vitamin B_{12} and folate deficiencies[107] but, as a practical test to evaluate these deficiencies, appear unlikely. A recent report would suggest that the level of ^{14}C-formate incorporation into aminoimidazolecarboxamide ribotide by red blood cells may prove to be a useful technique for evaluating folacin nutritional status.[108] The incorporation of ^{14}C-formate into serine by the lymphocytes has also been proposed as a test for folacin deficiency.[138]

In addition to a dietary deficiency of folacin, a number of other factors may influence folate metabolism.[1-3,7-10,12,13,15,17-24,113,152] As noted above, in patients with vitamin B_{12} deficiency (pernicious anemia), a folate deficiency of secondary origin may exist. The vitamin B_{12} deficiency impairs, in a manner not fully understood, the utilization of folacin giving rise to an apparent folate deficiency.[12,20,39,109] Thus, in the diagnosis of a primary folacin deficiency, the possible involvement of a vitamin B_{12} deficiency must be determined. Numerous drugs will interfere in the absorption and/or utilization of folacin.[12,110,149] Included are the folate antagonists, diphenylhydantoin dilantin, primidone, alcohol, and oral contraceptive agents.[113-122,125,127-129,136,139] A folacin deficiency may also occur due to malabsorption of folates from the diet in conditions of tropical sprue, idiopathic steatorrhoea, and intestinal disease.[12,124,129] A folate deficiency occurs frequently in hemolytic diseases such as sickle cell anemia and thalassaemia where the high rate of hemopoiesis imposes an increased demand for folacin.[12,111,112]

In summary, measurement of folate levels in serum and red blood cells is the most practical procedure to evaluate folacin nutritional status in population groups and clinical patients. Subjects with a suspected folacin deficiency should, however, be evaluated further to eliminate the possibility of pernicious anemia or a dietary vitamin B_{12} deficiency. Serum vitamin B_{12} analyses can be useful for this purpose. If facilities are available, FIGLU tests can provide additional diagnostic information in clinical situations.

REFERENCES

1. Requirements of Ascorbic acid, Vitamin D, Vitamin B_{12}, Folate, and Iron, Report of a Joint FAO/WHO Expert Group, FAO nutrition meetings report series No. 47, Food and Agriculture Organization of The United Nations, Rome, 1970.

2. Nutritional Anemias, Report of a WHO Scientific Group, WHO technical report series No. 405, World Health Organization, Geneva, Switzerland, 1968.

3. Recommended Dietary Allowances, A report of the Food and Nutrition Board of the National Research Council, publication No. 1694, 7th revised ed., National Academy of Sciences, 2101 Constitution Ave., Washington, D.C., 1968.

4. **Forshaw, J., Moorhouse, E. H., and Harwood, L.,** Megaloblastic anemia due to dietary deficiency, *Lancet,* 1, 1004, 1964.

5. **Varadi, S. and Elwis, A.,** Megaloblastic anemia due to dietary deficiency, *Lancet,* 1, 1162, 1964.

6. **Alperin, J. B., Hutchison, H. T., and Levin, W. C.,** Studies of folic acid requirements in megaloblastic anemia of pregnancy, *A.M.A. Arch. Int. Med.,* 117, 681, 1966.

7. **Stokstad, E. L. R. and Oace, S. M.,** Folic acid, biotin, and pantothenic acid, in *Newer Methods of Nutritional Biochemistry,* Vol. II, Albanese, A. A., Ed., Academic Press, New York, 1965, 286.

8. **Chow, B. F.,** The B vitamins: B_6, B_{12}, folic acid, pantothenic acid, and biotin, in *Nutrition. A Comprehensive Treatise,* Beaton, G. H. and McHenry, E. W., Eds., Academic Press, New York, 1964, 229.

9. **Herbert, V.,** Nutritional requirements for vitamins B_{12} and folic acid, *Am. J. Clin. Nutr.,* 21, 743, 1968.

10. **Baker, H. and Frank, O.,** Folates, *Clinical Vitaminology,* Interscience Publishers, New York, 1968, 87.

11. **Wagner, A. F. and Folkers, K.,** Pteroylglutamic acid group, in *Vitamins and Coenzymes,* Interscience Publishers, New York, 1964, 113.

12. **Blakley, R. L.,** *The Biochemistry of Folic Acid and Related Pteridines. Frontiers of Biology,* Vol. 13, Neuberger, A. and Tatum, E. L., Eds., North-Holland Publishing Co., Amsterdam (J. Wiley and Sons, Inc., New York, distributors), 1969.

13. **Herbert, V.,** Biochemical and hematologic lesions in folic acid deficiency, *Am. J. Clin. Nutr.,* 20, 562, 1967.

14. **Butterworth, C. E., Jr.,** The availability of food folate, *Br. J. Haematol.,* 14, 339, 1968.

15. **Luhby, A. L. and Cooperman, J. M.,** Folic acid deficiency in man and its interrelationship with vitamin B_{12} metabolism, in *Advances in Metabolic Disorders,* Vol. 1, Academic Press, New York, 1964, 263.

16. **Usdin, E.,** Blood folic acid studies. VI. Chromatographic resolution of folic acid-active substances obtained from blood, *J. Biol. Chem.,* 234, 2373, 1959.

17. **Stokstad, E. L. R. and Koch, J.,** Folic acid metabolism, *Physiol. Revs.,* 47, 83, 1967.

18. **Sullivan, L. W.,** Folates in human nutrition, in *Newer Methods of Nutritional Biochemistry,* Vol. III, Albanese, A. A., Ed., Academic Press, New York, 1967, 365.

19. **Streiff, R. R.,** Folic acid deficiency anemia, *Semin. Hematol.,* 7, 23, 1970.

20. **Johns, D. G. and Bertino, J. R.,** Folates and megaloblastic anemia: A review, *Clin. Pharmacol. Ther.,* 6, 372, 1965.

21. **Rowe, P. B.,** Inborn errors of folic acid metabolism — the regulation of the interconversion of active derivatives of folic acid, *Minn. Med.,* 54, 391, 1971.

22. **Doscherholmen, A.,** Folate deficiency, absolute and relative, *Minn. Med.,* 54, 909, 1971.

23. **Herbert, V.,** Folic acid, *Ann. Rev. Med.,* 16, 359, 1965.

24. **Hoffbrand, A. V., Newcombe, B. F. A., and Mollin, D. L.,** Method of assay of red cell folate activity and the value of the assay as a test for folate deficiency, *J. Clin. Pathol.,* 19, 17, 1966.

25. **Herbert, V.,** Experimental nutritional folate deficiency in man, *Trans. Assoc. Am. Physicians Phila.,* 75, 307, 1962.

26. **Herbert, V.,** Studies of folate deficiency in man, *Proc. R. Soc. Med.,* 57, 377, 1964.

27. **Chanarin, I., Rothman, D., and Berry, V.,** Iron deficiency and its relation to folic-acid in pregnancy: Results of a clinical trial, *Br. Med. J.,* 1, 480, 1965.

28. **Varadi, S., Abbot, D., and Elwis, A.,** Correlation of peripheral white cell and bone marrow changes with folate levels in pregnancy and their clinical significance, *J. Clin. Pathol.,* 19, 33, 1966.

29. **Lowenstein, L., Brunton, L., and Hsieh, Y-S.,** Nutritional anemia and megaloblastosis in pregnancy, *Can. Med. Assoc. J.,* 94, 636, 1966.

30. **Herbert, V.,** Minimal daily adult folate requirement, *Arch. Intern. Med.,* 110, 649, 1962.

31. **Hansen, H. A. and Weinfeld, A.,** Metabolic effects and diagnostic value of small doses of folic acid and B_{12} in megaloblastic anemias, *Acta Med. Scand.,* 172, 427, 1962.

32. **Zalusky, R. and Herbert, V.,** Megaloblastic anemia in scurvy with response to 50 micrograms of folic acid daily, *N. Engl. J. Med.,* 265, 1033, 1961.

33. **Herbert, V., Baker, H., Frank, O., Pasher, I., Sobotka, H., and Wasserman, L. R.,** The measurement of folic acid activity in serum: A diagnostic aid in the differentiation of the megaloblastic anemias, *Blood,* 15, 228, 1960.

34. **Chanarin, I.,** Studies on urinary formiminoglutamic acid excretion, *Proc. R. Soc. Med.,* 57, 384, 1964.

35. **Cooperman, J. M., Luhby, A. L., and Avery, C. M.,** Serum folic acid activity by improved *L. casei* assay, *Proc. Soc. Exp. Biol. Med.,* 104, 536, 1960.

36. **Cooper, B. A. and Lowenstein, L.,** Vitamin B_{12}-folate interrelations in megaloblastic anemia, *Br. J. Haematol.,* 12, 283, 1966.

37. Nomenclature policy: Generic descriptors and trivial names for vitamins and related compounds, *J. Nutr.,* 103, 159, 1973.

38. **Temperley, I. J., Meehan, M. M. M., and Gatenby, P. B. B.,** Serum folic acid levels in pregnancy and their relationship to megaloblastic marrow changes, *Br. J. Haematol.,* 14, 13, 1968.

39. **Herbert, V. and Zalusky, R.,** Interrelations of vitamin B_{12} and folic acid metabolism: Folic acid clearance studies, *J. Clin. Invest.,* 41, 1263, 1962.

40. **Herman, Y. F. and Sauberlich, H. E.,** *Lactobacillus casei* micro-assay procedure for determining folacin (folate) activity in serum or plasma and red blood cells, *U.S. Army Med. Res. and Nutr. Lab. Rep.,* 1972.

41. *Ten-State Nutrition Survey Reports, I–V,* Center for Disease Control, Atlanta, GA 30330, 1972.

42. **Izak, G., Rachmilewitz, M., Zan, S., and Grossowicz, N.,** The effect of small doses of folic acid in nutritional megaloblastic anemia, *Am. J. Clin. Nutr.,* 13, 369, 1963.

43. **Lowenstein, L., Cantlie, G., Ramos, O., and Brunton, L.,** The incidence and prevention of folate deficiency in a pregnant clinic population, *Can. Med. Assoc. J.,* 95, 797, 1966.

44. **O'Neal, R. M., Johnson, O. C., and Schaefer, A. E.,** Guidelines for classification and interpretation of group blood and urine data collected as part of the National Nutrition Survey, *Pediatr. Res.,* 4, 103, 1970.

45. **Herbert, V.,** Aseptic addition method for *Lactobacillus casei* assay of folate activity in human serum, *J. Clin. Pathol.,* 19, 12, 1966.

46. *Nutritional Evaluation of the Population of Central America and Panama,* Nutrition Program, Center for Disease Control, Atlanta, Georgia, U.S. Dept. of Health, Education and Welfare Publication No. (HSM) 72 – 8120, 1972.

47. **Baker, H., Herbert, V., Frank, O., Pasher, I., Hutner, S. H., Wasserman, L. R., and Sobotka, H.,** A microbiologic method for detecting folic acid deficiency in man, *Clin. Chem.,* 5, 275, 1959.

48. **Hoffbrand, A. F. and Newcombe, B. F. A.,** Leucocyte folate in vitamin B_{12} and folate deficiency and in leukaemia, *Br. J. Haematol.,* 13, 954, 1967.

49. **Chanarin, I., Hutchinson, M., McLean, A., and Moule, M.,** Hepatic folate in man, *Br. Med. J.,* 1, 396, 1966.

50. **Leevy, C. M., Cardi, L., Frank, O., Gellene, R., and Baker, H.,** Incidence and significance of hypovitaminemia in a random selected municipal hospital population, *Am. J. Clin. Nutr.,* 17, 259, 1965.

51. **Leevy, C. M., Baker, H., TenHove, W., Frank, O., and Cherrick, G. R.,** B-complex vitamins in liver disease of the alcoholic, *Am. J. Clin. Nutr.,* 16, 339, 1965.

52. **Vilter, R. W., Will, J. J., Wright, T., and Rullman, D.,** Interrelationships of vitamin B_{12}, folic acid and ascorbic acid in the megaloblastic anemias, *Am. J. Clin. Nutr.,* 12, 130, 1963.

53. **Lossy, F. T., Goldsmith, G. A., and Sarett, H. P.,** A study of test dose excretion of five B complex vitamins in man, *J. Nutr.,* 45, 213, 1951.

54. **Pace, J. K., Stier, L. B., Taylor, D. D., and Goodman, P. S.,** Metabolic patterns in preadolescent children. V. Intake and urinary excretion of pantothenic acid and of folic acid, *J. Nutr.,* 74, 345, 1961.

55. **Baker, H., Frank, O., Feingold, S., Ziffer, H., Gellene, R. A., Leevy, C. M., and Sobotka, H.,** The fate of orally and parenterally administered folates, *Am. J. Clin. Nutr.,* 17, 88, 1965.

56. **Cooperman, J. M., Pesci-Bourel, A., and Luhby, A. L.,** Urinary excretion of folic acid activity in man, *Clin. Chem.,* 16, 375, 1970.

57. **Register, U. D. and Sarett, H. P.,** Urinary excretion of vitamin B_{12}, folic acid and citrovorum factor in human subjects on various diets, *Proc. Soc. Exp. Biol. Med.,* 77, 837, 1953.

58. **Santini, R., Jr., Sheehy, T. W., Aviles, J., and Davilia, I.,** Daily urinary excretion of folic acid in normal subjects and in patients with tropical sprue, *Am. J. Trop. Med.,* 11, 421, 1962.

59. **Girdwood, R. H.,** Folic-acid-excretion studies in the investigation of malignant disease, *Br. Med. J.,* 2, 741, 1953.

60. **Girdwood, R. H.,** The megaloblastic anaemias. Their investigation and classification, *Q. J. Med.,* 25, 87, 1956.

61. **Girdwood, R. H.,** Microbiological assay methods in clinical medicine with particular reference to the investigation of deficiency of vitamin B_{12} and folic acid, *Scott. Med. J.,* 5, 10, 1960.

62. **Butterworth, C. E., Jr., Nadel, H., Perez-Santiago, E., Santini, R., Jr. and Gardner, F. H.,** Folic acid absorption, excretion, and leukocyte concentration in tropical sprue, *J. Lab. Clin. Med.,* 50, 673, 1957.

63. **Cox, E. V., Meynell, M. J., Cooke, W. T., and Gaddie, R.,** The folic acid excretion test in the steatorrhea syndrome, *Gastroenterology,* 35, 390, 1958.

64. **Girdwood, R. H.,** Folic acid, its analogs and antagonists, *Adv. Clin. Chem.,* 3, 235, 1960.

65. **Girdwood, R. H., and Delamore, I. W.,** Observations on tests of folic acid absorption and clearance, *Scott. Med. J.,* 6, 44, 1961.

66. **Anderson, B., Belcher, E. H., Chanarin, I., and Mollin, D. L.,** The urinary and faecal excretion of radioactivity after oral doses of ^{3}H-folic acid, *Br. J. Haematol.,* 6, 439, 1960.

67. **Kinnear, D. G., Johns, D. G., MacIntosh, P. C., Burgen, A. S. V., and Cameron, D. G.,** Intestinal absorption of tritium-labeled folic acid in idiopathic steatorrhea. Effect of a gluten-free diet, *Can. Med. Assoc. J.,* 89, 975, 1963.

68. **Klipstein, F. A.,** The urinary excretion of orally administered tritium-labeled folic acid as a test of folic acid absorption, *Blood,* 21, 626, 1963.

69. Chanarin, I., Mollin, D. L., and Anderson, B. B., The clearance from plasma of folic acid injected intravenously in normal subjects and patients with megaloblastic anemia, *Br. J. Haematol.*, 4, 435, 1958.

70. Chanarin, I., Mollin, D. L., and Anderson, B. B., Folic acid deficiency and the megaloblastic anaemias, *Proc. R. Soc. Med.*, 51, 757, 1958.

71. Metz, H., Stevens, K., Krawitz, S., and Brandt, V., The plasma clearance of injected doses of folic acid as an index of folic acid deficiency, *J. Clin. Pathol.*, 14, 622, 1961.

72. Baker, H., Frank, O., Sobotka, H., Ho, P. P., Chen, N., Janowitz, H., Ziffer, H., and Leevy, C. M., Mechanisms of folic acid deficiency in non-tropical sprue, *J.A.M.A.*, 187, 159, 1964.

73. Herbert, V. and Bertino, J. R., Folic acid, in *The Vitamins*, 2nd ed., György, P. and Pearson, W. N., Eds., Academic Press, New York, 1967, 243.

74. Baker, H. and Frank, O., IV. A microbiological assay for folate activity, in *The Vitamins*, 2nd ed., György, P. and Pearson, W. N., Eds., Academic Press, New York, 1967, 269.

75. Cooperman, J. M., Microbiological assay of serum and whole-blood folic acid activity, *Am. J. Clin. Nutr.*, 20, 1015, 1967.

76. *Difco Supplementary Literature*, May 1972, Difco Laboratories, Detroit, Michigan 48232, p. 444.

77. Temperley, I. J. and Horner, N., Effect of ascorbic acid on the serum folic estimation, *J. Clin. Pathol.*, 19, 43, 1966.

78. Feming, A. F., Comley, L., and Stenhouse, N. S., Assay of serum and whole blood folate by a modified aseptic addition technique, *Am. J. Clin. Nutr.*, 24, 1257, 1971.

79. Davis, R. E., Nicol, D. J., and Kelly, A., An automated method for the measurement of folate activity, *J. Clin. Pathol.*, 23, 47, 1970.

80. Millbank, L., Davis, R. E., Rawlins, M., and Waters, A. H., Automation of the assay of folate in serum and whole blood, *J. Clin. Pathol.*, 23, 54, 1970.

81. Chanarin, I. and Berry, V., Estimation of serum *L. casei* activity, *J. Clin. Pathol.*, 17, 111, 1964.

82. Frank, O., Baker, H., and Hutner, S. H., Microbiological assay of serum and whole-blood folic acid activity, *Am. J. Clin. Nutr.*, 21, 327, 1968.

83. Streeter, A. M. and O'Neill, B. J., Effect of incubation time on the *L. casei* bioassay of folic acid in serum, *Blood*, 34, 216, 1969.

84. Spray, G. H., Microbiological assay of folic acid activity in human serum, *J. Clin. Pathol.*, 17, 660, 1964.

85. Rae, P. G. and Robb, P. M., Megaloblastic anemia of pregnancy: a clinical and laboratory study with particular reference to the total and labile serum folate levels, *J. Clin. Pathol.*, 23, 379, 1970.

86. Cooper, B. A. and Lowenstein, L., Evaluation of assessment of folic-acid deficiency by serum folic-acid activity measured by *L. casei*, *Can. Med. Assoc. J.*, 85, 987, 1961.

87. Bird, O. D., McGlohon, V. M., and Vaitkus, J. W., A microbiological assay system for naturally occurring folates, *Can. J. Microbiol.*, 15, 465, 1969.

88. Noronha, J. M. and Aboobaker, V. S., Studies on the folate compounds of human blood, *Arch. Biochem. Biophys.*, 101, 445, 1963.

89. Cowan, J. D., Hoffbrand, A. V., and Mollin, D. L., Effect of serum-factors other than folate on the *Lactobacillus casei* assay, *Lancet*, 2, 11, 1966.

90. Luhby, A. L., Cooperman, J. M., and Teller, D. N., Histidine metabolic loading test to distinguish folic acid deficiency from vitamin B_{12} in megaloblastic anemias, *Proc. Soc. Exp. Biol. Med.*, 101, 350, 1959.

91. Mohamed, S. D. and Roberts, M., Relative importance of formiminoglutamic acid and urocanic acid excretion after a histidine load, *J. Clin. Pathol.*, 19, 37, 1966.

92. Hoffbrand, A. V., Neale, G., Hines, J. D., and Mollin, D. L., The excretion of formiminoglutamic acid and urocanic acid after partial gastrectomy, *Lancet*, 1, 1231, 1966.

93. Luhby, A. L. and Cooperman, J. M., Histidine metabolic loading and folic acid deficiency in pernicious anemia, *Am. J. Clin. Nutr.*, 16, 394, 1965.

94. Chanarin, I., Bennett, M. C., and Berry, V., Urinary excretion of histidine derivatives in megaloblastic anaemia and other conditions and a comparison with the folic acid clearance test, *J. Clin. Pathol.*, 15, 269, 1962.

95. Zalusky, R. and Herbert, B., Urinary formiminoglutamic acid as a test of folic-acid deficiency, *Lancet*, 2, 108, 1962.

96. Spector, I., Falcke, H. C., Yoffe, Y., and Metz, J., Observations on urocanic acid and formiminoglutamic acid excretion in infants with protein malnutrition, *Am. J. Clin. Nutr.*, 18, 426, 1966.

97. Arakawa, T., Congenital defects in folate utilization, *Am. J. Med.*, 48, 594, 1970.

98. Merritt, A. D., Rucknagel, D. L., Silverman, M., and Gardiner, R. C., Urinary urocanic acid in man: The identification of urocanic acid and the comparative excretion of urocanic acid and N-formiminoglutamic acid after oral histidine in patients with liver disease, *J. Clin. Invest.*, 41, 1472, 1962.

99. Chanarin, I. and Bennett, M. C., A spectrophotometric method for estimating formiminoglutamic and urocanic acid, *Br. Med. J.*, 1, 27, 1962.

100. Luhby, L. and Cooperman, J., Aminoimidazole-carboxamide excretion in vitamin B_{12} and folic acid deficiencies, *Lancet*, 2, 1381, 1962.

101. Herbert, V., Streiff, R., Sullivan, L., and McGreer, P., Accumulation of a purine intermediate (aminoimidazolecarboxamide) (AIC) in megaloblastic anemias associated with vitamin B_{12} deficiency, folate deficiency with alcoholism, and liver disease, *Fed. Proc.*, 23, 188, 1964.

102. **Herbert, V., Streiff, R. R., Sullivan, L. W., and McGreer, P. L.,** Deranged purine metabolism manifested by aminoimidazole carboxamide excretion in megalobastic anemias, hemolytic anemia and liver disease, *Lancet,* 2, 45, 1964.

103. **Sullivan, L. W., Liu, Y. K., and McGreer, P. L.,** The effect of methionine on the urinary excretion of aminoimidazolecarboxamide in megaloblastic anemia, *Blood,* 28, 991, 1966.

104. **Middleton, J. E., Coward, R. F., and Smith, P.,** Urinary excretion of A.I.C. in vitamin B_{12} and folic-acid deficiencies, *Lancet,* 2, 258, 1964.

105. **Hiatt, H. H., Rabinowitz, J. C., Toch, R., and Goldstein, M.,** Effects of folic acid antagonist therapy on urinary excretion of formic acid by humans, *Proc. Soc. Exp. Biol. Med.,* 98, 144, 1958.

106. **Fish, M. B., Pollycove, M., and Feichtmeir, T. V.,** Differentiation between vitamin B_{12}-deficient megaloblastic anemias with C^{14}-histidine, *Blood,* 21, 447, 1963.

107. **McCarthy, C. F., Fraser, I. D., and Read, A. E.,** Plasma lactate dehydrogenase in megaloblastic anaemia, *J. Clin. Pathol.,* 19, 51, 1966.

108. **Sauberlich, H. E., Rebouche, C., and Judd, J. H., Jr.,** Influence of folic acid on ^{14}C-formate incorporation by blood and blood components of the rat and human, *Fed. Proc. Abstr.,* 31, 712, 1972.

109. **Nixon, P. F. and Bertino, J. R.,** Interrelationships of vitamin B_{12} and folate in man, *Am. J. Med.,* 48, 555, 1970.

110. **Waxman, S., Corcino, J. J., and Herbert, V.,** Drugs, toxins and dietary amino acids affecting vitamin B_{12} or folic acid absorption or utilization, *Am. J. Med.,* 48, 599, 1970.

111. **Lindenbaum, J. and Klipstein, F. A.,** Folic acid deficiency in sickle-cell anemia, *N. Engl. J. Med.,* 269, 875, 1963.

112. **Hogan, J. A., Maniatis, A., and Moloney, W. C.,** The serum *Lactobacillus casei* folate clearance test in various hematologic disorders, *Blood,* 24, 187, 1964.

113. **Vitale, J. J.,** Present knowledge of folacin, *Nutr. Rev.,* 24, 289, 1966.

114. **Spray, G. H.,** Oral contraceptives and serum folate levels, *Lancet,* 2, 110, 1968.

115. **Paton, A.,** Oral contraceptives and folate deficiency, *Lancet,* 1, 418, 1969.

116. **Streiff, R. R.,** Folate deficiency and oral contraceptives, *J.A.M.A.,* 214, 105, 1970.

117. **Roe, D. A.,** Drug-induced deficiency of B vitamins, *N.Y. State J. Med.,* 2770, Dec. 1, 1971.

118. **Theuer, R. C.,** Effect of oral contraceptive agents on vitamin and mineral needs: A review, *J. Reprod. Med.,* 8, 13, 1972.

119. **Kahn, S. B., Fein, S., Rigberg, S., and Brodsky, I.,** Correlation of folate metabolism and socioeconomic status in pregnancy and in patients taking oral contraceptives, *Am. J. Obstet. Gynecol.,* 108, 931, 1970.

120. **Pritchard, J. A., Scott, D. E., and Whalley, P. J.,** Maternal folate deficiency and pregnancy wastage. IV. Effects of folic acid supplements, anticonvulsants, and oral contraceptives, *Am. J. Obstet. Gynecol.,* 109, 341, 1971.

121. **Sheehy, T. W. and Dempsey, H.,** Methotrexate therapy for *Plasmodium vivax* malaria, *J.A.M.A.,* 214, 109, 1970.

122. **Maxwell, J. D., Hunter, J., Stewart, D. A., Ardeman, S., and Williams, R.,** Folate deficiency after anticonvulsant drugs: An effect of hepatic enzyme induction?, *Br. Med. J.,* 1, 297, 1972.

123. **Bazzano, G., Thompson, P., Jr., and Hauser, R.,** Folic acid metabolism and complications of pregnancy, *Miss. Med.,* 11, 795, 1970.

124. **Lanzkowsky, P.,** Congenital malabsorption of folate, *Am. J. Med.,* 48, 580, 1970.

125. **Bertino, J. R., Ed.,** Folate antagonists as chemotherapeutic agents, *Ann. N.Y. Acad. Sci.,* 186, 5, 1971.

126. **Avery, B. and Ledger, W. J.,** Folic acid metabolism in well-nourished pregnant women, *Obstet. Gynecol.,* 35, 616, 1970.

127. **Newbauer, C.,** Mental deterioration in epilepsy due to folate deficiency, *Br. Med. J.,* 2, 759, 1970.

128. **Strickland, G. T. and Kostinas, J. E.,** Folic acid deficiency complicating malaria, *Am. J. Trop. Med. Hyg.,* 19, 910, 1970.

129. **Bernstein, L. H., Gutstein, S., Weiner, S., and Efron, G.,** The absorption and malabsorption of folic acid and its polyglutamates, *Am. J. Med.,* 48, 570, 1970.

130. **Elwood, P. C., Shinton, N. K., Wilson, C. I. D., Sweetnam, P., and Frazer, A. C.,** Haemoglobin, vitamin B_{12} and folate levels in the elderly, *Br. J. Haematol.,* 21, 557, 1971.

131. **Hla-Pe, U. and Aug-Than-Batu,** A new colorimetric method for determination of formiminoglutamic acid in urine, *Anal. Biochem.,* 20, 432, 1967.

132. **McCall, M. S., White, J. D., and Frenkel, E. P.,** Bacteria as specific binding agents for an isotopic assay of serum folate, *Proc. Soc. Exp. Biol. Med.,* 134, 536, 1970.

133. **Newcombe, D. S.,** The urinary excretion of aminoimidazolecarboxamide in the Lesch-Nyhan syndrome, *Pediatrics,* 46, 508, 1970.

134. **Yoshino, T.,** The clinical and experimental studies on the metabolism of folic acid using tritiated folic acid. I. Absorption tests of tritiated folic acid in man, *J. Vitaminol.,* 14, 21, 1968.

135. **Yoshino, T.,** The clinical and experimental studies on the metabolism of folic acid using tritiated folic acid. III. Plasma clearance in man and organ distribution in rat following intravenous administration of tritiated folic acid, *J. Vitaminol.,* 14, 49, 1968.

136. **Rothman, D.,** Folic acid in pregnancy, *Am. J. Obstet. Gynecol.,* 108, 149, 1970.

137. **Hibbard, B. M. and Hibbard, E. D.,** Neutrophil hypersegmentation and defective folate metabolism in pregnancy, *J. Obstet. Gynaecol. Br. Commonw.,* 78, 776, 1971.

138. **Ellegaard, J. and Esmann, V.,** A sensitive test for folic-acid deficiency, *Lancet,* 1, 308, 1970.
139. **Halsted, C. H., Griggs, R. C., and Harris, J. W.,** The effect of alcoholism on the absorption of folic acid (H^3-PGA) evaluated by plasma levels and urine excretion, *J. Lab. Clin. Med.,* 69, 116, 1967.
140. **Kahn, S. B.,** Recent advances in the nutritional anemias, *Med. Clin. North Am.,* 54, 631, 1970.
141. **Harris, J. W. and Kellermeyer, R. W.,** *The Red Cell,* Harvard University Press, Cambridge, Mass., 1970, 334.
142. **Eigen, E. and Shockman, G. D.,** The folic acid group, in *Analytical Microbiology,* Kavanagh,, E., Ed., Academic Press, New York, 1963, 431.
143. **Saraya, A. K., Singla, P. N., Ramchandran, K., and Ghai, O. P.,** Nutritional macrocytic anemia of infancy and childhood, *Am. J. Clin. Nutr.,* 23, 1378, 1970.
144. **Chanarin, I.,** *The Megaloblastic Anaemias,* Blackwell Scientific Publ., Oxford, England, 1969.
145. **Arroyave, G.,** Standards for the diagnosis of vitamin deficiency in man, in *Metabolic Adaptation and Nutrition,* Pan American Health Organization Scientific Publication No. 222, 1971, 88, Pan American Health Organization, Washington, D.C. 22037.
146. **Traill, M. A.,** When does a serum folate determination indicate folate deficiency?, *Lab Pract.,* 18, 154, 1969.
147. **Waxman, S., Schreiber, C., and Herbert, V.,** Radioisotopic assay for measurement of serum folate levels, *Blood,* 38, 219, 1971.
148. **Waxman, S.,** (Mt. Sinai School of Medicine, New York, N.Y.), Measurements of Serum, Whole Blood Folate Levels and Folic Acid Binding Protein Using Commercially Available ^{3}HPGA and β-lactoglobulin, presented at the 20th Anniversary Conference on Intestinal Absorption and Allied Disorders, January 23—26, 1973, San Juan, Puerto Rico.
149. **Herbert, V.,** The five possible causes of all nutrient deficiency: illustrated by deficients of vitamin B_{12} and folic acid, *Am. J. Clin. Nutr.,* 26, 77, 1973.
150. **Rothenberg, S. P., DaCosta, M., and Rosenberg, Z.,** Radioassay for serum folate, *N. Engl. J. Med.,* 286, 1335, 1972.
151. **Cook, J. D., Alvarado, J., Gutnisky, A., Jamra, M., Labardini, J., Layrisse, M., Linares, J., Loria, A., Maspes, V., Restrepo, A., Reynafarje, C., Sánchez-Medal, L., Vélez, H., and Viteri, F.,** Nutritional deficiency and anemia in Latin America: a collaborative study, *Blood,* 38, 591, 1971.
152. **Alter, H. J., Zvaifler, N. J., and Rath, C. E.,** Interrelationship of rheumatoid arthritis, folic acid, and aspirin, *Blood,* 38, 405, 1971.
153. Folic acid radioassay kits, available from Diagnostic Products Corporation, 9325 Venice Blvd., Culver City, California 90230.

Vitamin B_{12} (Cyanocobalamin, Corrinoids)

Vitamin B_{12} deficiency results in a megaloblastic anemia.[1-5,105] However, a vitamin B_{12} deficiency due to a lack of dietary intake of the nutrient is relatively rare.[1-6,17,18,110,113,120] Vitamin B_{12} is obtained through the ingestion of animal products (meat, milk, eggs, and cheese) with less than 1 μg of the vitamin required per day to maintain normal hematopoiesis.[1,2,4-6,15,29] Nevertheless, nutritional deficiencies in vitamin B_{12} do occur in India and other areas among vegans (vegetarians) who subsist exclusively on vegetables.[2,4-14,16,110,128] Such persons may have low serum levels of vitamin B_{12}, develop a sore tongue, paresthesias, amenorrhea, neurologic changes, and other signs of a vitamin B_{12} deficiency.[7-14] In some instances, megaloblastic anemia may occur.[10,11,13,14,128]

In the United States, most cases of vitamin B_{12} deficiency are the result of an impaired absorption of the vitamin due to lack of the intrinsic factor in the gastric secretions (pernicious anemia).[1-3,5,34,121,168] Thus, vitamin B_{12} deficiency is more a clinical consideration than a nutritional problem. Nevertheless, the incidence of readily diagnosable pernicious anemia in the United Kingdom is 0.13%, while the incidence of pernicious anemia that is not clinically evident may be considerably higher.[4] The biochemical procedures employed to evaluate vitamin B_{12} status are designed to establish whether a deficiency exists and, if so, whether the deficiency is due to an impaired absorption of the vitamin.[1-3,5,168]

As noted in the section on folacin, a close interrelationship exists between vitamin B_{12} and folacin.[1-3,5,19-21] Hence, vitamin B_{12} nutritional status must be evaluated also in terms of folacin nutrition. Several articles and reviews are referred to for details concerning the chemistry, functions and metabolism of vitamin B_{12} and its interrelationship with folacin.[1-3,5,20-33,36,42,111,112,114,116,121,129]

A deficiency in either vitamin B_{12} or folacin causes a morphologically identical macrocytic anemia.[1,5,21,25,27,105,121,129,159] Both deficiencies are associated with megaloblastic bone marrow changes and hypersegmented polymorphonuclear neutrophils in the peripheral blood with a lobe average greater than 2.8 to 3.4.[1-3,5,105] In pernicious anemia as in folate deficiency, the number of cells with four lobes increases significantly, and cells with five or more lobes may become common. Thus, histological examinations of the bone marrow and peripheral blood do not permit a differentiation between vitamin B_{12} and folacin deficiency. Several biochemical tests can be employed for this purpose.[1-3,5,105,129]

The most common procedure useful for the diagnosis of a vitamin B_{12} deficiency has been the determination of the serum vitamin B_{12} level. Low serum vitamin B_{12} levels have been observed to be associated with low body contents of the vitamin.[130] Microbiological assay methods may be used for this purpose.[1-3,36-42] The test organisms used in the microbiological assays for vitamin B_{12} have included *Lactobacillus lactis* Dorner (ATCC 8000),[40,83] *L. leichmannii* (ATCC 7830),[37-39,41,44,127] *L. leichmannii* (ATCC 4797),[37,41,44,123] *Euglena gracilis* Z strain,[41-43,45,51,71,110,125,127] and *Ochromonas malhamensis*.[41-43] Of these organisms, *L. leichmannii* (ATCC 7830) is the least troublesome and appears to be most commonly employed in the assay for vitamin B_{12} in serum. Detailed procedures using this organism are available.[37-39,41,44] The micro-methods require only 0.1 to 0.2 ml of serum or plasma. Serum samples stored at $-20°C$ were stable for at least 10 months.[83]

Vitamin B_{12} levels may be determined also in serum with the use of the radioactive vitamin B_{12} isotope methods.[37,46,47,49,50,105,172,173] Several methods have been outlined by Skeggs.[37] Additional improvements in the methods have been reported in recent years.[49,50,124-127,160,174] With experience, the isotope methods are reasonably fast, reliable, and reproducible. The values obtained are similar to those obtained by microbiological assays[124-127] but tend to be slightly higher.[127] The methods have the advantage over the microbiological assay procedures in that they are not influenced by inhibitory substances, such as antibiotics, which may be present in serum samples.[45,122] On the other hand, the isotope methods have the disadvantage of requiring the use of radioisotopes, larger sample volumes, and expensive counting equipment.[124]

The normal fasting serum vitamin B_{12} level ranges from 150 pg ($\mu\mu$g) to 900 pg/ml, with a mean of about 475 pg/ml.[1,2,51,105,110,117,124-127] In vitamin B_{12} deficiency, serum levels of the vitamin are usually less than 100 pg/ml.[1,2,47,61,105,124-127] Suggested guidelines that have been used to evaluate serum vitamin B_{12} data are presented in Table 13 (Figures 20 and 21). Low or borderline serum vitamin B_{12} values should be interpreted with a degree of flexibility and caution in order to allow for differences in analytical procedures. Further, an occasional normal subject may have a serum vitamin B_{12} level between 120 and 150 pg/ml without any other abnormality revealed. Low serum vitamin B_{12} levels have been observed in the elderly with no apparent harmful effects.[106,107] Similarly, a small number of pernicious anemia patients may have serum vitamin B_{12} levels as high as 170 pg/ml.[52,83] Such may occur in pernicious anemia patients suffering also with liver disease.[86,87]

In folacin deficiency, serum vitamin B_{12} levels may be low, but in the majority of the patients the serum vitamin B_{12} levels are still above those found in patients with pernicious anemia (Figures 20 and 21).[27,62] These patients do not appear to have any defect in the ability to absorb vitamin B_{12} and, after folate treatment, serum vitamin B_{12} levels return to normal.[27,63] In contrast, in pernicious anemia, serum folate levels may be elevated while red blood cell folate levels may be low (Figure 18).[21,25,28,31,65-69,108]

Elevated urinary excretions of aminoimidazole-carboxamide (AIC), urocanic acid, formimino-glutamic acid (FIGLU), and other histidine metabolites, as also observed in a folate deficiency, may occur in patients with a vitamin B_{12} deficiency.[20,27,30,70,108,121,158,166,167] Where the primary deficiency is vitamin B_{12}, these abnormalities are corrected by the administration of vitamin B_{12}.[27,29-31,65,69] Serum vitamin B_{12} levels may be low in iron deficiency and slowly return to normal following iron therapy.[64] Serum vitamin B_{12} levels may decrease also during pregnancy and increase again after delivery; this pattern may not change with vitamin B_{12} supplementation.[26,72,109,156,169]

Red blood cells have been reported to have a mean of 155 to 195 pg of vitamin B_{12}/ml of cells.[48,51,53,54,117-119] In pernicious anemia, lower levels of vitamin B_{12} were noted (mean of 53 to 91 pg/ml of red blood cells).[51,53,117] In folacin deficiency, however, low red blood cell levels of vitamin B_{12} were also found (mean of 80

TABLE 13

Guidelines for the Interpretation of Serum Vitamin B_{12} Levels[a,b]

(all age groups)

	Less than acceptable (at risk)		
Reference	Deficient (high risk) pg ($\mu\mu$g)/ml	Low (medium risk) pg ($\mu\mu$g)/ml	Acceptable[c] (low risk) pg ($\mu\mu$g)/ml
1. World Health Organization[16]	< 150	150 to 200	⩾ 200
2. Others			
(A)[46,106,125,159]	< 100	100 to 149	⩾ 150
(B)[124,126]	< 100	100 to 159	⩾ 160

[a]Adapted from the reports of WHO[16] and others.[46,106,124-127,159,162]

[b]Guidelines should be regarded as suggested and must be considered in terms of the microbiological assay or radioassay method employed.[127]

[c]Levels above 1000 pg/ml are suggestive of liver disease or a myeloproliferative disorder (e.g., polycythemia vera, granulocytic leukemia or myeloid metaplasia).[129,175,176]

to 95 pg/ml).[51,118] Following folacin therapy, the vitamin B_{12} levels in the red blood cells returned toward normal.[118] Thus, red blood cell vitamin B_{12} determinations do not appear to provide any advantages over serum vitamin B_{12} measurements as an index of vitamin B_{12} status (Figure 21). Leucocytes have been reported to contain relatively high levels of vitamin B_{12} (0.5 to 4.3 ng/g or 2.45 to 6.65 pg/10^6 cells).[55] Leucocyte vitamin B_{12} levels have not been used to assess vitamin B_{12} status and would not appear to have any practical advantage over serum vitamin B_{12} measurements. Liver stores of vitamin B_{12} are low in patients with pernicious anemia. However, liver biopsy procedures are likewise not practical as a routine diagnostic procedure.[56-60,83]

The urinary excretion of methylmalonic acid (MMA) is increased in the majority of patients with a vitamin B_{12} deficiency.[73-77,99,171] Methylmalonyl coenzyme A is isomerized by the vitamin B_{12} activated methylmalonyl-CoA carbonylmutase (mutase; isomerase) enzyme to form succinyl coenzyme A.[78,99] In a vitamin B_{12} deficiency, this reaction is believed to be impaired giving rise to methylmalonate excretion.[90] Methylmalonic aciduria may also occur as a result of an inborn error of metabolism.[91,99,115,116] In these patients, a qualitative or quantitative abnormality exists in the methylmalonyl-CoA mutase enzyme giving rise to a block in the

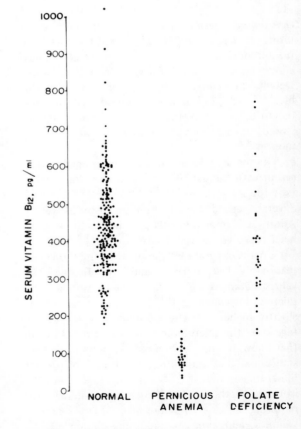

FIGURE 20. Serum vitamin B_{12} levels in normal subjects and in patients with pernicious anemia or folate deficiency. (From Wagstaff and Broughton.[126])

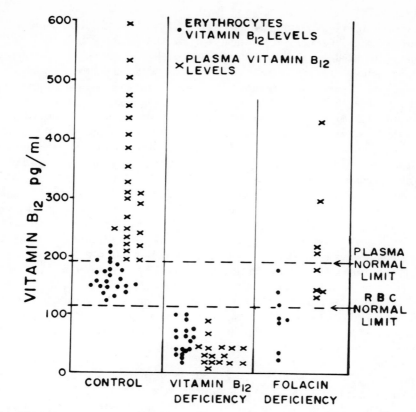

FIGURE 21.   Plasma and erythrocyte vitamin B_{12} levels in normal subjects and in patients with vitamin B_{12} deficiency or folacin deficiency. (From Omer et al.[51])

metabolism of methylmalonyl-CoA.[92,93,115]

Normal subjects usually excrete less than 12 mg of methylmalonic acid in 24 hr,[73,77,79-81,83,90,171] while patients with pernicious anemia may excrete levels in excess of 500 mg in 24 hr.[81] Vitamin B_{12} therapy corrects the condition.[73,79,131,171] Since valine may serve as a precursor of methylmalonic acid, the use of an oral load of L-valine (5 to 10 g) has been employed as means to increase the urinary excretion of methylmalonic acid in a vitaimin B_{12} deficiency.[80,83,84,99,100,110,157,165] The megaloblastic anemia of folate deficiency is not accompanied by an increased urinary excretion of methylmalonic acid.[99,101] Hence a vitamin B_{12} deficiency can be distinguished from a folacin deficiency by this determination. However, the level of methylmalonic acid excretion does not necessarily provide information as to the severity of the vitamin B_{12} deficiency.[94]

Various procedures are available for the measurement of methylmalonic acid, including paper and thin-layer chromatography,[76,79,82,171] colorimetric,[81,83,88,96,104,163,165] gas chromatography,[77,89,90,97,98,101-103] and column chromatography.[95] The simplest procedure to measure urinary methylmalonic acid in urine appears to be the method of Giorgio and Luhby.[81,88,96,163,165] However, the method lacks sensitivity and has limited use for detecting vitamin B_{12} deficiency except where markedly elevated excretions of methylmalonic acid occur or in conjunction with a valine load test. Thin-layer chromatography can be useful as a semiquantitative screening procedure.[82,171] The gas-liquid-chromatography (GLC) procedure of Cox and White[77,97] is considerably more sensitive and reliable, but the method is rather involved and difficult to perform in the clinical laboratory. A more simplified GLC method has been provided by Sprinkle et al.[103] Recently, Giorgio et al.[89] have reported on a simple, specific and sensitive

GLC method for measuring urinary methylmalonic acid using boron trifluoride methylation of the acid. In addition to the need for a GLC instrument, each analysis required approximately an hour to complete.[89] Although urinary methylmalonic acid determinations can be of value as a diagnostic aid in the clinical laboratory and in research studies, the lack of a simple sensitive quantitative method limits the application of the test as a practical index for the evaluation of vitamin B_{12} nutritional status.[99]

Formiminoglutamic acid (FIGLU), urocanic acid and aminoimidazolecarboxamide (AIC) are often excreted in increased amounts in vitamin B_{12} deficiency.[21,28,30,158] Unfortunately, the excretion of these compounds is also increased in folacin deficiency and, hence, their measurement cannot serve as a means to distinguish between these two deficiencies (see section on *Folacin*).

The rate of plasma disappearance of intravenously injected vitamin B_{12} is slower in vitamin B_{12} deficient patients than in normal subjects.[85] However, this procedure has seldom been used as an index of vitamin B_{12} deficiency.[83] Low urinary uropepsin excretion has also been employed to screen for vitamin B_{12} deficiency.[132] However, the majority of subjects with abnormally low uropepsin excretion values did not prove to have a vitamin B_{12} deficiency.[132]

Once biochemical measurements have been established confirming an existing megaloblastic anemia due to a deficiency of vitamin B_{12} and not of folacin, vitamin B_{12} absorption tests can be employed to determine whether the condition is a result of (a) lack of intrinsic factor (pernicious anemia), (b) other forms of malabsorption, or (c) nutritional deficiency of vitamin B_{12}. Pernicious anemia can be readily diagnosed by measuring the oral absorption of vitamin B_{12} given without and with intrinsic factor.[1-3,36,129,148,149] For this purpose, the Schilling test[36,133,138,148-150,170] or modifications of it, such as the double-tracer test using ^{57}Co and ^{60}Co[134] or ^{57}Co and ^{58}Co,[135-137] are usually employed. The basic principle of the procedures is to orally administer a tracer dose of radioactively labeled vitamin B_{12}, usually 0.5 to 2.0 μg. In the following 24 hr, in conjunction with an intramuscularly administered "flushing" dose of 1 mg of unlabeled vitamin B_{12}, a normal person will excrete in the urine 10 to 40% of the administered radioactivity, while patients with pernicious anemia will excrete 0 to 7% of the administered dose.[1,36,146-148] If a source of intrinsic factor is administered simultaneously with the radioactively labeled vitamin B_{12} to the pernicious anemia patient, the amount of radioactivity excreted in the urine will approach that of the normal subject. Where whole body monitors are available, the amount of the administered radioactivity retained in the body can serve as a diagnosis of pernicious anemia.[137,139,144,170] Normal subjects absorb 45 to 80% of the administered vitamin B_{12} in comparison to 0 to 17% by patients with pernicious anemia.[137,139,144] The rise in serum radioactivity following the oral administration of radioactively labeled vitamin B_{12} has also been useful as an index of vitamin B_{12} absorption.[145-147,170] Although this procedure overcomes the problems associated with obtaining reliable urine collections, a disadvantage exists in that the low levels of radioactivity present in the serum require long counting periods.

If the vitamin B_{12} deficiency is the result of malabsorption other than of the pernicious anemia type, conducting the Schilling test in the presence of intrinsic factor may produce little or no improvement in the absorption of the orally administered radioactively labeled vitamin B_{12}.[1,150,161] In these cases, the malabsorption of vitamin B_{12} may be due to forms of tropical and nontropical sprue, ileitis, ileal resection, gastrectomy, specific vitamin B_{12} malabsorption syndromes, parasites or drugs.[1,105,151,152,159,161,168] Vitamin B_{12} malabsorption has been associated with the use of neomycin, colchicine, p-amino salicylic acid, ethanol, phenothiazines and metformin.[1,120,149,152-155,164,168] Subjects with an uncomplicated primary nutritional deficiency of vitamin B_{12} would be expected to have a normal absorption test.

In summary, it is essential in patients with megaloblastic anemia that the precise deficiency be established (folacin and/or vitamin B_{12}) before therapy is initiated. Serum vitamin B_{12} and serum folacin levels should be determined as a minimum. If a normal vitamin B_{12} level is observed in the presence of a low serum folate level, a diagnosis of pernicious anemia is most unlikely. Low serum vitamin B_{12} levels are indicative of pernicious anemia and can be precisely established with the use of a Schilling test.

REFERENCES

1. Harris, J. W. and Kellermeyer, R. W., *The Red Cell,* Harvard University Press, Cambridge, 1970, 334.
2. Baker, S. J., Human vitamin B_{12} deficiency, *World Rev. Nutr. Diet.,* 8, 62, 1967.
3. Reisner, E. H., XI. Deficiency effects and physiology in man, in *The Vitamins* Vol. II, 2nd ed., Sebrell, W. H., Jr. and Harris, R. S., Eds., Academic Press, Inc., New York, 1968, 220.
4. Requirements of Ascorbic Acid, Vitamin D, Vitamin B_{12}, Folate, and Iron, Report of a joint FAO/WHO Expert Group. FAO nutrition meetings report series No. 47. Food and Agriculture Organization of the United Nations, Rome, 1970.
5. Sullivan, L. W., Vitamin B_{12} metabolism and megaloblastic anemia, *Semin. Hematol.,* 7, 6, 1970.
6. *Recommended dietary allowances,* 7th revised ed., A report of the Food and Nutrition Board of the National Research Council. Publication No. 1694, National Academy of Sciences, 2101 Constitution Ave., Washington, D.C., 1968.
7. Jadhav, M., Webb, J. K. G., Vaishnava, S., and Baker, S. J., Vitamin B_{12} deficiency in Indian infants: A clinical syndrome, *Lancet,* 2, 903, 1962.
8. Winawer, S. J., Streiff, R., and Zamchek, N., Gastric and hematological abnormalities in a vegan with nutritional vitamin B_{12} deficiency: Effect of oral vitamin B_{12}, *Gastroenterology,* 53, 130, 1967.
9. Mehta, B. M., Rege, D. W., and Satoskar, R. S., Serum Vitamin B_{12} and folic acid activity in lactovegetarian and nonvegetarian healthy adult Indians, *Am. J. Clin. Nutr.,* 15, 77, 1964.
10. Majumdar, S., Agarwal, K. N., Gupta, S., and Chandhuri, S. N., Serum vitamin B_{12} and/or folic acid deficiency in childhood anaemias, *Indian Pediatr.,* 7, 455, 1970.
11. Singla, P. N., Saraya, A. K., and Ghai, O. P., Vitamin B_{12} and folic acid deficiency in nutritional megaloblastic anaemia of infancy and childhood, *Indian J. Med. Res.,* 58, 599, 1970.
12. Smith, A. D. M., Veganism: A clinical survey with observations on vitamin B_{12} metabolism, *Br. Med. J.,* 1, 1655, 1962.
13. Hines, J. D., Megaloblastic anemia in an adult vegan, *Am. J. Clin. Nutr.,* 19, 260, 1966.
14. Baker, S. J., Jacob, E., Rajan, K. T., and Swaminathan, S., Vitamin B_{12} deficiency in pregnancy and the puerperium, *Br. Med. J.,* 1, 1658, 1962.
15. Darby, W. J., Bridgforth, E. B., LeBrocquy, J., Clark, S. L., Jr., Dutra de Oliveira, J., Kevany, J., McGanity, W. J., and Pérez, C., Vitamin B_{12} requirement of adult man, *Am. J. Med.,* 25, 726, 1958.
16. Nutritional Anaemias, Report of a WHO Scientific Group, World Health Organization Technical Report Series No. 405. World Health Organization, Geneva, Switzerland, 1968.
17. Bengoa, J. M., Nutrition activities of the World Health Organization, *J. Am. Diet. Assoc.,* 55, 228, 1969.
18. Herbert, V., Megaloblastic anemia as a problem in world health, *Am. J. Clin. Nutr.,* 21, 1115, 1968.
19. Herbert, V. and Zalusky, R., Interrelations of vitamin B_{12} in folic acid metabolism: Folic acid clearance studies, *J. Clin. Invest.,* 41, 1263, 1962.
20. Luhby, A. L. and Cooperman, J. M., Folic acid deficiency in man and its interrelationship with vitamin B_{12} metabolism, in *Advances in Metabolic Disorders,* Vol. 1, Academic Press, Inc., New York, 1964, 263.
21. Nixon, P. F. and Bertino, J. R., Interrelationships of vitamin B_{12} and folate in man, *Am. J. Med.,* 48, 555, 1970.
22. Chow, B. F., The B vitamins: B_6, B_{12}, folic acid, pantothenic acid, and biotin, in *Nutrition. A Comprehensive Treatise,* Beaton, G. H. and McHenry, E. W., Eds., Academic Press, Inc., New York, 1964, 219.
23. Moore, H. W. and Folkers, K., Vitamin B_{12} II. Chemistry, in *The Vitamins,* Vol. II, 2nd ed., Sebrell, W. H., Jr. and Harris, R. S., Eds., Academic Press, Inc., New York, 1968, 121.
24. Barker, H. A., Vitamin B_{12} IX. Biochemical systems, in *The Vitamins,* Vol. II, 2nd ed., Sebrell, W. H., Jr. and Harris, R. S., Eds., Academic Press, Inc., New York, 1968, 184.
25. Johns, D. G. and Bertino, J. R., Folates and megaloblastic anemia: A review, *Clin. Pharmacol. Ther.,* 6, 372, 1965.
26. Lowenstein, L., Brunton, L., and Hsieh, Y.-S., Nutritional anemia and megaloblastosis in pregnancy, *Can. Med. Assoc. J.,* 94, 636, 1966.
27. Sullivan, L. W., Folates in human nutrition, in *Newer Methods of Nutritional Biochemistry,* Vol. III, Albanese, A. A., Ed., Academic Press, Inc., New York, 1967, 365.
28. Herbert, V., Studies of folate deficiency in man, *Proc. R. Soc. Med.,* 57, 377, 1964.
29. Herbert, V., Nutritional requirements for vitamin B_{12} and folic acid, *Am. J. Clin. Nutr.,* 21, 743, 1968.
30. Herbert, V., Biochemical and hematologic lesions in folic acid deficiency, *Am. J. Clin. Nutr.,* 20, 562, 1967.
31. Blakley, R. L., *The Biochemistry of Folic Acid and Related Pteridines. Frontiers of Biology,* Vol. 13, Neuberger, A. and Tatum, E. L., Eds., North-Holland Publishing Co., Amsterdam (J. Wiley and Sons, Inc., New York, Distributors), 1969.
32. Vilter, R. W., Will, J. J., Wright, T., and Rullman, D., Interrelationships of vitamin B_{12}, folic acid, and ascorbic acid in the megaloblastic anemias, *Am. J. Clin. Nutr.,* 12, 130, 1963.
33. Vilter, R. W., Interrelationships between folic acid, vitamin B_{12} and ascorbic acid in the megaloblastic anemias, *Medicine,* 43, 727, 1964.
34. Castle, W. B., Current concepts of pernicious anemia, *Am. J. Med.,* 48, 541, 1970.

35. **Edwin, E.,** The segmentation of polymorphonuclear neutrophils. The conditions in hypovitaminosis B_{12} and hypersegmentation, *Acta Med. Scand.,* 182, 401, 1967.

36. **Gräsbeck, R.,** Physiology and pathology of vitamin B_{12} absorption, distribution, and excretion, *Adv. Clin. Chem.,* 3, 299, 1960.

37. **Skeggs, H. R.,** Vitamin B_{12}, in *The Vitamins,* Vol. VII, 2nd ed., György, P. and Pearson, W. N., Eds., Academic Press, Inc., New York, 1967, 277.

38. *The Pharmacopeia of the United States of America,* 17th revision, Mack Publ., Easton, Pennsylvania, 1965, 864.

39. *Official Methods of Analysis of the Association of Official Agricultural Chemists,* 9th ed., Horowitz, W., Ed., Assoc. Offic. Agr. Chemists, Washington, D.C., 1960, 665.

40. **Cooperman, J. M., Luhby, A. L., Teller, D. M., and Marley, J. F.,** Distribution of radioactive and nonradioactive vitamin B_{12} in the dog, *J. Biol. Chem.,* 235, 191, 1960.

41. *Difco Supplementary Literature,* Difco Laboratories, Detroit, 1972, 20, 439.

42. **Baker, H. and Frank, O.,** *Clinical Vitaminology,* Vitamin B_{12}, Interscience Publishers, New York, 1968, 116.

43. **Guttman, H. N.,** Vitamin B_{12} and congeners, in *Analytical Microbiology,* Kavanagh, E., Ed., Academic Press, Inc., New York, 1963, 527.

44. **Skeggs, H. R.,** *Lactobacillus leichmannii* assay for vitamin B_{12} in *Analytical Microbiology,* Kavanagh, E., Ed., Academic Press, Inc., New York, 1963, 551.

45. **Anderson, B.,** Investigations into the *Euglena* method for the assay of the vitamin B_{12} in serum, *J. Clin. Pathol.,* 17, 14, 1964.

46. **Grossowicz, N., Sulitzeanu, D., and Merzbach, D.,** Isotopic determination of vitamin B_{12} binding capacity and concentration, *Proc. Soc. Exp. Biol. Med.,* 109, 604, 1962.

47. **Lau, K., Gottlieb, C., Wasserman, L. R., and Herbert, V.,** Measurement of serum vitamin B_{12} level using radioisotope dilution and coated charcoal, *Blood,* 26, 202, 1965.

48. **Kato, N.,** Location of vitamin B_{12} in human erythrocytes, *J. Vitaminol.,* 4, 226, 1958.

49. **Hillman, R. S., Oakes, M., and Finholt, C.,** Hemoglobin-coated charcoal radioassay for serum vitamin B_{12}. A simple modification to improve intrinsic factor reliability, *Blood,* 34, 385, 1969.

50. **Raven, J. L., Robson, M. B., Walker, P. L., and Barkan, P.,** Improved method for measuring vitamin B_{12} in serum using intrinsic factor, $^{57}Co\ B_{12}$, and activated charcoal, *J. Clin. Pathol.,* 22, 205, 1969.

51. **Omer, A., Finlayson, N. D. C., Shearman, D. J. C., Samson, R. R., and Girdwood, R. H.,** Erythrocyte vitamin B_{12} activity in health, polycythemia, and in deficiency of vitamin B_{12} and folate, *Blood,* 35, 73, 1970.

52. **Ardeman, S., Chanarin, I., Krafchik, B., and Singer, W.,** Addisonian pernicious anemia and intrinsic factor antibodies in thyroid disorder, *Q. J. Med.,* 35, 421, 1966.

53. **Sobotka, H., Baker, H., and Ziffer, H.,** Distribution of vitamin B_{12} between plasma and cells, *Am. J. Clin. Nutr.,* 8, 283, 1960.

54. **Biggs, J. C., Mason, S. L. A., and Spray, G. H.,** Vitamin-B_{12} activity in red cells, *Br. J. Haematol.,* 10, 36, 1964.

55. **Molin, D. L. and Ross, G. I. M.,** Serum vitamin B_{12} concentrations in leukaemia and in some other haematological conditions, *Br. J. Haematol.,* 1, 155, 1955.

56. **Swendseid, M. E., Hvolboll, E., Shick, G., and Halsted, J. A.,** The vitamin B_{12} content of human liver tissue and its nutritional significance. A comparison study of various age groups, *Blood,* 12, 24, 1957.

57. **Nelson, R. S. and Doctor, V. M.,** The vitamin B_{12} content of human liver as determined by bio-assay of needle biopsy material, *Ann. Intern. Med.,* 49, 1361, 1958.

58. **Pitney, W. R. and Onesti, P.,** Vitamin B_{12} and folic acid concentrations of human liver with reference to the assay of needle biopsy material, *Aust. J. Exp. Biol. Med. Sci.,* 39, 1, 1961.

59. **Joske, R. A.,** The vitamin B_{12} content of human liver tissue obtained by aspiration biopsy, *Gut,* 4, 231, 1963.

60. **Kelly, A. and Davis, R. E.,** The determination of liver vitamin B_{12} and folate activity in a single extract, *J. Vitaminol.,* 11, 68, 1965.

61. **Mollin, D. L.,** The megaloblastic anaemias, *Ann. Rev. Med.,* 11, 333, 1960.

62. **Sullivan, L. W. and Herbert, V.,** Suppression of hematopoiesis by ethanol, *J. Clin. Invest.,* 43, 2048, 1964.

63. **Johnson, S., Swaminathan, S. P., and Baker, S. J.,** Changes in serum vitamin B_{12} levels in patients with megaloblastic anemia treated with folic acid, *J. Clin. Pathol.,* 15, 274, 1962.

64. **Cox, E. V., Meynell, M. J., Gaddie, R., and Cooke, W. T.,** Inter-relation of vitamin B_{12} and iron, *Lancet,* 2, 998, 1959.

65. **Herbert, V. and Zalusky, R.,** Interrelations of vitamin B_{12} and folic acid metabolism: Folic acid clearance studies, *J. Clin. Invest.,* 41, 1263, 1962.

66. **Hansen, H. A. and Weinfeld, A.,** Metabolic effects and diagnostic value of small doses of folic acid and B_{12} in megaloblastic anemias, *Acta Med. Scand.,* 172, 427, 1962.

67. **Cooper, B. A. and Lowenstein, L.,** Relative folate deficiency of erythroid cells in vitamin B_{12} deficiency, *Clin. Res.,* 11, 191, 1963.

68. **Cooper, B. A. and Lowenstein, L.,** Vitamin B_{12}-folate interrelationship in megaloblastic anemia, *Br. J. Haematol.,* 12, 283, 1966.

69. **Cooper, B. A. and Lowenstein, L.,** Relative folate deficiency of erythrocytes in pernicious anaemia and its correction with cyanocobalamin, *Blood,* 24, 502, 1964.

70. **Chanarin, I., Bennett, M. C., and Berry, V.,** Urinary excretion of histidine derivatives in megaloblastic anaemia and other conditions and a comparison with folic acid clearance test, *J. Clin. Pathol.,* 15, 269, 1962.

71. **Shinton, N. K.,** Total serum vitamin B_{12} concentration in normal human adult serum assayed by *Euglena gracilis, Clinical Sci.,* 18, 389, 1959.

72. **Metz, J., Festenstein, H., and Welch, P.,** Effect of folic acid and vitamin B_{12} supplementation on tests of folate and vitamin B_{12} nutrition in pregnancy, *Am. J. Clin. Nutr.,* 16, 472, 1965.

73. **White, A. M.,** Vitamin B_{12} deficiency and the excretion of methylmalonic acid by the human, *Biochem. J.,* 84, 41P, 1962.

74. **White, A. M.,** The effect of vitamin B_{12} deficiency on the excretion of propionic acid by the human, *Biochem. J.,* 95, 17P, 1965.

75. **White, A. M. and Cox, E. V.,** Methylmalonic acid excretion and vitamin B_{12} deficiency in the human, *Ann. N.Y. Acad. Sci.,* 112, 915, 1964.

76. **Barness, L. A., Young, D., Mellman, W. J., Kahn, S. B., and Williams, W. J.,** Methylmalonate excretion in a patient with pernicious anemia, *N. Engl. J. Med.,* 268, 144, 1963.

77. **Cox, E. V. and White, A. M.,** Methylmalonic acid excretion: An index of vitamin B_{12} deficiency, *Lancet,* 2, 853, 1962.

78. **Mazumder, R., Sasakawa, T., and Ochoa, S.,** Metabolism of propionic acid in animal tissues. X. Methylmalonyl coenzyme A mutase holoenzyme, *J. Biol. Chem.,* 238, 50, 1963.

79. **Kahn, S. B., Williams, W. J., Barness, L. A., Young, D., Shafer, B., Vivacqua, R. J., and Beaupre, E. M.,** Methylmalonic acid excretion: A sensitive indicator of vitamin B_{12} deficiency in man, *J. Lab. Clin. Med.,* 66, 75, 1965.

80. **Gompertz, D., Jones, J. H., and Knowles, J. P.,** Metabolic precursors of methylmalonic acid in vitamin B_{12} deficiency, *Clin. Chim. Acta,* 18, 197, 1967.

81. **Giorgio, A. J. and Plaut, G. W. E.,** A method for the colorimetric determination of urinary methylmalonic acid in pernicious anemia, *J. Lab. Clin. Med.,* 66, 667, 1965.

82. **Dreyfus, P. M. and Dubé, V. E.,** The rapid detection of methylmalonic acid in urine – a sensitive index of vitamin B_{12} deficiency, *Clin. Chim. Acta,* 15, 525, 1967.

83. **Luhby, A. L., Cooperman, J. M., Lopez, R., and Giorgio, A. J.,** Vitamin B_{12} metabolism in thalassemia major, *Ann. N.Y. Acad. Sci.,* 165, 443, 1969.

84. **Luhby, A. L., Giorgio, A. J., and Cooperman, J. M.,** Metabolic loading for urinary methylmalonate (MMA) in B_{12} deficiency in man, *Fed. Proc.,* 27, 359, 1968.

85. **Mollin, D. L., Pitney, W. R., Baker, S. J., and Bradley, J. E..,** The plasma clearance and urinary excretion of parenterally administered ^{58}Co B_{12}, *Blood,* 11, 31, 1956.

86. **Rachmilewitz, M., Aronovitich, J., and Grossowicz, N.,** Serum concentrations of vitamin B_{12} in acute and chronic liver disease, *J. Lab. Clin. Med.,* 48, 339, 1956.

87. **Jones, P. N., Mills, E. H., and Capps, R. B.,** The effect of liver disease on serum vitamin B_{12} concentrations, *J. Lab. Clin. Med.,* 49, 910, 1957.

88. **Giorgio, A. J.,** The colorimetric measurement of urinary methylmalonic acid, in *Methods in Enzymology (Vitamins and Co-Enzymes),* Vol. XVIII, Part C, McCormick, D. B., and Wright, L., Eds., Academic Press, Inc., New York, 1971, 103.

89. **Giorgio, A. J., Malloy, E., and Black, T.,** A clinical laboratory GLC method for urine methylmalonic acid, *Anal. Lett.,* 5, 13, 1972.

90. **Contreras, E. and Giorgio, A. J.,** Leukocyte methylmalonyl-Co A mutase, I. Vitamin B_{12} deficiency, *Am. J. Clin. Nutr.,* 25, 695, 1972.

91. **Oberholzer, V. G., Levin, B., Burgess, E. A., and Young, W. F.,** Methylmalonic aciduria. An inborn error of metabolism leading to chronic metabolic acidosis, *Arch. Dis. Child.,* 42, 492, 1967.

92. **Morrow, G., III and Barness, L. A.,** Studies in a patient with methylmalonic acidemia, *J. Pediatr.,* 74, 691, 1969.

93. **Rosenberg, L. E., Lilljeqvist, A., Hsia, Y. E.,** Methylmalonic aciduria. Metabolic block localization and vitamin B_{12} dependency. *Science,* 162, 805, 1968.

94. **Neumann, E.,** Methylmalonsäureausscheidung und megaloblastische Blutbidungsstörung, *Wiener klinische Wochenschrift,* 20, 373, 1970.

95. **Barness, L. A., Morrow, G., III, Nocho, R. E., and Maresca, R. A.,** Silicic acid chromatography of organic acids in blood cells and biological fluids, *Clin. Chem.,* 16, 20, 1970.

96. **Giorgio, A. J. and Luhby, A. L.,** A rapid screening test for the detection of congenital methylmalonic aciduria in infancy, *Am. J. Clin. Pathol.,* 52, 374, 1969.

97. **White, A. M.,** (215) Detecting vitamin B_{12} deficiency in humans by measuring urinary excretion of methylmalonic acid, in *Methods in Enzymology,* Vol. XVIII, Part C, McCormick, D. B. and Wright, L., Eds., Academic Press, Inc., New York, 1971, 101.

98. **Hoffman, N. E. and Barboriak, J. J.,** Gas chromatographic determination of urinary methylmalonic acid, *Anal. Biochem.,* 18, 10, 1967.

99. **Gompertz, D. and Hoffbrand, A. V.,** Methylmalonic aciduria, *Br. J. Haematol.,* 18, 377, 1970.

100. **Green, A. E. and Pegrum, G. D.,** Value of estimating methylmalonic acid excretion in anaemia, *Br. Med. J.,* 3, 591, 1968.

101. **Brozović, M., Hoffbrand, A. V., Dimitriadore, A., and Mollin, D. L.,** The excretion of methylmalonic acid and succinic acid in vitamin B_{12} and folate deficiency, *Br. J. Haematol.,* 13, 1021, 1967.

102. **Gomertz, D.,** The measurement of urinary methylmalonic acid by a combination of thin-layer and gas chromatography, *Clin. Chim. Acta,* 19, 477, 1968.

103. **Sprinkle, T. J., Porter, A. H., Greer, M., and Williams, C. M.,** A simple method for the determination of methylmalonic acid by gas chromatography, *Clin. Chim. Acta,* 24, 476, 1969.

104. **Williams, D. L., Spray, G. H., Newman, G. E., and O'Brien, J. R. P.,** Dietary depletion of vitamin B_{12} and the excretion of methylmalonic acid in the rat, *Br. J. Nutr.,* 23, 343, 1969.

105. **Kahn, S. B.,** Recent advances in the nutritional anemias, *Med. Clin. of North Am.,* 54, 631, 1970.

106. **Elwood, P. C., Shinton, N. K., Wilson, C. I. D., Sweetnam, P., and Frazier, A. C.,** Haemoglobin, vitamin B_{12} and folate levels in the elderly, *Br. J. Haematol.,* 21, 557, 1971.

107. **Hughes, D., Elwood, P. C., Shinton, N. K., and Wrighton, R. J.,** Clinical trial of the effect of vitamin B_{12} in elderly subjects with low serum B_{12} levels, *Br. Med. J.,* 2, 458, 1970.

108. **Hoffbrand, A. V., Newcombe, B. F. A., and Mollin, D. L.,** Method of assay of red cell folate activity and the value of the assay as a test for folate deficiency, *J. Clin. Pathol.,* 19, 17, 1966.

109. **Tasker, P. W. G.,** Folic acid and vitamin B_{12}. Effects of graded doses in the treatment of tropical nutritional megaloblastic anaemia, *Trans. R. Soc. Trop. Med. Hyg.,* 54, 578, 1960.

110. **Stewart, J. S., Roberts, P. D., and Hoffbrand, A. V.,** Response of dietary vitamin-B_{12} deficiency to physiological oral doses of cyanocobalamin, *Lancet,* 2, 542, 1970.

111. **Weissbach, H. and Dickerman, H.,** Biochemical role of vitamin B_{12}, *Physiol. Rev.,* 45, 80, 1965.

112. **Stadtman, T. C.,** Vitamin B_{12}, *Science,* 171, 859, 1971.

113. **Britt, R. P., Harper, C., and Spray, G. H.,** Response of dietary vitamin-B_{12} deficiency to physiological oral doses of cyanocobalamin, *Lancet,* 2, 670, 1970.

114. **Silber, R. and Moldow, C. F.,** The biochemistry of B_{12}-mediated reactions in man, *Am. J. Med.,* 48, 549, 1970.

115. **Hsia, Y. E., Lilljeqvist, A. C., and Rosenberg, L. E.,** Vitamin B_{12}-dependent methylmalonicaciduria: Amino acid toxicity, long chain ketonuria, and protective effect of vitamin B_{12}, *Pediatrics,* 46, 497, 1970.

116. **Mahoney, M. J. and Rosenberg, L. E.,** Inherited defects of B_{12} metabolism, *Am. J. Med.,* 48, 584, 1970.

117. **Harrison, R. J.,** Vitamin B_{12} levels in erythrocytes in normal subjects and in pernicious anaemia, *J. Clin. Path.,* 23, 219, 1970.

118. **Harrison, R. J.,** Vitamin B_{12} levels in erythrocytes in anaemia due to folate deficiency, *Brit. J. Haematol.,* 20, 623, 1971.

119. **Kelly, A. and Herbert, V.,** Coated charcoal assay of erythrocyte vitamin B_{12} levels, *Blood,* 29, 139, 1967.

120. **Isaksson, A., Myrstener, A., and Ottosson, J. O.,** Screening for vitamin B_{12} deficiency in psychiatric patients, *Acta Psychiatr. Scand.,* Suppl.No. 221, p. 133, 1971.

121. **Sullivan, L. W.,** Differential diagnosis and management of the patient with megaloblastic anemia, *Am. J. Med.,* 48, 609, 1970.

122. **Herbert, V., Gottlieb, C. W., and Altschule, M. D.,** Apparent low serum-vitamin B_{12} levels associated with chlorpromazine, *Lancet,* 2, 1052, 1965.

123. **Stuart, J. and Sklaroff, S. A.,** Rapid microbiological assay of serum vitamin B_{12} by electronic counter, *J. Clin. Path.,* 19, 46, 1966.

124. **Britt, R. P., Bolton, F. G., Cull, A. C., and Spray, G. H.,** Experience with a simplified method of radio-isotopic assay of serum vitamin B_{12}, *Br. J. Haematol.,* 16, 457, 1969.

125. **Wide, J. and Killander, A.,** A radiosorbent technique for the assay of serum vitamin B_{12}, *Scand. J. Clin. Lab. Invest.,* 27, 151, 1971.

126. **Wagstaff, M. and Broughton, A.,** A simple routine radioisotopic method for the estimation of serum vitamin B_{12} using DEAE cellulose and human serum binding agent, *Br. J. Haematol.,* 21, 581, 1971.

127. **Raven, J. L., Robson, M. B., Morgan, J. O., and Hoffbrand, A. V.,** Comparison of three methods for measuring vitamin B_{12} in serum: Radioisotopic, *Euglena gracilis* and *Lactobacillus leichmannii, Br. J. Haematol.,* 22, 21, 1972.

128. **Saraya, A. K., Singla, P. N., Ramachandran, K., and Ghai, O. P.,** Nutritional macrocytic anemia of infancy and childhood, *Am. J. Clin. Nutr.,* 23, 1378, 1970.

129. **Chanarin, I.,** *The megaloblastic anaemias,* Blackwell Scientific Publications, Oxford, England, 1969.

130. **Boddy, K. and Adams, J. F.,** The long-term relationship between serum vitamin B_{12} and total body vitamin B_{12}, *Am. J. Clin. Nutr.,* 25, 395, 1972.

131. **Barness, L. A.,** Vitamin B_{12} deficiency with emphasis on methylmalonic acid as a diagnostic aid, *Am. J. Clin. Nutr.,* 20, 573, 1967.

132. **Trowbridge, M., Jr., Wadsworth, R. C., and Moffitt, E. L.,** Evaluation of the Segal uropepsin test in screening for hypovitaminosis B_{12}, *Am. J. Clin. Nutr.,* 25, 282, 1972.

133. **Schilling, R. F.,** Intrinsic factor studies. II. The effect of gastric juice on the urinary excretion of radioactivity after the oral administration of radioactive vitamin B_{12}, *J. Lab. Clin. Med.,* 42, 860, 1953.

134. **Katz, J. H., Dimase, J., and Donaldson, R. M.,** Simultaneous administration of gastric juice-bound and free radioactive cyanocobalamin: rapid procedure for differentiating between intrinsic factor deficiency and other causes of vitamin B_{12} malabsorption, *J. Lab. Clin. Med.,* 61, 266, 1963.

135. **Bell, T. K., Bridges, J. M., and Nelson, M. G.,** Simultaneous free and bound radioactive vitamin B_{12} urinary excretion test, *J. Clin. Pathol.,* 18, 611, 1965.

136. **Bell, T. K. and Lee, D.,** Evaluation of a dual radioisotope urinary excretion test in the diagnosis of pernicious anaemia, *Acta Haematol.,* 42, 183, 1969.

137. **Boddy, K., Mahaffy, M. E., and Will, G.,** A double-tracer test of the oral absorption of ^{57}Co- and ^{58}Co-vitamin B_{12} using a whole-body monitor: clinical experience and technical factors, *Am. J. Clin. Nutr.,* 25, 703, 1972.

138. **Schilling, R. F., Clatanoff, D. V., and Korst, D. R.,** Intrinsic factor studies: III. Further observations utilizing the urinary radioactivity test in subjects with achlorhydria, pernicious anemia or a total gastrectomy, *J. Lab. Clin. Med.,* 45, 926, 1955.

139. **Bozian, R. C., Ferguson, J. L., Heyssel, R. M., Meneely, G. R., and Darby, W. J.,** Evidence concerning the human requirement for vitamin B_{12}. Use of the whole body counter for determination of absorption of vitamin B_{12}, *Am. J. Clin. Nutr.,* 12, 117, 1963.

140. **Reizenstein, P. G., Cronkite, E. P., and Cohn, S. H.,** Measurement of absorption of vitamin B_{12} by whole-body gamma spectrometry, *Blood,* 18, 95, 1961.

141. **Naversten, Y., Liden, K., Stahlberg, K. G., and Norden, A.,** The study of ^{57}Co-vitamin B_{12} absorption using a whole-body counter, *Phys. Med. Biol.* 14, 441, 1969.

142. **Tappin, J. W., Rahman, I. A., and Rogers K.,** A study of absorption of vitamin B_{12} using a whole-body spectrometer, *Br. J. Radiol.,* 39, 295, 1966.

143. **Finlayson, N. D. C., Simpson, J. D., Tothill, P., Sampson, R. R., Girdwood, R. H., and Shearman, D. J. C.,** Application of whole body counting to the measurement of vitamin B_{12} absorption wtih reference to achlorhydria, *Scand. J. Gastroenterol.,* 4, 397, 1969.

144. **Irvine, W. J., Cullen, D. R., Scarth, L., Simpson, J. D., and Davies, S. H.,** Total body counting in the assessment of vitamin B_{12} absorption in patients with pernicious anemia, achlorhydria without pernicious anemia and in acid secretors, *Blood,* 36, 20, 1970.

145. **Armstrong, B. K. and Woodliff, H. J.,** Studies on the ^{57}Co vitamin B_{12} plasma level absorption test, *J. Clin. Pathol.,* 23, 569, 1970.

146. **Donaldson, D., Blight, B. J. N., and Lascelles, P. T.,** An assessment of serum ^{57}Co cyanocobalamin as an index of vitamin B_{12} absorption, *J. Clin. Pathol.,* 23, 558, 1970.

147. **Donaldson, D. and Lascelles, P. T.,** Vitamin B_{12} absorption in some neurological and neuroendocrine disorders, *J. Clin. Pathol.,* 23, 563, 1970.

148. **Lamar, C., McCracken, B. H., Miller, O. N., and Goldsmith, G. A.,** Experiences with the Schilling test as a diagnostic tool, *Am. J. Clin. Nutr.,* 16, 402, 1965.

149. **Corcino, J. J., Waxman, S., and Herbert, V.,** Absorption and malabsorption of vitamin B_{12}, *Am. J. Med.,* 48, 562, 1970.

150. **Ellenbogen, L. and Williams, W. L.,** Quantitative assay of intrinsic factor by urinary excretion of radioactive vitamin B_{12}, *Blood,* 13, 582, 1958.

151. **Rivera, J. V., de La Obra, F. R., and Maldonado, M. M.,** Anemia due to vitamin B_{12} deficiency after treatment with folic acid in tropical sprue, *Am. J. Clin. Nutr.,* 18, 110, 1966.

152. **Waxman, S., Corcino, J. J., and Herbert, V.,** Drugs, toxins and dietary amino acids affecting vitamin B_{12} or folic acid absorption or utilization, *Am. J. Med.,* 48, 599, 1970.

153. **Roe, D. A.,** Drug-induced deficiency of B vitamins, *N.Y. State J. Med.,* p. 2770, Dec. 1, 1971.

154. **Stowers, J. M. and Smith, O. A. O.,** Vitamin B_{12} and metformin, *Brit. Med. J.,* 2, 246, 1971.

155. **Tomkin, G. H., Hadden, D. R., Weaver, J. A., and Montgomery, D. A. D.,** Vitamin B_{12} status of patients on long-term metformin therapy, *Brit. Med. J.,* 2, 685, 1971.

156. **Lowenstein, L., Lalonde, M., Deschenes, E. B., and Shapiro, L.,** Vitamin B_{12} in pregnancy and the puerperium, *Am. J. Clin. Nutr.,* 8, 265, 1960.

157. **Gompertz, D., Jones, J. H., and Knowles, J. P.,** Metabolic precursors of methylmalonic acid in vitamin-B_{12} deficiency, *Lancet,* 1, 424, 1967.

158. **Middleton, J. E., Coward, R. F., and Smith, P.,** Urinary excretion of A.I.C. in vitamin-B_{12} and folic-acid deficiencies, *Lancet,* 2, 258, 1964.

159. **Hibbard, B. M. and Hibbard, E. D.,** Neutrophil hypersegmentation and defective folate metabolism in pregnancy, *J. Obstet. Gynaecol. Br. Commonw.,* 78, 776, 1971.

160. **Frenkel, E. P., McCall, M. S., and White, J. D.,** Recognition and resolution of errors in the radioisotopic assay of serum vitamin B_{12}, *Am. J. Clin. Pathol.,* 53, 891, 1970.

161. **Mahmud, K., Ripley, D., and Doscherholmen, A.,** Vitamin B_{12} absorption tests. Their unreliability in postgastrectomy states, *J.A.M.A.,* 216, 1167, 1971.

162. **Arroyave, G.,** Standards for the diagnosis of vitamin deficiency in man, in *Metabolic Adaptation and Nutrition,* American Health Organization Scientific Publication No. 222, Pan American Health Organization, 525 Twenty-third Street, N.W., Washington, D.C. 20037, 1971, 88.

163. **Gawthorne, J. M., Watson, J., and Stokstad, E. L. R.,** Automated methylmalonic acid assay, *Anal. Biochem.,* 42, 555, 1971.

164. **Voogd, C. E. and Burg, P. V. D.,** Serum vitamin B_{12} levels and chlorpromazine, *Clin. Chim. Acta,* 37, 533, 1972.

165. **Dale, R. A.,** The assay of methylmalonic acid in urine, *Clin. Chim. Acta,* 41, 141, 1972.

166. **Middleton, J. E.,** Detection by paper chromatography of imidazoles, including hydantoin-5-propionic acid, in urine after histidine dosage, *J. Clin. Pathol.,* 18, 605, 1965.

167. **Van Roon-Djordjevic, B. and Van Staalen, I. C.,** Urinary excretion of histidine metabolites as an indication for folic acid and vitamin B_{12} deficiency, *Clin. Chim. Acta,* 41, 55, 1972.

168. **Herbert, V.,** The five possible causes of all nutrient deficiency: illustrated by deficiencies of vitamin B_{12} and folic acid, *Am. J. Clin. Nutr.,* 26, 77, 1973.

169. **Cook, J. D., Alvarado, J., Gutnisky, A., Jamra, M., Labardini, J., Layrisse, M., Linares, J., Loria, A., Maspes, V., Restrepo, A., Reynafarje, C., Sánchez-Medal, L., Vélez, H., and Viteri, F.,** Nutritional deficiency and anemia in Latin America: A collaborative study, *Blood,* 38, 591, 1971.

170. **Cottrall, M. F., Wells, D. G., Trott, N. G., and Richardson, N. E. G.,** Radioactive vitamin B_{12} absorption studies: comparison of the whole-body retention, urinary excretion, and eight-hour plasma levels of radioactive vitamin B_{12}, *Blood,* 38, 604, 1971.

171. **Bashir, H. V., Hinterberger, H., and Jones, B. P.,** Methylmalonic acid excretion in vitamin B_{12} deficiency, *Br. J. Haematol.,* 12, 704, 1966.

172. **Herbert, V., Gottlieb, C. W., and Lau, K.-S.,** Hemoglobin-coated charcoal assay for serum vitamin B_{12}, *Blood,* 28, 180, 1966.

173. **Matthews, D. M., Gunasegaram, R., and Linnell, J. C.,** Results with radioisotopic assay of serum B_{12} using serum binding agent, *J. Clin. Pathol.,* 20, 683, 1967.

174. **Shum, H.-Y., Streeter, A. M., and O'Neill, B. J.,** A modified isotopic dilution method for measuring the serum vitamin B_{12} level, *Med. J. Aust.,* 1, 1144, 1970.

175. **Herbert, V.,** Diagnostic and prognostic values of measurement of serum vitamin B_{12}-binding proteins, *Blood,* 32, 305, 1968.

176. **Gilbert, H. S., Krauss, S., Pasternack, B., Herbert, V., and Wasserman, L. R.,** Serum vitamin B_{12} in binding capacity (UBBC) in myeloproliferative disease. Value in differential diagnosis and as parameters of disease activity, *Ann. Intern. Med.,* 71, 719, 1969.

Niacin (Nicotinic Acid)

Although pellagra is now relatively rare in the United States, niacin deficiency continues to occur in certain maize-eating populations of other areas of the world, such as in Yugoslavia, Egypt, and among the Bantu of South Africa.[1,2,5,6,20,41] Nevertheless, clinical cases of pellagra occur, such as those in association with alcoholism. Pellagra is usually a complex disease often involving deficiencies of proteins, calories, and other members of the vitamin B-complex besides niacin. Niacin nutrition is further complicated by the ability of the amino acid, tryptophan, to serve as a precursor of nicotinic acid, and by the uncertainty of the biological availability of the bound forms of the vitamin in foods.[3-6,16,40,43]

Although it has been shown that 60 mg of tryptophan can be converted by the human body into approximately 1 mg of nicotinic acid,[7-9,43] much of the nicotinic acid in foods such as miaze is in a bound form frequently unavailable to man (e.g., niacytin).[4,5,40,43] Unless these factors are carefully considered and nicotinic acid intakes calculated in terms of biologically available nicotinic acid equivalents, dietary surveys can be misleading with respect to niacin nutrition. Since such dietary data are difficult to obtain, biochemical information has been considered more useful for evaluating niacin nutritional status.[39]

Despite the long-standing knowledge concerning the human requirement for nicotinic acid, biochemical procedures for assessing the nutritional status of this vitamin still remain uncertain. The two major metabolites of niacin are N^1-methylnicotinamide and N^1-methyl-2-pyridone-5-carboxylamide (2-pyridone). Under normal circumstances, adults excrete 20 to 30% of their nicotinic acid as the N^1-methylnicotinamide form and 40 to 60% as the 2-pyridone.[10-12,28,31] Thus, a ratio of 1.3 to 4 exists between 2-pyridone/N^1-methylnicotinamide excretion under normal conditions.[11,12] Du Plessis[10] and Lange and Joubert[12] consider a ratio value of less than 1.0 to be indicative of latent nicotinic acid deficiency.

Subjects on a daily intake of about 5 mg of nicotinic acid and 200 mg of tryptophan show clinical signs of pellagra and excrete N^1-methylnicotinamide at the rate of only 0.2 mg in 6 hr or 0.5 mg/g of creatinine.[8,13-15,19] When intakes of nicotinic acid are 8 to 10 mg and above/day, the excretion of nicotinic acid metabolites increases rapidly.[8,15] In pregnancy, N-methylnicotinamide excretion is elevated, particularly in the third trimester.[18],[45]

In nutrition surveys, including those conducted by the Interdepartmental Committee on Nutrition for National Defense (ICNND), the measurement of urinary excretion levels of N^1-methylnicotinamide has been commonly employed for evaluating niacin nutrition. This measurement has been the only practical procedure available for survey studies, although the value and interpretation of the data have been uncertain and less than satisfactory.[39] Part of the difficulty relates to the poor reproducibility observed in the methods employed and to interfering compounds present in urine. More recently, measurements for 2-pyridone have been reported to provide a more satisfactory criterion of niacin status than N^1-methylnicotinamide assays.[10],[28] However, in the past the measurement of N^1-methylnicotinamide has been favored because the assay procedure for 2-pyridone is considerably more cumbersome.[28] Both procedures are beset with the problem of interpretation of results. Usually it is not practical to collect 24-hr urine samples, or even 2- or 6-hr samples; hence, random fasting samples are employed with the metabolite levels expressed per gram of creatinine. Since the level of creatinine excretion differs in children from that of adults,

interpretation of nicotinic acid metabolite excretion data expressed in terms of creatinine has been difficult. Data are limited on the excretion of nicotinic acid metabolites in small children. Nevertheless, information available on 7 to 15-year-old children shows with increasing age a pronounced fall in both 2-pyridone and N^1-methylnicotinamide excretion when expressed in terms of creatinine (Figure 22). In the ICNND nutrition surveys, interpretation guides for niacin status were limited to N^1-methylnicotinamide excretion by adults (Table 14).

The most promising procedure for evaluating niacin status appears to be the use of the 2-pyridone/N^1-methylnicotinamide excretion ratio. Urinary-2-pyridone can be measured by the method of Joubert and de Lange[12],[28] or Price,[24],[46] and N^1-methylnicotinamide can be determined by several methods.[12],[21-23],[47],[49] While N^1-methylnicotinamide excretion falls to a minimum at about the time of appearance of clinical symptoms of pellagra or niacin deficiency,[8],[19] the excretion of 2-pyridone is essentially absent for weeks before the clinical changes are noted.[19],[24],[36] Hence, the excretion ratio of these metabolites has been observed to be a useful and probably the best criteria for evaluating niacin nutritional status under survey conditions.[10],[12],

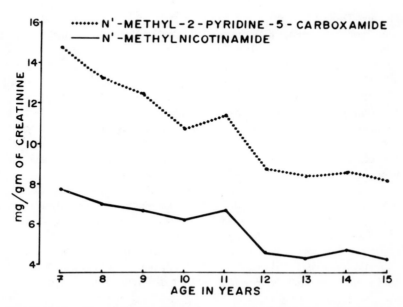

FIGURE 22. The relationship between age and urinary excretion of N-methyl-2-pyridone-5-carbox(yl)amide (2-pyridone) and N′-methylnicotinamide in white Pretoria children. (Adapted from studies of DuPlessis.[10])

71

TABLE 14

ICNND Suggested Guide to Interpretation N¹-methylnicotinamide Excretion Data[17]

Subjects	Deficient	Low	Acceptable	High
Adults:				
(males and nonpregnant				
nonlactating females)				
mg/g creatinine	< 0.5	0.5 to 1.59	1.6 to 4.29	⩾ 4.3
mg/6 hr	< 0.2	0.2 to 0.59	0.6 to 1.59	⩾ 1.6
Pregnant women:[18]				
(mg/g creatinine)				
1st trimester	< 0.5	0.5 to 1.59	1.6 to 4.29	⩾ 4.3
2nd trimester	< 0.6	0.6 to 1.99	2.0 to 4.99	⩾ 5.0
3rd trimester	< 0.8	0.8 to 2.49	2.5 to 6.49	⩾ 6.5
All age groups:				
2-pyridone/N¹-methylnicotinamide				
ratio[10,12,36]		< 1.0	1.0 to 4.0	

[27,36,48] With the age range studied (7 to 15 years), age did not appear to have a significant influence on the 2-pyridone/N¹-methylnicotinamide ratio.[10] In another report, similar ratios were noted for children less than 1 year of age and for adults.[25] Thus, apparently a single guide value can be used for all age groups in the application of the metabolite ratio procedure to evaluate niacin nutritional status. In addition, the ratio is uninfluenced by level of creatinine excretion or accuracy of collection period and is therefore particularly useful in field studies. Tentatively, a ratio value of less than 1.0 has been considered as indicative of latent niacin deficiency (Table 14).[10,12,27,36,48] Under special circumstances, erroneous deductions could occur. Such may exist when insufficient methyl groups are available to carry out the methylation of nicotinic acid or impairment or insufficiency of enzymes responsible for the formation of N¹-methylnicotinamide and 2-pyridone.[29,42] Such impairment appears rare, even in pellagra patients.[26,27]

Few additional biochemical procedures are available for evaluation of niacin nutritional status. For example, the sum or levels of N¹-methylnicotinamide and 2-pyridone excreted/24 hr appears to be a reasonably accurate reflection of niacin status.[27] Expressing the results on a 24-hr basis is preferred to expressing the values on a per gram of creatinine basis. Although not practical under field conditions, such is feasible in clinical or research situations. In the case of clinical patients suspected of having pellagra, load tests using nicotinic acid, nicotinamide or tryptophan have been proposed to aid in their diagno-

sis.[14,19,27,30-32] These load tests are based on the principle that a high retention of dose or low production of niacin metabolites indicates a state of tissue depletion. For the most part, the value of these load tests has been questioned, and their use has been limited. However, the procedure of Goldsmith and associates[14,32] may be of value in special research studies.

Only very small amounts of nicotinic acid are excreted as such in the urine. Even these amounts are relatively uninfluenced by dietary intakes of niacin or tryptophan.[8,19,29] Similarly, urinary excretion levels of tryptophan or quinolinic acid, a metabolite of nicotine acid, are of little use as an index of niacin nutritional status.[8,19]

Although little niacin is present in plasma, appreciable quantities are present in the erythrocytes and leucocytes as nicotinamide adenine dinucleotide (NAD).[28,33] In the normal adult, the following levels of NAD were observed:[34] whole blood, 30 μg/ml; erythrocytes, 90 μg/ml; serum, 0.5 μg/ml; and leucocytes, 70 μg/ml. Earlier reports indicated that NAD levels in blood of niacin-deficient subjects were not depressed.[33,35] Later it was observed that whole-blood NAD values decreased almost 40% in adults after 3 weeks on a low-niacin, low-tryptophan diet.[36] Raghuramulu et al.,[37] however, reported that the concentration of nicotinamide nucleotides in the erythrocytes of subjects suffering from pellagra was not different from that in normal subjects. More recently, Srikantia et al.[38] observed that the concentration of the individual nucleotides differed between pellagrins and normal subjects. The erythrocytes of pellagrins had significantly higher amounts of nicotinamide mononucleotide (NMN) than the erythrocytes of normal subjects, while levels of NAD and NADP tended to be lower in the pellagrins as compared to normals. At present, however, measurement of niacin compounds in blood or its components does not appear to be a reliable or satisfactory method for evaluating niacin status.

In summary, biochemical procedures for evaluating niacin status are not entirely satisfactory. A functional biochemical test has not been developed for assessing body reserves of nicotinic acid. The only practical index available is the measurement of urinary levels of N-methylnicotinamide and 2-pyridone and expressing the results in terms of creatinine excretion and their ratio.

REFERENCES

1. Scrimshaw, N. S., Progress in solving world nutrition problems, *J. Am. Diet. Assoc.*, 35, 441, 1959.
2. Darby, W. J., Nutritional deficiencies today, *J. Am. Diet. Assoc.*, 33, 17, 1957.
3. Kodicek, E., Braude, R., Kon, S. K., and Mitchell, K. G., The effect of alkaline hydrolysis of maize on the availability of its nicotinic acid to the pig, *Br. J. Nutr.*, 10, 51, 1956.
4. Pearson, W. N., Stempfel, S. J., Valenzuela, J. S., Hutley, M. H., and Darby, W. J., The influence of cooked vs. raw maize on the growth of rats receiving a 9% casein ration, *J. Nutr.*, 62, 445, 1957.
5. Kodicek, E., Nicotinic acid and the pellagra problem, *Nutr. Dieta*, 4, 109, 1962.
6. May, J. M., *Studies in Medical Geography. The Ecology of Malnutrition*, Vols. 1-11, Hafner Publ. Co., New York, 1961–1972.
7. Goldsmith, G. A., Miller, O. N., and Unglaub, W. G., Efficiency of tryptophan as a niacin precursor in man, *J. Nutr.*, 73, 172, 1961.
8. Horwitt, M. K., Harvey, C. C., Rothwell, W. S., Cutler, J. L., and Haffron, D., Tryptophan-niacin relationships in man, *J. Nutr.*, Suppl. 1, 60, 1956.
9. Vivian, V. M., Relationship between tryptophan-niacin metabolism and changes in nitrogen balance, *J. Nutr.*, 82, 395, 1964.
10. Du Plessis, J. P., An evaluation of biochemical criteria for use in nutrition status surveys, Council for Scientific and Industrial Research Report No. 261, National Nutrition Research Institute, Pretoria, South Africa, 1967.
11. Holman, W. I. M. and de Lange, D. J., Metabolism of nicotinic acid and related compounds by humans, *Nature (Lond.)*, 165, 604, 1950.
12. de Lange, D. J. and Joubert, C. P., Assessment of nicotinic acid status of population groups, *Am. J. Clin. Nutr.*, 15, 169, 1964.
13. Goldsmith, G. A., Rosenthal, H. L., Gibbens, J., and Unglaub, W. G., Studies on niacin requirement in man. II. Requirement on wheat and corn diets low in tryptophan, *J. Nutr.*, 56, 371, 1955.
14. Unglaub, W. G. and Goldsmith, G. A., Evaluation of vitamin adequacy: Urinary excretion tests, in Methods for Evaluation of Nutritional Adequacy and Status – A Symposium, Advisory Board on Quartermaster Research and Development, Committee on Foods, National Academy of Sciences, National Research Council, Washington, D.C., 1954, 73.
15. Frazier, E. I., Prather, M. E., and Hoene, E., Nicotinic acid metabolism in humans. I. The urinary excretion of nicotinic acid and its metabolic derivatives on four levels of dietary intake, *J. Nutr.*, 56, 501, 1955.
16. Goldsmith, G. A., Gibbens, J., Unglaub, W. G., and Miller, O. N., Studies of niacin requirement in man. III. Comparative effects of diets containing lime-treated and untreated corn in the production of experimental pellagra, *Am. J. Clin. Nutr.*, 4, 151, 1956.
17. Manual for Nutrition Surveys, 2nd ed., Interdepartmental Committee on Nutrition for National Defense, U.S. Govt. Printing Office, Washington, D.C. 20402, 1963.
18. Darby, W. J. et al., The Vanderbilt cooperative study of maternal and infant nutrition. IV. Dietary, laboratory and physical findings in 2,129 delivered pregnancies, *J. Nutr.*, 51, 565, 1953.
19. Goldsmith, G. A., Sarett, H. P., Register, U. D., and Gibbens, J., Studies of niacin requirement in man. I. Experimental pellagra in subjects on corn diets low in niacin and tryptophan, *J. Clin. Invest.*, 31, 533, 1952.
20. Potgieter, J. F., Fellingham, S. A., and Nesser, M. L., Incidence of nutritional diseases upon the Bantu and coloured population in South Africa as reflected by the results of a questionnaire survey, *S. Afr. Med. J.*, 40, 504, 1966.
21. Carpenter, K. J. and Kodicek, E., The fluorometric estimation of N^1-methylnicotinamide and its differentiation from coenzyme I, *Biochem. J.*, 46, 42, 1950.
22. Hochberg, M. D., Melnick, D., and Oser, B. L., Chemical determination and urinary excretion of the metabolite N^1-methylnicotinamide, *J. Biol. Chem.*, 158, 265, 1945.
23. Pelletier, O. and Campbell, J. A., A rapid method for the determination of N^1-methylnicotinamide in urine, *Anal. Biochem.*, 3, 60, 1962.

24. Walters, C. J., Brown, R. R., Kaihara, M., and Price, J. M., The excretion of N-methyl-2-pyridone-5-carboxamide by man following ingestion of several known or potential precursors, *J. Biol. Chem.,* 217, 489, 1955.

25. Careddu, P., Mainardi, L., Sacchetti, G., and Tenconi, L. T., Urinary excretion of N^1-methyl-2-pyridone-5-carbox-amide in children 3 to 12 months, *Acta Vitaminol. Milano,* 19, 135, 1965.

26. El Ridi, M. S., Abdelkader, M. M., Habib, A., Hasaballa, A., Hazzi, C., Zaki, M., and Riad, Y., The role of the liver and kidney in the metabolism of nicotinic acid amide in pellagrins, *Acta Physiol. Acad. Sci. Hung.,* 4, 429, 1960.

27. Prinsloo, J. G., Du Plessis, J. P., Kruger, H., de Lange, D. J., and de Villiers, L. S., Protein nutrition status in childhood pellagra. Evaluation of nicotinic acid status and creatinine excretion, *Am. J. Clin. Nutr.,* 21, 98, 1968.

28. Joubert, C. P. and de Lange, J., A modification of the method for the determination of N^1-methyl-2-pyridone-carboxylamide in human urine and its application in the evaluation of nicotinic acid status, *Proc. Nutr. Soc. Southern Africa,* 3, 60, 1962.

29. Gabuzda, G. J. and Davidson, C. S., Tryptophan and nicotinic acid metabolism in patients with cirrhosis of the liver, *Am. J. Clin. Nutr.,* 11, 502, 1962.

30. Lossy, F. T., Goldsmith, G. A., and Sarett, H. P., A study of test dose excretion of five B complex vitamins in man, *J. Nutr.,* 45, 213, 1951.

31. Rosenthal, H. L., Goldsmith, G. A., and Sarett, H. P., Excretion of N^1-methylnicotinamide and the 6-pyridone of N^1-methylnicotinamide in urine of human subjects, *Proc. Soc. Exp. Biol. Med.,* 84, 208, 1953.

32. Goldsmith, G. A., Miller, O. N., Unglaub, W. G., and Gibbens, J., Procedures for evaluating niacin nutrition, *Fed. Proc.,* 14, 434, 1955.

33. Klein, J. R., Perlzweig, W. A., and Handler, P., Determination of nicotinic acid in blood cells and plasma, *J. Biol. Chem.,* 145, 27, 1942.

34. Burch, H. B., Storvick, C. A., Bicknell, L., Kung, H. C., Alejo, L. G., Everhart, W. A., Lowry, O. H., King, C. G., and Bessey, O. A., Metabolic studies of precursors of pyridine nucleotides, *J. Biol. Chem.,* 212, 897, 1955.

35. Carter, C. W. and O'Brien, J. R. P., The nicotinic acid content of blood in health and disease, *Q. J. Med.,* 14, 197, 1945.

36. Vivian, V. M., Chaloupka, M. M., and Reynolds, M. S., Some aspects of tryptophan metabolism in human subjects. I. Nitrogen balances, blood pyridine nucleotides and urinary excretion of N^1-methylnicotinamide and N^1-methyl-2-pyridone-5-carboxamide on a low-niacin diet, *J. Nutr.,* 66, 587, 1958.

37. Raghuramula, N., Srikantia, S. G., Narasinga Rao, B. S., and Gopalan, C., Nicotinamide nucleotides in the erythrocytes of patients suffering from pellagra, *Biochem. J.,* 96, 837, 1965.

38. Srikantia, S. G., Narasinga Rao, B. S., Raghuramulu, N., and Gopalan, C., Pattern of nicotinamide nucleotides in the erythrocytes of pellagrins, *Am. J. Clin. Nutr.,* 21, 1306, 1968.

39. Pearson, W. N., Assessment of nutritional status: Biochemical Methods, in *Nutrition,* Vol. III, Beaton, G. H. and McHenry, E. W., Eds., Academic Press, New York, 1966, 265.

40. Harper, A. E., Punekar, B. D., and Elvehjem, C. A., The effect of alkali treatment on the availability of niacin and amino acids in maize, *J. Nutr.,* 66, 163, 1958.

41. Du Plessis, J. P., Wittmann, W., Louw, M. E. J., and Nel, A., The clinical and biochemical effects of riboflavin and nicotinamide supplementation upon Bantu school children using maize meal as carrier medium, *S. Afr. Med. J.,* 45, 530, 1971.

42. Tabaqchali, S. and Pallis, C., Reversible nicotinamide-deficiency encephalopathy in a patient with jejunal diverticulosis, *Gut,* 11, 1024, 1970.

43. Goldsmith, G. A., Niacin: Antipellagra factor, hypocholesterolemic agent, *J.A.M.A.,* 194, 167, 1965.

44. Goldsmith, G. A., The B vitamins: Thiamine, riboflavin, niacin, in *Nutrition,* Vol. II, Beaton, G. H. and McHenry, E. W., Eds., Academic Press, New York, 1964, 109.

45. Lojkin, M. E., Wertz, A. W., and Dietz, C. G., Metabolism of nicotinic acid in pregnancy, *J. Nutr.,* 46, 335, 1952.

46. Price, J. M., The determination of N^1-methyl-2-pyridone-5-carboxamide in human urine, *J. Biol. Chem.,* 211, 117, 1954.

47. Huff, J. W. and Perlzweig, W. A., The fluorescent condensation product of N^1-methylnicotinamide and acetone. II. A sensitive method for the determination of N^1-methylnicotinamide in urine, *J. Biol. Chem.,* 167, 157, 1947.

48. Perlzweig, W. A., Rosen, F., and Pearson, P. B., Comparative studies in niacin metabolism. The fate of niacin in man, rat, dog, pig, rabbit, guinea pig, goat, sheep and calf, *J. Nutr.,* 40, 453, 1950.

49. Vivian, V. M., Reynolds, M. S., and Price, J. M., Use of ion-exchange resins for the determination of N^1-methylnicotinamide in human urine, *Anal. Biochem.,* 10, 274, 1965.

Vitamin E (Tocopherol)

The precise biochemical mechanism whereby vitamin E functions in the body remains to be elucidated.[1,17,29,42,73,83] Although a vitamin E deficiency in humans is uncommon,[17,29] it has been reported to occur in some newborn infants,[2-10,24,25,29,36,73,74,84] in patients with acanthocytosis,[11,12] in some cases with malabsorption of fats,[4,13,26,29] in association with protein-calorie malnutrition,[7,30] and in certain other diseases.[17,38-40,59,60] There has been some suggestion that vitamin E requirements are related to the dietary intake of polyunsaturated fatty acids.[1,10,14-19,33,73,76] Vitamin E deficiency has been associated with anemia,[6-8,17,22-25,32,33-37,73] low plasma levels of tocopherol,[17,20,21,29,31,45,78] creatinuria,[7,29,39] and susceptibility of erythrocytes to hemolysis in vitro by dilute solutions of hydrogen peroxide.[26,27-29,31-35,41,45,77,78,84]

The extensive and lengthy study conducted by Horwitt and associates[15,33,34,42-44] on vitamin E deficiency in adult males has provided considerable information concerning the biochemical changes that occur with low intakes of tocopherol. Their investigation demonstrated a relationship of decreasing plasma tocopherol levels to increased susceptibility of erythrocytes to hemolysis in the presence of hydrogen peroxide (Figure 23).[33] Their work also established that the requirement for vitamin E is a function of the tissue content of polyunsaturated fatty acids.[15,33,34,42,43] Thus, when the intake of linoleic acid from corn oil was increased from 16.5 g to 33 g daily, the supplement of d-a-tocopherol was doubled to 27.2 mg daily in order to prevent a decrease in plasma tocopherol levels.

In the earlier studies of György and associates[5,27,41] and others,[2,26,35] it was observed that red blood cells from vitamin E-deficient rats and from certain infants and children were susceptible to the hemolyzing effects of dilute solutions of hydrogen peroxide or dialuric acid. The hemolysis could be prevented by in vitro or in vivo supplements of vitamin E.[2,5,26,35] The hemolysis test for vitamin E deficiency has evolved from these studies.

The erythrocyte hemolysis test represents an indirect in vitro measurement of vitamin E nuriture which correlates quite well with serum and plasma levels of tocopherol (Figures 23 and 24).[5,26,29,34] Binder and Spiro[29] concluded from their studies that there was an excellent correlation between serum tocopherol levels and the hydrogen peroxide hemolysis test. They observed that almost every subject with an elevated hydrogen peroxide hemolysis test had a low serum tocopherol level and that most subjects with normal hemolysis tests had normal serum tocopherol levels (Figure 24).

Various erythrocyte hemolysis tests have been developed[2,5,27,28,34,47-49,53,70,74,77,78] using either hydrogen peroxide, dialuric acid or isotonic saline-phosphate buffer as the hemolyzing agent. However, the hydrogen peroxide erythrocyte hemolysis test has been used most commonly.[2,5,27,28,35,77,78] The procedure is relatively simple, involving the incubation of washed ery-

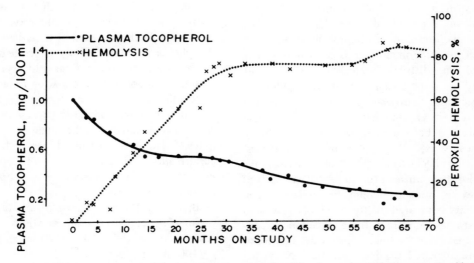

FIGURE 23. Relationship of average plasma tocopherol levels to average hydrogen peroxide hemolysis of red blood cells from experimental human subjects on vitamin E deficient diets. (From Horwitt.[33])

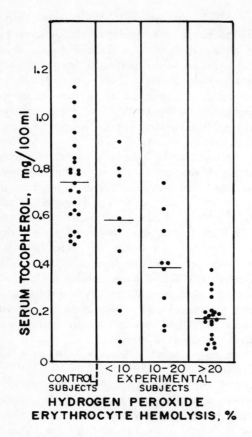

FIGURE 24. Relationship between serum tocopherol levels and hydrogen peroxide hemolysis of red blood cells in human subjects. (From Binder and Spiro.[29])

throcytes in a 2 to 2.4% hydrogen peroxide solution for a period of 3 hr. The amount of hemoglobin produced by hemolysis during the hydrogen peroxide incubation is compared to that produced in distilled water and the result expressed as a percentage. Tentative guides for evaluating the hydrogen peroxide erythrocyte hemolysis test are indicated in Table 15. The procedure has been used in civilian and military nutrition surveys[28,50] as well as in clinical studies.

The dialuric acid test[47,48,70] and the isotonic saline-phosphate buffer procedure[49] have received little use in human vitamin E studies.[59] The authors have compared the three hemolysis tests in human studies and from these experiences concluded that the hydrogen peroxide hemolysis procedure appeared the most practical. Nevertheless, the hydrogen peroxide hemolysis procedure must be performed in a standardized manner with caution exercised with regard to sample handling,

time lapse between sample collection and test performance, preparation of reagents, and incubation temperature.

Recently, the measurement of blood-cell fragility with the use of a Fragiligraph (Kalmedic Instruments, Inc., 425 Park Avenue, New York, N.Y. 10022) has been proposed for evaluating vitamin E nutritional status.[51,52] Although the procedure may have application, further investigations are required to establish its usefulness in vitamin E nutritional assessments.[51]

As noted above, erythrocyte hemolysis tests provide indirect information concerning vitamin E status. More direct information can be obtained by measuring tocopherol levels in the serum or plasma.[3,8,10,17,21,26,29,71,75-78] A number of chemical methods have been employed to determine the tocopherols in blood and blood components.[16,21,54-59,61-69] However, the Emmerie-Engel reaction is the basis for most of the commonly used methods for the measurement of tocopherols.[16,21,54-56,59,61,68,72,75] More recently, gas-liquid chromatography procedures have been applied to tocopherol measurements.[55,62,63] In these methods, the a-tocopherol in a total lipid extract is oxidized with ferric chloride-bipyridyl to a-tocopherol quinone which is purified by thin-layer chromatography and quantified by gas-liquid chromatography.[55]

Both plasma (serum) and erythrocytes have been analyzed for their tocopherol content as an index of vitamin E status. The rat studies of Bieri and Poukka did not indicate that the erythrocyte content of a-tocopherol would serve as a more accurate indicator of vitamin E status than would the plasma content.[48] They concluded that, due to the relatively constant ratio of erythrocyte to plasma a-tocopherol over a wide range of blood levels, the determination of plasma a-tocopherol should be preferred primarily because of its ease of analysis compared to the analysis of erythrocytes.[48] However, in some types of human lipid abnormalities, plasma levels of a-tocopherol may be misleading and erythrocyte a-tocopherol may be more informative.[59]

Bieri and Poukka reported the red cell and plasma a-tocopherol concentrations of normal subjects to be 230 ± 13 μg/100 ml and 984 ± 91 μg/100 ml, respectively.[59] The variation in the a-tocopherol of the red cell was considerably less than the variation in plasma. The ratio of red cell: plasma a-tocopherol ranged from 0.123 to 0.418

TABLE 15

Tentative Guidelines for Interpreting Vitamin E Data[28]

(for all age groups)

Classification category	Determination	
	Serum a-tocopherol level* mg/100 ml	Erythrocyte H_2O_2 hemolysis %
Deficient	< 0.50	> 20
Low	0.50 to 0.70	10 to 20
Acceptable	> 0.70	< 10

*Serum (plasma) a-tocopherol levels will vary according to the method of analysis.[55,59,75,77,78]

with an average of 0.254. Bieri and associates[46] had previously observed that normal adult males and females in the Washington, D.C. area had an average serum tocopherol level of 1.06 mg/100 ml, while the average serum tocopherol levels of adult males and females of East Pakistan (Bangladesh) were only 0.76 and 0.73 mg/100 ml, respectively.[37] Harris and co-workers[20] found a mean plasma tocopherol level of 1.05 ± 0.32 mg/100 ml in Rochester, N.Y. factory workers which was similar to the values noted in previous reports.[20] Similar plasma tocopherol levels have been observed by other investigators for children and young adults.[79-82] Herting and Drury reported considerably lower plasma tocopherol levels in normal adult subjects.[21] The lower values may be related to the analytical methods employed as noted by Bieri and Poukka.[48,55,59] In the study of Lewis et al.,[76] all adult subjects and all normal children had plasma tocopherol levels above 0.6 mg/100 ml.

Nevertheless, simultaneous determinations of plasma tocopherol and erythrocyte hydrogen peroxide hemolysis indicate that, when the tocopherol level was above 0.5 mg/100 ml of plasma, appreciable hemolysis was rarely observed (Figures 23 and 24; Table 15).[4,26,29,77] What is not certain is whether vitamin E status, as determined by plasma tocopherol levels or by in vitro erythrocyte hemolysis, is indicative of the a-tocopherol status of the other tissues of the body.[59] Information on the tocopherol content of human adipose tissue has not appeared useful in this respect.[19,72]

In view of these limitations, vitamin E nutritional status should be evaluated, whenever feasible, by performing both plasma tocopherol level measurements and erythrocyte hemolysis tests. However, measurement of plasma tocopherol is rather technically difficult and, for this reason, the erythrocyte hemolysis test has been more commonly employed in nutrition surveys to evaluate vitamin E status.

REFERENCES

1. *The Fat-Soluble Vitamins,* De Luca, H. F. and Suttie, J. W., Eds., The University of Wisconsin Press, Madison, 1969, 293.
2. **Gordon, H. H., Nitowsky, H. M., and Cornblath, M.,** Studies of tocopherol deficiency in infants and children. I. Hemolysis of erythrocytes in hydrogen peroxide, *Am. J. Dis. Child.,* 90, 669, 1955.
3. **Nitowsky, H. M., Hsu, K. S., and Gordon, H. H.,** Vitamin E requirements of human infants, *Vitam. Horm.,* 20, 559, 1962.
4. **Binder, H. J., Herting, D. C., Hurst, V., Finch, S. C., and Spiro, H. M.,** Tocopherol deficiency in man, *N. Engl. J. Med.,* 273, 1289, 1965.
5. **György, P., Cogan, G., and Rose, C. S.,** Availability of vitamin E in the newborn infant, *Proc. Soc. Exp. Biol. Med.,* 81, 536, 1952.

6. **Gordon, H. H., Nitowsky, H. M., Tildon, H. M., and Levin, S.,** Studies of tocopherol deficiency in infants and children, *Pediatrics,* 21, 673, 1958.

7. **Majaj, A. S., Dinning, J. S., Azzam, S. A., and Darby, W. J.,** Vitamin E responsive megaloblastic anemia in infants with protein-calorie malnutrition, *Am. J. Clin. Nutr.,* 12, 374, 1963.

8. **Asfour, R. Y. and Firzli, S.,** Hematologic studies in undernourished children with low serum vitamin E levels, *Am. J. Clin. Nutr.,* 17, 158, 1965.

9. **Horwitt, M. K. and Bailey, P.,** Cerebellar pathology in an infant resembling chick nutritional encephalomalacia, *A. M. A. Arch. Neurol.,* 1, 312, 1959.

10. **Hassan, H., Hashim, S. A., Van Itallie, B., and Sebrell, W. H.,** Syndrome in premature infants associated with low plasma vitamin E levels and high polyunsaturated fatty acid diet, *Am. J. Clin. Nutr.,* 19, 147, 1966.

11. **Siber, R. and Kayden, H. J.,** Vitamin E deficiency and autohemolysis in acanthocytosis, *Blood,* 26, 895, 1965.

12. **Kayden, H. J. and Silber, R.,** The role of vitamin E deficiency in the abnormal autohemolysis of acanthocytosis, *Trans. Assoc. Am. Physicians Phila.,* 78, 334, 1965.

13. **Darby, W. J., Cherrington, M. E., and Ruffin, J. M.,** Plasma tocopherol levels in sprue, *Proc. Soc. Exp. Biol. Med.,* 63, 310, 1946.

14. **Dayton, S., Hashimoto, S., Rosenblum, D., and Pearce, M. L.,** Vitamin E status of humans during prolonged feeding of unsaturated fats, *J. Lab. Clin. Med.,* 65, 739, 1965.

15. **Horwitt, M. K.,** Interrelations between vitamin E and polyunsaturated fatty acids in adult men, *Vitam. Horm.,* 20, 541, 1962.

16. **Hashim, S. A. and Schuttringer, G. R.,** Rapid determination of tocopherol in macro- and microquantities of plasma. Results obtained in various nutrition and metabolic studies, *Am. J. Clin. Nutr.,* 19, 137, 1966.

17. **Herting, D. C.,** Perspective on vitamin E, *Am. J. Clin. Nutr.,* 19, 210, 1966.

18. **Harris, P. L. and Embree, N. D.,** Quantitative consideration of the effect of polyunsaturated fatty acid content of the diet upon the requirements for vitamin E, *Am. J. Clin. Nutr.,* 13, 385, 1963.

19. **Imaichi, K. K., Cox, S., Kinsell, L. W., Schelstraete, M., and Olcott, H. S.,** Tocopherol content of human adipose tissue, *Am. J. Clin. Nutr.,* 16, 347, 1965.

20. **Harris, P. L., Hardenbrook, E. G., Dean, F. P., Cusack, E. R., and Jensen, J. L.,** Blood tocopherol values in normal human adults and incidence of vitamin E deficiency, *Proc. Soc. Exp. Biol. Med.,* 107, 381, 1961.

21. **Herting, D. C. and Drury, E. J. E.,** Plasma tocopherol levels in man, *Am. J. Clin. Nutr.,* 17, 351, 1965.

22. **Melhorn, D. K. and Gross, S.,** Vitamin E-dependent anemia in the premature infant. I. Effects of large doses of medicinal iron, *J. Pediatr.,* 79, 569, 1971.

23. **Melhorn, D. K. and Gross, S.,** Vitamin E-dependent anemia in the premature infant. II. Relationship between gestational age and absorption of vitamin E, *J. Pediatr.,* 79, 581, 1971.

24. **Oski, F. A. and Barness, L. A.,** Vitamin E deficiency: A previously unrecognized cause of hemolytic anemia in the premature infant, *J. Pediatr.,* 70, 211, 1967.

25. **Ritchie, J. H., Fish, M. B., McMasters, V., and Grossman, M.,** Edema and hemolytic anemia in premature infants, *N. Engl. J. Med.,* 27, 1185, 1969.

26. **Nitowsky, H. M., Cornblath, M., and Gordon, H. H.,** Studies of tocopherol deficiency in infants and children. II. Plasma tocopherol and erythrocyte hemolysis in hydrogen peroxide, *Am. J. Dis. Child.,* 92, 164, 1956.

27. **Rose, C. S. and György, P.,** Specificity of hemolytic reaction in vitamin E deficient erythrocytes, *Am. J. Physiol.,* 168, 414, 1952.

28. Interdepartmental Committee on Nutrition for National Defense, *Union of Burma Nutrition Survey Report,* U.S. Govt. Printing Office, Washington, D.C., May 1963, 171.

29. **Binder, H. J. and Spiro, H. M.,** Tocopherol deficiency in man, *Am. J. Clin. Nutr.,* 20, 594, 1967.

30. **Majaj, A. S.,** Vitamin E-responsive macrocytic anemia in protein-calorie malnutrition. Measurements of vitamin E, folic acid, vitamin C, vitamin B_{12} and iron, *Am. J. Clin. Nutr.,* 18, 362, 1966.

31. **Tulloch, J. A. and Sood, N. K.,** Vitamin deficiency in Uganda, *Am. J. Clin. Nutr.,* 20, 384, 1967.

32. **Oski, F. A. and Barness, L. A.,** Hemolytic anemia in vitamin E deficiency, *Am. J. Clin. Nutr.,* 21, 45, 1968.

33. **Horwitt, M. K.,** Vitamin E and lipid metabolism in man, *Am. J. Clin. Nutr.,* 8, 451, 1960.

34. **Horwitt, M. K., Harvey, C. C., Duncan, G. D., and Wilson, W. C.,** Effects of limited tocopherol intake in man with relationship to erythrocyte hemolysis and lipid oxidations, *Am. J. Clin. Nutr.,* 4, 408, 1956.

35. **Gordon, H. H. and DeMetry, J. P.,** Hemolysis in hydrogen peroxide of erythrocytes of premature infants. Effects of alpha-tocopherol, *Proc. Soc. Exp. Biol. Med.,* 79, 446, 1952.

36. **Darby, W. J., Ferguson, M. E., Furman, R. H., Lemley, J. M., Ball, C. T., and Meneely, G. R.,** Plasma tocopherols in health and disease, *Ann. N.Y. Acad. Sci.,* 52, 328, 1949.

37. **Rahman, M. M., Hossain, S., Talukdar, S. A., Ahmad, K., and Bieri, J. G.,** Serum vitamin E levels in the rural population of East Pakistan, *Proc. Soc. Exp. Biol. Med.,* 117, 113, 1964.

38. **Higashi, O. and Fujiwara, T.,** Vitamin E deficiency in a child with intestinal lymphangiectasia, *Tohoku J. Exp. Med.,* 102, 169, 1970.

39. **Nitowsky, H. M., Gordon, H. H., and Tildon, J. T.,** Studies of tocopherol deficiency in infants and children. IV. The effect of alpha tocopherol on creatinuria in patients with cystic fibrosis of the pancreas and biliary atresia, *Bull. Johns Hopkins Hosp.,* 98, 361, 1956.

40. **Molenaar, I., Hommes, F. A., Bramms, W. G., and Polman, H. A.,** Effect of vitamin E on membranes of the intestinal cell, *Proc. Natl. Acad. Sci.,* 61, 982, 1968.

41. **György, P. and Rose, C. S.,** Tocopherol and hemolysis in vivo and in vitro, *Ann. N.Y. Acad. Sci.,* 52, 231, 1949.

42. **Horwitt, M. K.,** Vitamin E in human nutrition — an interpretative review, *Borden's Rev. Nutr. Res.,* 22, 1, 1961.

43. **Horwitt, M. K., Harvey, C. C., Century, B., and Witting, L. A.,** Polyunsaturated lipids and tocopherol requirements, *J. Am. Diet. Assoc.,* 38, 231, 1961.

44. **Horwitt, M. K., Century, B., and Zeman, A. A.,** Erythrocyte survival time and reticulocyte levels after tocopherol depletion in man, *Am. J. Clin. Nutr.,* 12, 99, 1963.

45. **Mackenzie, J. B.,** Relation between serum tocopherol and hemolysis in hydrogen peroxide of erythrocytes in premature infants, *Pediatrics,* 13, 346, 1954.

46. **Bieri, J. G., Teets, L., Belavady, B., and Andrews, E. L.,** Serum vitamin E levels in a normal adult population in the Washington, D.C. area, *Proc. Soc. Exp. Biol. Med.,* 117, 133, 1964.

47. **Friedman, L., Weiss, W., Wherry, F., and Klive, O. L.,** Bioassay of vitamin E by the dialuric acid hemolysis test, *J. Nutr.,* 65, 143, 1958.

48. **Bieri, J. G. and Poukka, R. K. H.,** In vitro hemolysis as related to rat erythrocyte content of α-tocopherol and polyunsaturated fatty acids, *J. Nutr.,* 100, 557, 1970.

49. **Draper, H. H. and Csallany, A. S.,** A simplified hemolysis test for vitamin E deficiency, *J. Nutr.,* 98, 390, 1969.

50. **Canham, J. E.,** U.S. Army Medical Research and Nutrition Laboratory, Fitzsimons Army Medical Center, Denver, Colorado 80240, personal communication.

51. **Brin, M.,** Hoffmann-La Roche, Nutley, New Jersey, personal communication.

52. **Stadin, R.,** Blood-cell fragility measurement, *Medical Electronics and Data,* Jan — Feb 1970, 89.

53. **Bliss, C. I. and György, P.,** VII. Bioassays of vitamin E, in *The Vitamins,* Vol. VI, 2nd ed., György, P. and Pearson, W. N., Eds., Academic Press, New York, 1967, 306.

54. **Bunnell, R. H.,** Vitamin E assay by chemical methods, in *The Vitamins,* Vol. VI, 2nd ed., György, P. and Pearson, W. N., Eds., Academic Press, New York, 1967, 261.

55. **Bieri, J. G., Poukka, R. K. H., and Prival, E. L.,** Determination of α-tocopherol in erythrocytes by gas-liquid chromatography, *J. Lipid Res.,* 11, 118, 1970.

56. **Bieri, J. G.,** Chromatography of tocopherols, in *Lipid Chromatographic Analysis,* Vol. 2, Marinetti, G. V., Ed., M. Dekker, Inc., New York, 1969, 459.

57. **Emmerie, A. and Engle, C.,** Colorimetric determination of *dl-α*-tocopherol (vitamin E), *Nature,* 142, 873, 1938.

58. **Quaife, M. L. and Harris, P. L.,** Chemical estimation of tocopherols in blood plasma, *J. Biol. Chem.,* 156, 499, 1944.

59. **Bieri, J. G. and Poukka, R. K. H.,** Red cell content of vitamin E and fatty acids in normal subjects and patients with abnormal lipid metabolism, *Int. J. Vitam. Nutr. Res.,* 40, 344, 1970.

60. **Dodge, J. T., Cohen, G., Kayden, H. J., and Phillips, G. B.,** Peroxidative hemolysis of red blood cells from patients with abetalipoproteinemia (acanthocytosis), *J. Clin. Invest.,* 46, 357, 1967.

61. **Quaife, M. L., Scrimshaw, N. S., and Lowry, O. H.,** Micromethod for assay of total tocopherols in blood serum, *J. Biol. Chem.,* 18, 1229, 1949.

62. **Nair, P. P. and Turner, D. A.,** The application of gas-liquid chromatography to the determination of vitamins E and K, *J. Am. Oil Chem. Soc.,* 40, 353, 1963.

63. **Bieri, J. G. and Andrews, E. L.,** The determination of α-tocopherol in animal tissues by gas-liquid chromatography, *Iowa State J. Sci.,* 38, 3, 1963.

64. **Sturm, P. A., Parkhurst, R. M., and Skinner, W. A.,** Quantitative determination of individual tocopherols by thin-layer chromatographic separation and spectrophotometry, *Anal. Chem.,* 38, 1244, 1966.

65. **Fabianek, J., De Filippi, J., Rickards, T., and Herp, A.,** Micromethod for tocopherol determination in blood serum, *Clin. Chem.,* 14, 456, 1968.

66. **Duggan, D. E.,** Spectrofluorometric determination of tocopherols, *Arch. Biochem. Biophys.,* 84, 116, 1959.

67. **Herting, D. C. and Drury, E. J. E.,** Thin-layer chromatography with precoated alumina sheets. II. Application to tocopherols, *J. Chromatogr.,* 30, 502, 1967.

68. **Hansen, L. G. and Warwick, W. J.,** A fluorometric micro-method for serum tocopherol, *Am. J. Clin. Pathol.,* 46, 133, 1966.

69. **Bayfield, R. F., Falk, R. H., and Barrett, J. D.,** The separation and determination of α-tocopherol and carotenoids in serum and plasma by paper chromatography, *J. Chromatogr.,* 36, 54, 1968.

70. **Tsen, C. C. and Collier, H. B.,** The protective action of tocopherol against hemolysis of rat erythrocytes by dialuric acid, *Can. J. Biochem. Physiol.,* 38, 957, 1960.

71. **Gross, S. and Guilford, M. V.,** Vitamin E relationship in premature infants, *J. Nutr.,* 100, 1099, 1970.

72. **McMasters, V., Lewis, J. K., Kinsell, L. W., Van Der Veen, J., and Olcott, H. S.,** Effect of supplementing the diet of man with tocopherol on the tocopherol levels of adipose tissue and plasma, *Am. J. Clin. Nutr.,* 17, 357, 1965.

73. **Nair, P. P. and Kayden, H. J., Eds.,** Vitamin E and its role in cellular metabolism, *Ann. N.Y. Acad. Sci.,* 203, 3, 1972.

74. **Younkin, S., Oski, F. A., and Barness, L. A.,** Mechanism of the hydrogen peroxide hemolysis test and its reversal with phenols, *Am. J. Clin. Nutr.,* 24, 7, 1971.

75. **McMasters, V., Howard, T., Kinsell, L. W., Van Der Veen, J., and Olcott, H. S.,** Tocopherol storage and depletion in adipose tissue and plasma of normal and diabetic human subjects, *Am. J. Clin. Nutr.,* 20, 622, 1967.

76. **Lewis, J. S., Pian, A. K., Baer, M. T., Acosta, P. B., and Emerson, G. A.,** Effect of long-term ingestion of polyunsaturated fat, age, plasma cholesterol, diabetes mellitus and supplemental tocopherol upon plasma tocopherol, *Am. J. Clin. Nutr.,* 26, 136, 1973.

77. **Horwitt, M. K., Harvey, C. C., and Harmon, E. M.,** Lipids, α-tocopherol and erythrocyte hemolysis, *Vitam. Horm.,* 26, 487, 1968.

78. **Leonard, P. J. and Losowsky, M. S.,** Relationship between plasma vitamin E level and peroxide hemolysis test in human subjects, *Am. J. Clin. Nutr.,* 20, 795, 1967.

79. **Muller, D. P. R. and Harries, J. T.,** Vitamin E studies in children with malabsorption, *Biochem. J.,* 112, 28, 1969.

80. **Bennett, M. J. and Medwadowski, B. F.,** Vitamin A, vitamin E, and lipids in serum of children with cystic fibrosis or congenital heart defects compared with normal children, *Am. J. Clin. Nutr.,* 20, 415, 1967.

81. **Baker, H., Frank, O., Feingold, S., Christakis, G., and Ziffer, H.,** Vitamins, total cholesterol, and triglycerides in 642 New York City school children, *Am. J. Clin. Nutr.,* 20, 850, 1967.

82. **Desai, I. D.,** Plasma tocopherol levels in normal adults, *Can. J. Physiol. Pharmacol.,* 46, 819, 1968.

83. **Green, J.,** Tocopherols IX. Biochemical systems, in *The Vitamins,* Vol. V, 2nd ed., Sebrell, W. H., Jr. and Harris, R. S., Eds., Academic Press, New York, 1972, 259.

84. **Mason, K. E. and Horwitt, M. K.,** Tocopherols XI. Effects of deficiency in man, in *The Vitamins,* Vol. V, 2nd ed., Sebrell, W. H., Jr. and Harris, R. S., Eds., Academic Press, New York, 1972, 293.

Vitamin D

Vitamin D is required by humans of all ages for maintenance of skeletal integrity and proper utilization of calcium.[1-3,29,47,48] Since the requirement can be met by the ingestion of vitamin D_2 or vitamin D_3 or in part or entirely by skin exposure to sunlight, biochemical procedures used to evaluate vitamin D nutriture cannot be correlated with dietary intake of the nutrient.

The greatest need for vitamin D appears to exist in infants and children in whom rickets may develop in the presence of inadequate intakes of the vitamin. Hence, it is within these age groups that biochemical procedures to assess vitamin D nutriture would be most useful. Unfortunately, at present no fully acceptable specific measurement is available to assess the adequacy of vitamin D nutriture. Methods currently available for the measurement of vitamin D or its metabolic products preclude direct measurements in blood or urine as a routine means of evaluating vitamin D nutritive status.[3-6,25,43] Consequently, indirect measurements, such as serum alkaline phosphatase activity, are employed.

Serum alkaline phosphatase activity measurements have been the most reliable and useful biochemical determination for the confirmation of clinically diagnosed rickets.[7-8,25,29,31,38,43] Alkaline phosphatase activity generally rises early with the onset of rickets, even before clinical manifestations, and the increase tends to be proportional to the severity of the vitamin D deficiency. The enzyme activity can be easily measured using manual or automated procedures that require only a very small quantity of serum.[9,10,23,24,42,44] Hence, alkaline phosphatase serum activity measurements are a practical means for evaluating vitamin D nutritional status in nutrition surveys.[19,31-36] However, serum alkaline phosphatase data must be interpreted with caution since the enzyme activity is susceptible to alteration by a variety of other disease processes.[11,16] Thus, serum alkaline phosphatase levels may be reduced in cases with kwashiorkor[12,13,22] or protein-calorie malnutrition,[14] and this may mask the rise induced by a vitamin D deficiency. In general, the use of serum alkaline phosphatase activity measurements to detect subclinical states of a vitamin D deficiency has not been a satisfactory index.[31,35] This is largely due to the fact that the relationship of the level of serum alkaline phosphatase to states of subclinical vitamin D deficiency has not been clearly established. Thus, the measurement of this enzyme may not in itself be a sole index for diagnosing subclinical vitamin D deficiency but may be useful as a screening procedure.

In osteomalacia of adults, which may occur as a result of a vitamin D deficiency, serum alkaline phosphatase activity may increase.[29,37,39,40,43] The increase in alkaline phosphatase is not specific and may occur in a number of other conditions such as metastatic carcinoma, Paget's disease, hyperparathyroidism, and osteogenic sarcoma.[11,15,16,38]

Serum alkaline phosphatase levels are usually

expressed in terms of Bodansky units although international units, King-Armstrong units, Kind-King units and other units are sometimes used.[23,42] The normal level in the child is 5 to 15 Bodansky units/100 ml of serum,[20] while for the normal adult it ranges from 3 to 5 units.[11] In the child with clinically active rickets, the serum alkaline phosphatase level usually increases to above 20 Bodansky units (Table 16).

Some useful information concerning vitamin D deficiency status may be obtained from serum calcium and phosphorus measurements.[30,38,39,43,45] Rickets are generally associated with a decrease in blood levels of inorganic phosphorus and usually, but not always, with low calcium levels. However, these changes are not entirely specific to vitamin D deficiency since, for example, in cases of parathyroid hyperactivity, serum calcium is generally elevated and serum phosphorus decreased. Osteomalacia in adults is usually associated with a decrease in the concentration of serum calcium.[43]

Serum calcium levels in the normal infant and adult range from 9.5 to 10.5 mg/100 ml. The serum inorganic phosphorus concentration in the normal adult is 3.0 to 4.5 mg/100 ml with an average of about 3.8 mg. The serum inorganic phosphorus level in the infant is much higher and more variable with a range of 5 to 8 mg/100 ml and an average of about 6.5 mg. Except in the possible case of patients with renal failure, a reduced serum Ca x P product (in mg percent) is associated with all types of rickets and osteomalacia, and that elevation of the product by whatever means cures the disease.[7,21,49] A product below 30 usually indicates that rickets is present or will develop while such will not occur when it is above 40. Children, as well as adults, with vitamin D deficiency rickets are often observed to have low urinary excretion of calcium, elevated excretions of phosphorus and an associated aminoaciduria with excess urinary proline and hydroxyproline.[25,38,43]

Recently, Wittle et al.[43] used the serum-phosphate response to intravenous vitamin D as a method for detecting clinical or subclinical vitamin D deficiency. Adult control and patient subjects were given an intravenous dose of 1 mg (40,000 I.U.) of vitamin D_3. During the following 5 days, fasting blood samples were obtained for serum or plasma phosphate determinations. Changes in the serum or plasma phosphate levels were expressed as a percentage difference above or below the basal value. The results of the study suggested that a significant increase in the fasting serum phosphate level after intravenous vitamin D administration may provide a sensitive and convenient index of vitamin D deficiency in the human.[43] Additional studies appear warranted to establish the reliability and usefulness of the procedure.

A phosphorus load test has also been suggested as a means of detecting a mild state of vitamin D deficiency. This was based on the observed decrease in plasma calcium in vitamin D deficiency

TABLE 16

Approximate Serum Levels of Alkaline Phosphatase, Calcium and Phosphorus in Normal and in Various Disease States

Serum alkaline phosphatase

Condition	Bodansky units (per 100 ml)	King-Armstrong units (per 100 ml)	International units* ($\mu M/min/\ell$)	Serum Ca mg/100 ml	Serum P mg/100 ml
Normal					
Infant	5 to 15	14 to 42	26 to 80	10	5 to 8
Adult	3 to 5	8 to 14	16 to 26	10	3 to 4.5
Rickets (children)	> 20	> 55	>115	8 to 9	3
Osteomalacia	15	42	80	9	2 to 3
Hyperparathyroidism	4 to 20	11 to 55	20 to 120	12 to 16	2 to 8
Osteoporosis	2	5	10	10 to 12	4 to 5
Paget's disease	50	140	268	10	4
Neoplasm:osteoblastic	30	85	160	10	4

*Based on use of Bodansky values. Somewhat different values may be obtained depending upon the methods or conditions used.

states 24 hr after an oral administration of standard doses of sodium phosphate.[45] This procedure appears to have received little acceptance for detecting vitamin D deficiency.

An epiphysometer has been suggested for use for the measurement of epiphyseal enlargement at the wrist as a simple objective method for the diagnosis of rickets in the field.[17] Although the measurement of wrist width or girth may be useful in the clinic, this technique appears to be of limited value in surveys on rickets.[18] Similarly,

x-ray examinations are usually not feasible in field surveys but are useful and essential for the diagnosis of clinical patients with active or healing rickets.

Thus, whenever a clinical case of active rickets or abnormal calcium metabolism is encountered or suspected, the diagnosis is usually supplemented with radiographic examinations[46] and, if warranted, with calcium-47 space measurements,[26] calcium-45 absorption tests[27] and bone biopsy studies.[28,41]

REFERENCES

1. *Recommended Dietary Allowances,* 1968, 7th ed., Food and Nutrition Board, National Academy of Sciences-National Research Council, Washington, D.C., Publ. 1964.

2. **Arnstein, A. R., Framne, R., and Frost, H. M.,** Recent progress in osteomalacia and rickets, *Ann. Int. Med.,* 67, 1296, 1967.

3. **Hoffenberg, F. H. and Black, E.,** Calcium kinetics in vitamin D deficiency rickets, *Metabolism,* 14, 1101, 1965.

4. **Kodicek, E. and Lawson, D. E. M.,** Vitamin D, in *The Vitamins,* Vol. VI, 2nd ed., György, P. and Pearson, W. N., Eds., Academic Press, New York, 1967, 211.

5. **Thomas, W. C., Jr., Morgan, H. G., Connor, T. B., Haddock, L., Bills, C. E., and Howard, J. E.,** Studies of antiricketic activity in sera from patients with disorders of calcium metabolism and preliminary observations on the mode of transport of vitamin D in human serum, *J. Clin. Invest.,* 38, 1078, 1959.

6. **DeLuca, H. F. and Suttie, J. W.,** Eds., *The Fat-Soluble Vitamins,* The University of Wisconsin Press, Madison, 1970.

7. **Yendt, E. R., DeLuca, H. F., Garcia, D. A., and Cohanim, M.,** Clinical aspects of vitamin D, in *The Fat-Soluble Vitamins,* De Luca, H. F. and Suttie, J. W., Eds., The University of Wisconsin Press, Madison, 1970, 125.

8. **Bessey, O. A.,** in *Methods for Evaluation of Nutritional Adequacy and Status,* Quartermaster Food and Container Institute for the Armed Forces, Chicago, Washington, D.C.: National Research Council, 1954, 59.

9. **Wootton, I. D. P.,** *Micro-Analyses in Medical Biochemistry,* 4th ed., King, E. J., Ed., Grune and Stratton, New York and London, 1964.

10. **Bessey, O. A., Lowry, O. H., and Brock, M. J.,** A method for the rapid determination of alkaline phosphatase with five cubic millimeters of serum, *J. Biol. Chem.,* 164, 321, 1946.

11. **Hoffman, W. S.,** *The Biochemistry of Clinical Medicine,* 4th ed., Year Book Medical Publishers, Inc., Chicago, 1970, 609.

12. **Dean, R. F. A. and Schwartz, R.,** The serum chemistry in uncomplicated kwashiorkor, *Br. J. Nutr.,* 7, 131, 1953.

13. **Scrimshaw, N. S., Béhar, M., Arroyave, G., Viteri, F., and Tejada, C.,** Characteristics of kwashiorkor (Sindrome pluricarencial de la infancia), *Fed. Proc.,* 15, 977, 1956.

14. **Mannheimer, E.,** Programs for combating malnutrition in the pre-school child in Ethiopia, in *Pre-School Child Malnutrition: Primary Deterrent to Human Progress,* National Academy of Sciences Publication No. 1282, Washington, D.C., 1966.

15. **Goldsmith, G. A.,** in *Nutritional Diagnosis,* Thomas Publishers, Springfield, Ill., 1959.

16. **Woodhouse, N. J. Y., Doyle, F. H., and Joplin, G. F.,** Vitamin-D deficiency and primary hyperparathyroidism, *Lancet,* 2, 283, 1971.

17. **Jelliffe, D. B.,** An epiphysometer and the community diagnosis of nutritional rickets, *Lancet,* 2, 549, 1971.

18. **Richardson, B. D. and Walker, A. R. P.,** An epiphysometer and the community diagnosis of nutritional rickets, *Lancet,* 2, 1266, 1971.

19. **Guzman, M. A., Arroyave, G., and Scrimshaw, N. S.,** Serum ascorbic acid, riboflavin, carotene, vitamin A, vitamin E and alkaline phosphatase values in Central American school children, *Am. J. Clin. Nutr.,* 9, 164, 1961.

20. **Clark, L. C. and Beck, E.,** Plasma alkaline phosphatase activity, I. Normative data for growing children, *J. Pediatr.,* 36, 335, 1950.

21. **Nordin, B. E. C. and Smith, D. A.,** Pathogenesis and treatment of osteomalacia, in *L'Osteomalacie,* Hioco, D. J., Ed., Masson and Cie, Paris, 1967, 379.

22. **Béhar, M., Arroyave, G., Flores, M., and Scrimshaw, N. S.,** The nutritional status of children of pre-school age in the Guatemalan community of Amatitlan. II. Comparison of dietary, clinical and biochemical findings, *Br. J. Nutr.,* 14, 217, 1960.

23. **Morgenstern, S., Kessler, G., Auerback, J., Flor, R. V., and Klein, B.,** An automated p-nitrophenylphosphate serum alkaline phosphatase procedure for the AutoAnalyzer, *Clin. Chem.,* 11, 876, 1965.

24. Technicon AutoAnalyzer Methodology: Alkaline phosphatase, Method file No. N-6b I/II, Technicon Corp., Tarrytown, 1969.

25. **Teotia, S. P. S. and Teotia, M.,** Antirachitic activity in sera of patients with vitamin-D deficiency rickets, *Indian J. Pediatr.,* 38, 213, 1971.

26. **Joplin, G. F., Robinson, C. J., Melvin, K. E. W., Thompson, G. R., and Fraser, R.,** in *L'Osteomalacie,* Hioco, D. J., Ed., Masson and Cie, Paris, 1967, 249.

27. **Reiner, M., Nadarajah, A., Leese, B., and Gale, G. F.,** Measurement of calcium absorption by a double isotope method in patients with disorders of calcium metabolism, *Calcif. Tissue Res.,* Suppl., 4, 95, 1970.

28. **Ball, J.,** A simple method of defining osteoid in undecalcified sections, *J. Clin. Pathol.,* 10, 281, 1957.

29. **Thompson, G. R.,** Vitamin D deficiency after gastrectomy, *Sci. Basis Med. Annu. Rev.,* 260, 1970.

30. **Berthaux, P., Laurent, M., and Beck, H.,** Fréquence et causes de l'hypovitaminose D chez les personnes âgrées a l'Hospice, *J. Int. Vitaminol.,* 40, 489, 1970.

31. **Stephen, J. M. L. and Stephenson, P.,** Alkaline phosphatase in normal infants, *Arch. Dis. Child.,* 46, 185, 1971.

32. **Arneil, G. C. and Crosbie, J. C.,** Infantile rickets returns to Glasgow, *Lancet,* 2, 423, 1963.

33. **Arneil, G. C., McKilligin, H. R., and Lobo, E.,** Malnutrition in Glasgow children, *Scott. Med. J.,* 10, 480, 1965.

34. **Lapatsanis, P., Deliyanni, V., and Doxiadis, S.,** Vitamin D deficiency rickets in Greece, *J. Pediatr.,* 73, 195, 1968.

35. **Richards, I. D. G., Hamilton, F. M. W., Taylor, E. C., Sweet, E. M., Bremner, E., and Price, H.,** A search for sub-clinical rickets in Glasgow children, *Scott. Med. J.,* 12, 297, 1968.

36. **Richards, I. D. G., Sweet, E. M., and Arneil, G. C.,** Infantile rickets persists in Glasgow, *Lancet,* 1, 803, 1968.

37. **Anon.,** Hypophosphataemic osteomalacia in adults, *Lancet,* 1, 1343, 1971.

38. **Arnaud, C., Maijer, R., Reade, T., Scriver, C. R., and Whelan, D. T.,** Vitamin D dependency: An inherited postnatal syndrome with secondary hyperparathyroidism, *Pediatrics,* 46, 871, 1970.

39. **Condon, J. R., Nassim, J. R., and Rutter, A.,** Pathogenesis of rickets and osteomalacia in familial hypophosphataemia, *Arch. Dis. Child.,* 46, 269, 1971.

40. **Dent, C. E. and Smith, R.,** Nutritional osteomalcia, *Q. J. Med.,* NS38, 195, 1969.

41. **Fischer, J. A., Binswanger, U., Schenk, R. K., and Merz, W.,** Histological observations on bone in intestinal malabsorption and vitamin D deficiency, *Horm. Metab. Res.,* 2, 110, 1970.

42. **Kind, P. R. N. and King, E. J.,** Estimation of plasma phosphatase by determination of hydrolyzed phenol with aminoantipyrine, *J. Clin. Pathol.,* 7, 322, 1954.

43. **Whittle, H., Neale, G., McLaughlin, M., Peters, T. J., Blair, A., Thalassinos, N., Marsh, M. N., Wedzicha, B., and Thompson, G. R.,** Intravenous vitamin D in the detection of vitamin-D deficiency, *Lancet,* 1, 747, 1972.

44. **Roy, A. V.,** Rapid method for determining alkaline phosphatase activity in serum with thymolphthalein monophosphate, *Clin. Chem.,* 16, 431, 1970.

45. **Jonxis, J. H. P.,** Some investigations on rickets, *J. Pediatr.,* 59, 607, 1961.

46. **Doyle, F. H.,** Some quantitative radiological observations in primary and secondary hyperparathyroidism, *Br. J. Radiol.,* 39, 161, 1966.

47. **De Luca, H. F.,** Vitamin D group. IX. Biochemical systems, in *The Vitamins,* Vol. III, 2nd ed., Sebrell, W. H., Jr. and Harris, R. W., Eds., Academic Press, New York, 1971, 240.

48. **Kramer, B. and Gribetz, D.,** Vitamin D group. IX. Deficiency effects in humans, in *The Vitamins,* Vol. III, 2nd ed., Sebrell, W. H., Jr. and Harris, R. S., Eds., Academic Press, New York, 1971, 259.

49. **Howard, J. E., Thomas, W. C., Jr., Barker, L. M., Smith, L. H., and Wadkins, C. L.,** *Bull. Johns Hopkins Hosp.,* 120, 119, 1967.

Vitamin K

Vitamin K is required by the human to maintain prothrombin (factor II) and other factors (VII, IX, X) necessary for normal blood clotting.[1-3] Although the amount of vitamin K required for the adult man has not been established,[4,5] a dietary deficiency of the vitamin uncomplicated by other factors is considered to be rare.[2] A vitamin K deficiency may be encountered in the newborn, in patients with diseases affecting the metabolism or absorption of vitamin K, in patients receiving certain drugs (such as antibiotics) which interfere with the intestinal synthesis of vitamin K or anticoagulants which interfere with prothrombin synthesis. A vitamin K deficiency in the newborn infant can easily be prevented by the administration of small doses of the vitamin to the mother shortly before birth or to the newborn.[6] The process of blood clotting and the factors involved in bleeding disorders have been summarized in several recent reports.[1,3,7-10]

The clinical manifestation of a vitamin K deficiency is hemorrhage as a result of an increase in the time required for blood to clot. A deficiency of vitamin K produces a deficiency in prothrombin (factor II) and factor VII and to a lesser extent in factors IX and X. Since all of these factors are produced in the liver, severe liver disease may also cause their deficiency which is not correctable with vitamin K administration. When any of these factors are deficient, prothrombin time will be prolonged. The coagulation mechanism is exceedingly complex, as outlined in Figure 25, and has not been elucidated with complete certainty.[3,11-15] A simplistic version of the blood clotting reactions, representing the one-stage prothrombin time test, is as follows:

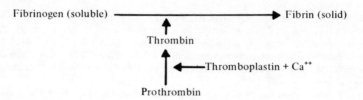

When bleeding disorders are suspected, including the presence of petechiae or purpura, a number of diagnostic tests are available to determine whether the problem is due to a vitamin K deficiency or is related to other hemorrhagic disorders.[1,3,16] The tests represent indirect measurements since direct analyses for vitamin K in biological samples are not feasible. The initial laboratory procedures should include a hemoglobin or hematocrit determination, establishing the presence of an adequate number of platelets through a blood smear, and a fecal examination of gross and occult blood.

In general, the laboratory tests most widely used to establish a bleeding disorder are those that reflect the overall clotting kinetics rather than a method that measures only a single clotting factor. For this purpose, the most commonly used procedure is the measurement of the speed of conversion of prothrombin to thrombin in a plasma sample. The Quick one-stage prothrombin time test which measures the activities of prothrombin and of factors VII and X is a simple and inexpensive procedure routinely used.[8,17-22,26] The procedure consists of the addition of excess thromboplastin and calcium to the plasma sample obtained from citrated or oxalated blood followed by the measurement of the velocity of clotting (prothrombin time). The prothrombin time may be determined on whole plasma or diluted plasma. Usually the dilution procedure is employed since it provides a more reliable and precise assay. The test plasma is diluted with adsorbed normal plasma, rather than with physiologic saline, to provide an optimum test.[25,26] Adsorbed plasma is prepared by treating normal plasma with barium sulfate to adsorb out factors II, VII, IX, and X but leave behind fibrinogen and factor V.

A relationship between prothrombin activity and prothrombin time is presented in Figure 26. A normal prothrombin time is considered to be 12 seconds.[26] However, due to the variety of modifications in the prothrombin time methods and other factors that may influence the prothrombin time, it is essential that a normal prothrombin time be established for each laboratory. A common and simple procedure is to standardize the conditions for the test so as to give a prothrombin time from 11 to 13 seconds for a normal or pooled normal plasma sample.

The "Thrombotest" developed by Owren[23,24,34] also measures factor IX and, theoretically, should be a more comprehensive procedure. In practice, however, the test appears to offer little advantage over the Quick test since, in a vitamin K deficiency, the reductions in factors II, VII, and X far exceed that which would occur in factor IX.[25] In only rare instances would inordinate depressions of factor IX contribute appreciably to a prolonged prothrombin time. The procedure can be performed, however, on capillary blood at the bedside.

The two-stage prothrombin time procedure is a method in which the prothrombin determination is made in two stages.[27-30] In the first stage, thromboplastin and calcium are mixed with an appropriately diluted plasma sample which converts all the prothrombin to thrombin. In the second stage, the amount of thrombin formed is measured by its clotting of a standardized fibrinogen solution. The method is specific for measuring prothrombin and, hence, has been of considerable use in coagulation research but has had less practical value in clinical situations.[33]

A whole blood prothrombin test, referred to as the bedside method, is of value for the general practitioner but probably receives limited use in the clinical laboratory.[31,32] The test is conducted

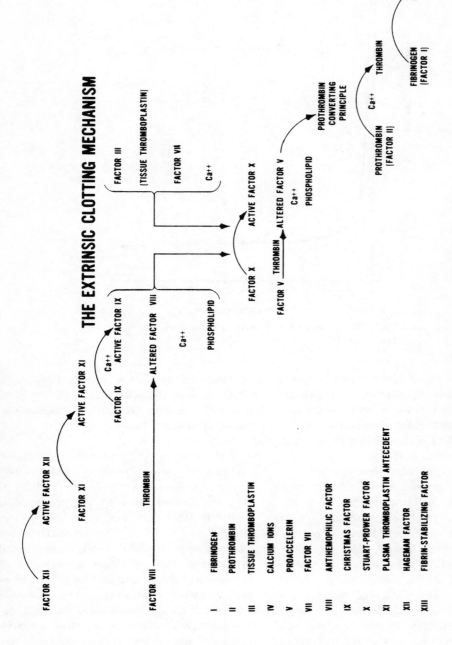

FIGURE 25. Cascade theory of blood coagulation.[12-15]

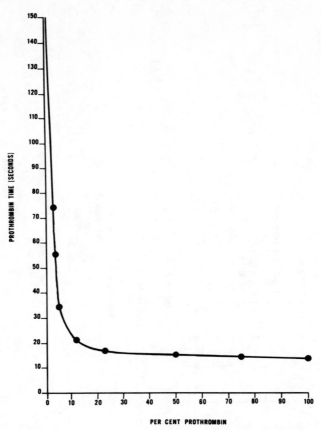

FIGURE 26. Relationship between prothrombin activity and prothrombin time.

by adding freshly drawn blood into a test tube containing a measured quantity of a standard thromboplastin solution. The contents of the tube are mixed and the tube tilted every second or so to observe when clotting occurs. With normal blood, a clot should form in 25 to 40 sec.

Clotting time (Lee-White) determinations are also employed in detecting hemorrhagic disorders.[16] The test is performed by placing freshly drawn blood into two clean test tubes to a calibrated volume mark, sealed with a paraffin cork and time noted. One tube is gently tilted once a minute until clotting occurs. The other tube is then tilted until a clot forms. This is the clotting time in minutes. Normal blood has a clotting time of approximately 10 min. Determination of the clotting time by the capillary tube method is considered less reliable than the regular test tube procedure. It should be noted, however, that serious clotting defects can be masked by a normal clotting time. The test does not reveal lesser, but nevertheless clinically serious, degrees of deficiency in clotting factors. Deficiencies of fibrinogen, prothrombin, factor V, or platelets have to be extreme before the clotting time of the blood is prolonged.

If a vitamin K deficiency exists, administration of the vitamin should result in prompt correction of an abnormal prothrombin or clotting time. However, in severe hepatitis or other liver diseases in which diminished production of prothrombin and factors VII, IX, and X may occur, vitamin K administration results in little improvement in prothrombin time. In other instances in which improvement in prothrombin time fails to occur with vitamin K treatment, the abnormal coagulation and resulting hemorrhagic disorders are the consequence of effects other than a vitamin K deficiency such as genetic, drug usage, etc. Special determinations, such as the prothrombin-consumption test and the thromboplastin generation test, will be required to diagnose the specific coagulation defect in these subjects.[1,3,7-9,16,34-36]

Although a vitamin K deficiency has been considered to occur rarely in the human, evidence of deficiency of the vitamin was found in a study on elderly patients.[34] Using the Thrombotest, Hazell and Baloch[34] found a low prothrombin time in nearly 75% of the 1,110 patients studied. When vitamin K was administered orally, a majority of the low Thrombotests returned to normal. Part of those who failed to respond were found to have hepatic damage or were on drugs with anticoagulant action. These results may suggest that increased attention should be given to the vitamin K nutritional status of the elderly and hospitalized patients.

REFERENCES

1. Owen, C. A., Jr., Bowie, E. J. W., Didisheim, P., and Thompson, J. H., Jr., *The Diagnosis of Bleeding Disorders,* Little, Brown and Co., Boston, 1969.
2. Vitamin K group, in *The Vitamins,* Vol. III, 2nd ed., Sebrell, W. H., Jr. and Harris, R. S., Eds., Academic Press, New York, 1971, 416.
3. Symposium on hemorrhagic disorders, in *The Medical Clinics of North America,* Vol. 56, Rossi, E. C., Ed., W. B. Saunders Co., Philadelphia, 1972.
4. *Recommended Dietary Allowances,* 7th ed., Food and Nutrition Board, National Academy of Sciences-National Research Council Publication No. 1694, Washington, D.C., 1968.
5. Frick, P. G., Riedler, G., and Brögli, H., Dose response and minimal daily requirement for vitamin K in man, *J. Appl. Physiol.,* 23, 387, 1967.
6. Committee on Nutrition, American Academy of Pediatrics, *Pediatrics,* 48, 483, 1971.
7. *Human Blood Coagulation, Biochemistry, Clinical Investigation and Therapy,* Hemker, H. C., Loeliger, E. A., and Veltkamp, J. J., Eds., Springer-Verlag New York Inc., New York, 1969.
8. Quick, A. J., *Bleeding Problems in Clinical Medicine,* W. B. Saunders Co., Philadelphia, 1970.
9. *Recent Advances in Blood Coagulation,* Poller, L., Ed., J. and A. Churchill Ltd., London, 1969.
10. Konttinen, Y. P., *Fibrinolysis: Chemistry, Physiology, Pathology and Clinics,* Oy STAR ab., Pharmaceutical Manufacturers, Tampere, Finland, 1968.
11. MacFarlane, R. G., An enzyme cascade in the blood clotting mechanism and its function as a biochemical amplifier, *Nature (Lond.),* 202, 498, 1964.
12. Davie, E. W. and Ratnoff, O. D., Waterfall sequence for intrinsic blood clotting, *Science,* 145, 1310, 1964.
13. Seegers, W. H., Basic enzymology of blood coagulation, *Thromb. Diath. Haemorrh.,* 14, 213, 1965.
14. McFarlane, R. G., The basis of the cascade hypothesis of blood clotting, *Thromb. Diath. Haemorrh.,* 15, 591, 1966.
15. Bennett, B. and Ratnoff, O. D., The normal coagulation mechanism. Symposium on Hemorrhagic Disorders, in *The Medical Clinics of North America,* Vol. 56, Rossi, E. C., Ed., W. B. Saunders Co., Philadelphia, 1972, 95.
16. Didisheim, P., Screening tests for bleeding disorders, *Am. J. Clin. Pathol.,* 47, 622, 1967.
17. Quick, A. J., Determination of prothrombin, *Proc. Soc. Exp. Biol. Med.,* 42, 788, 1939.
18. Hjort, P., Rapaport, S., and Owren, P. A., *J. Lab. Clin. Med.,* 46, 89, 1955.
19. Quick, A. J., *Hemorrhagic Diseases and Thrombosis,* 3rd ed., Lea & Febiger, Philadelphia, 1964.
20. Alexander, B., Goldstein, R., and Landwehr, G., The labile factor of prothrombin conversion: Its consumption under normal and pathological conditions affecting blood coagulation, *J. Clin. Invest.,* 30, 252, 1951.
21. Alexander, B., Goldstein, R., and Landwehr, G., The prothrombin conversion accelerator of serum (SPCA): Its partial purification and its properties compared with serum AC-globulin, *J. Clin. Invest.,* 29, 881, 1950.
22. Frommeyer, W. B., Determination of prothrombin by the dilution method and activity of human and bovine prothrombin-free plasma, *J. Lab. Clin. Med.,* 34, 1356, 1949.
23. Owren, P. A., Thrombotest. A new method for controlling anti-coagulant therapy, *Lancet,* 2, 754, 1959.
24. Shoshkes, M. and Odze, M., *Circulation,* 28, 58, 1963.
25. Alexander, B. and Wessler, S., A guide to anticoagulant therapy, *Circulation,* 24, 123, 1961.
26. Alexander, B., Thrombin and precursors. 1. Estimation of plasma prothrombin by one-stage method, in *Coagulation of Blood: Methods of Study,* Tocantins, L. M., Ed., Grune and Stratton, New York, 1955, 89.
27. Smith, H. P., Warner, E. D., and Brinkhous, K. M., Prothrombin deficiency and the bleeding tendency in liver injury, *J. Exp. Med.,* 66, 801, 1937.
28. Stewart, J. D. and Rourke, G. M., Prothrombin and vitamin K therapy, *N. Engl. J. Med.,* 221, 403, 1939.
29. Warner, E. D., Brinkhous, K. M., and Smith, H. P., Quantitative study on blood clotting, *Am. J. Physiol.,* 114, 667, 1936.
30. Herbert, F. K., The estimation of prothrombin in human plasma, *Biochem. J.,* 34, 1554, 1940.
31. Smith, H. P., Ziffren, S. E., Owen, C. A., and Hoffman, G. R., Clinical and experimental studies on vitamin K, *J.A.M.A.,* 113, 380, 1939.

32. **Ziffren, S. E., Owen, C. A., Hoffman, G. R., and Smith, H. P.,** Control of vitamin K therapy, *Proc. Soc. Exp. Biol. Med.,* 40, 595, 1939.
33. **Hemker, H. C., Muller, A. D., and Loeliger, E. A.,** Two types of prothrombin in vitamin K deficiency, *Thromb. Diath. Haemorrh.,* 23, 633, 1970.
34. **Hazell, K. and Baloch, K. H.,** Vitamin K deficiency in the elderly, *Gerontol. Clin.,* 12, 10, 1970.
35. **Beller, F. K. and Porges, R. F.,** Blood coagulation and fibrinolytic enzyme studies during cyclic and continuous application of progestational agents, *Am. J. Obstet. Gynecol.,* 97, 448, 1967.
36. **MacFarlane, R. G.,** Disease of the blood, in *Biochemical Disorders in Human Disease,* Thompson, R. H. S. and King, E. J., Eds., Academic Press, New York, 1964, 190.

Pantothenic Acid

Pantothenic acid is ubiquitous in nature and, hence little concern has been given to the occurrence of a pantothenic acid deficiency in the human.[1] Although pantothenic acid as a component of coenzyme A participates in numerous important enzymatic reactions, particularly in association with the synthesis and oxidation of fatty acids, a clearly defined deficiency of the vitamin has not been described for the human.[1] Nevertheless, in malnutrition, multiple deficiencies frequently exist and a deficiency in pantothenic acid may be an unrecognized part of the condition. Thus, chronic malnourished patients[2,3,35] and poorly nourished alcoholic patients[4] have been observed to have low blood, urine or serum levels of pantothenic acid. A pantothenic acid deficiency syndrome has been induced in human subjects who maintained a diet deficient in the vitamin and supplemented with the pantothenic acid antagonists, e.g., omega methyl pantothenic acid.[5-8] The study did not permit the development of suitable biochemical tests for the assessment of pantothenic acid nutritional status.

Because of the lack of interest concerning pantothenic acid requirements in the human, techniques for evaluating the nutriture of this vitamin are very limited. In the few studies in which attempts have been made to control dietary intakes of pantothenic acid, results indicate that the urinary excretion of the vitamin is related to its dietary intake.[9-21] The results of these studies are summarized in Table 17. Since little or no bound pantothenic acid appears in the urine, urinary values for the vitamin have been expressed usually as "free pantothenic acid"/24 hr.

Few attempts have been made to express the urinary excretion of pantothenic acid in terms of mg/g of creatinine. Cohenour and Calloway,[21] however, expressed their pantothenic acid excretion data in terms of both per day and per gram of urinary creatinine. Five nonpregnant girls with an average daily intake of 3.3 mg of pantothenic acid excreted a mean of 2.5 mg/day (range: 1.4 to 3.5) or 2.5 mg/g of urinary creatinine (range: 1.6 to 3.3). Eight young men with a constant intake of 12 mg of pantothenic acid/day excreted a mean of 7.4 mg/day (range: 4.2 to 9.6) or 5.3 mg/g of urinary creatinine (range: 2.7 to 7.2). Whether or not fasting random urine samples could be used in place of 24-hr collections and expressing the pantothenic acid excretion results on a creatinine basis remains for future consideration. At present, urinary excretions of pantothenic acid of less than 1.0 mg/day are considered abnormally low for the adult human, but the data to support this concept are very tenuous.

Both serum and erythrocytes contain relatively high levels of pantothenic acid.[13,20,21,23-30] Whether or not changes in these levels or their association with coenzyme A as an activator of a specific blood enzyme can be developed as an indicator of pantothenic acid nutriture remains uncertain.[13,20,21,23,26-30] Serum contains free pantothenic acid and no coenzyme A, while the majority of the vitamin is present in the red cells as coenzyme A. Blood samples following collection and held at room temperature will spontaneously autolyze to free quantities of the bound pantothenate giving rise to falsely high free pantothenic acid values in plasma or red cells.[22] Hence, it would appear that in order to avoid such possible errors, measurement of total blood pantothenic acid would be recommended. Moreover, the level of pantothenic acid in the red cells is considerably greater than that in the plasma and appears to be more responsive to changes in dietary intakes of pantothenic acid.[21] Cohenour and Calloway[21] found a mean value of free pantothenic acid in pregnant subjects, postpartum subjects, and nonpregnant subjects of 8, 8, and 6 μg/100 ml of blood, respectively. The total blood

TABLE 17

Urinary Excretion of Pantothenic Acid by Subjects on Known Intakes of the Vitamin

Subjects	Pantothenic acid (mg)		Reference
	Intake (per day)	Urinary excretion (per day)	
29 medical students		3.42	Wright[34]
40 medical students on hospital staff	—	3.52	Gordon[16]
3 young women	6.9*	6.0	Gardner et al.[17]
12 young women	2.1 to 4.8*	1.6 to 4.0	Oldham et al.[18]
7 young men	4.73*	3.04	Denko et al.[14]
5 young men	1.1*	1.0	Denko et al.[15]
10 children; 1 to 10 years	—	2.05	Schmidt[9]
10 children; 7 to 14 years	—	2.86	Schmidt[9]
17 children; 2 to 14 years	—	2.5	Schmidt[10]
56 adults; 16 to 45 years	—	2.7	Schmidt[10]
23 adults; 51 to 82 years	—	2.3	Schmidt[10]
8 college women	2.8**	3.2	Fox et al.[11,12]
	7.8**	4.5	
	12.8**	5.6	
6 men	0	0.78	Fox et al.[13]
4 men	10	5.53	
11 girls; 7 to 9 years	4.49**	2.85	Pace et al.[19]
12 girls; 7 to 9 years	5.00**	1.71	
12 girls; 7 to 9 years	2.79**	1.31	
Students	12.4**	6.2	Koyangi et al.[20]
8 men	12.0**	7.4	Cohenour and Calloway[21]
5 nonpregnant girls	3.3**	2.5	Cohenour and Calloway[21]
14 girls, postpartum	4.1**	3.5	Cohenour and Calloway[21]

*Food analyses were made with the use of only a single enzyme system for the liberation of bound pantothenic acid; therefore, values are probably low and do not represent total pantothenic acid intake.
**Double enzyme system used to determine total pantothenic acid intake (e.g., alkaline phosphatase and chicken liver enzyme[22-24]).

pantothenic acid values (free plus bound) for these same subjects were 103, 112, and 183 μg/100 ml of blood, respectively. Similar findings were reported by Ishiguro.[29] The number of subjects involved in these studies were too few to establish a level of blood pantothenic indicative of a pantothenic acid deficiency. Nevertheless, a total pantothenic acid level of less than 100 μg/100 ml of blood was suggestive of low or inadequate dietary intakes of the vitamin. In general, urinary pantothenic acid values appear to be a more sensitive indicator of intake than blood pantothenic acid levels.

Administering test loads of 10 to 50 mg of pantothenic acid and following resultant changes in blood or urine levels of the vitamin does not appear very useful in the diagnosis of a pantothenic acid deficiency.[31,32] The ability of coenzyme A in red cells to acetylate sulfanilimide has also been suggested as a technique to assess pantothenic acid nutriture.[30] Until additional controlled studies have been performed, the usefulness of the procedure cannot be established.

Pantothenic acid is usually measured in biological samples by microbiological procedures using either *Saccharomyces uvarum* (formerly known as *S. carlsbergensis*), *Lactobacillus casei* or *L. plantarum (L. arabinsus)* as the test organism.[1,22-25] The protozoan *Tetrahymena pyriformis* has also been used to measure pantothenic acid levels in biological fluids.[26] As noted above, care must be exercised in the handling of blood samples[21,22] and in the procedure used for the enzymatic release of bound forms of pantothenic acid[22-25] in order to avoid falsely high or low values.

Coenzyme A activity in red blood cells may be determined by the method of Novelli.[33] Normal values for coenzyme activity have been considered to be 4 Lipmann units/ml of red blood cells.

REFERENCES

1. **Sauberlich, H. E.,** Pantothenic acid, in *Modern Nutrition in Health and Disease,* 5th ed., Goodhart, R. S. and Shils, M. E., Eds., Lea and Febiger, Philadelphia, 1972.
2. **Mäkilä, E.,** The vitamin status of elderly denture wearers, *Int. Z. Vitaminforsch.,* 40, 81, 1970.
3. **Kerrey, E., Crispin, S., Fox, H. M., and Kies, C.,** Nutritional status of preschool children. I. Dietary and biochemical findings, *Am. J. Clin. Nutr.,* 21, 1274, 1968.
4. **Leevy, C. M., Baker, H., ten Hove, W., Frank, O., and Cherrick, G. R.,** B-complex vitamins in liver disease of the alcoholic, *Am. J. Clin. Nutr.,* 16, 339, 1965.
5. **Hodges, R. E., Bean, W. B., Ohlson, M. A., and Bleiler, R.,** Human pantothenic acid deficiency produced by omega-methyl pantothenic acid, *J. Clin. Invest.,* 38, 1421, 1959.
6. **Hodges, R. E., Bean, W. B., Ohlson, M. A., and Bleiler, R.,** Factors affecting human antibody response. III. Immunologic response of men deficient in pantothenic acid, *Am. J. Clin. Nutr.,* 11, 85, 1962.
7. **Hodges, R. E., Bean, W. B., Ohlson, M. A., and Bleiler, R.,** Factors affecting human antibody response. V. Combined deficiencies of pantothenic acid and pyridoxine, *Am. J. Clin. Nutr.,* 11, 187, 1962.
8. **Hodges, R. E., Ohlson, M. A., and Bean, W. B.,** Pantothenic acid deficiency in man, *J. Clin. Invest.,* 37, 1642, 1958.
9. **Schmidt, V.,** The excretion of pantothenic acid in young and other individuals, *Int. Z. Vitaminforsch.,* 21, 257, 1949-51.
10. **Schmidt, V.,** The excretion of pantothenic acid in young and other individuals, *J. Gerontol.,* 6, 132, 1951.
11. **Fox, H. M., Linkswiler, H., and Geschwender, D.,** Effect of altering the pantothenic acid intake on the urinary excretion of this vitamin, *Fed. Proc.,* 18, 2068, 1968.
12. **Fox, H. M. and Linkswiler, H.,** Pantothenic acid excretion on three levels of intake, *J. Nutr.,* 75, 451, 1961.
13. **Fox, H. M., Lee, S., and Chen, C. S. L.,** Response to alterations in pantothenic acid content of the diet, *Fed. Proc. Abstr.,* 23, 1964, Abs.
14. **Denko, C. W., Grundy, W. E., Porter, J. W., Berryman, G. H., Friedemann, T. E., and Youmans, J. B.,** The excretion of B-complex vitamins in the urine and feces of seven normal adults, *Arch. Biochem.,* 10, 33, 1946.
15. **Denko, C. W., Grundy, W. E., Wheeler, N. C., Henderson, C. R., Berryman, G. H., Friedemann, T. E., and Youmans, J. B.,** The excretion of B-complex vitamins by normal adults on a restricted intake, *Arch. Biochem.,* 11, 109, 1946.
16. **Gordon, E. S.,** Pantothenic acid in human nutrition, in *The Biological Actions of the Vitamins, a Symposium,* Evans, E. A., Ed., Univ. of Chicago Press, Chicago, 1942, 136.
17. **Gardner, J., Neal, A. L., Peterson, W. H., and Parsons, H. T.,** Biotin, pantothenic acid, and riboflavin balances of young women on a milk diet, *J. Am. Diet. Assoc.,* 19, 683, 1943.
18. **Oldham, H. G., Davis, M. V., and Roberts, L. J.,** Thiamine excretions and blood levels of young women on diets containing varying levels of the B vitamins, with some observations on niacin and pantothenic acid, *J. Nutr.,* 32, 163, 1946.
19. **Pace, J. K., Stier, L. R., Taylor, D. D., and Goodman, P. S.,** Metabolic patterns in preadolescent children. V. Intake and urinary excretion of pantothenic acid, *J. Nutr.,* 74, 345, 1961.
20. **Koyanagi, T., Hareyama, S., Kiruchi, R., Takanohaski, T., Oikawa, K., and Akazawa, N.,** Effect of administration of thiamine, riboflavin, ascorbic acid and vitamin A to students on their pantothenic acid contents in serum and urine, *Tohoku J. Exp. Med.,* 98, 357, 1969.
21. **Cohenour, S. H. and Calloway, D. H.,** Blood, urine, and dietary pantothenic acid levels of pregnant teenagers, *Am. J. Clin. Nutr.,* 25, 512, 1972.
22. **Hatano, M.,** Microbiological assay of pantothenic acid in blood and urine, *J. Vitaminol.,* 8, 134, 1962.
23. **Ishiguro, K., Kobayashi, S., and Kaneta, S.,** Pantothenic acid content of human blood, *Tohoku J. Exp. Med.,* 74, 65, 1961.
24. **Bird, O. D. and Thompson, R. Q.,** Pantothenic acid, in *The Vitamins,* Vol. VII, 2nd ed., György, P. and Pearson, W. N., Eds., Academic Press, New York, 1967, 209.
25. **Barton-Wright, E. C. and Elliot, W. A.,** The pantothenic acid metabolism of rheumatoid arthritis, *Lancet,* 2, 862, 1963.
26. **Baker, H. and Frank, O.,** *Clinical Vitaminology,* Interscience Publishers, New York, 1968.
27. **Denko, C. W., Grundy, W. E., and Porter, J. W.,** Blood levels in normal adults on a restricted dietary intake of B-complex vitamins and tryptophan, *Arch. Biochem.,* 13, 481, 1947.

28. **Koyanagi, T., Hareyama, S., Kikuchi, R., and Kimura, T.,** Effect of diet on the pantothenic acid content of serum and on the incidence of hypertension among villagers, *Tohoku J. Exp. Med.,* 88, 93, 1966.
29. **Ishiguro, K.,** Blood pantothenic acid content of pregnant women, *Tohoku J. Exp. Med.,* 78, 7, 1962.
30. **Ellestad, J. J., Nelson, R. A., Adson, M. A., and Palmer, W. M.,** Pantothenic acid and coenzyme A activity in blood and colinic mucosa from patients with chronic ulcerative colitis, *Fed. Proc.,* 29, 820, 1970, Abs.
31. **Spies, T. D., Stanbery, S. R., Williams, R. J., Jukes, T. H., and Babcock, S. H.,** Pantothenic acid in human nutrition, *J.A.M.A.,* 115, 523, 1940.
32. **Krahnke, H. and Gordon, E. S.,** Pantothenic acid in human nutrition, *J.A.M.A.,* 116, 2431, 1941.
33. **Novelli, G. D.,** Methods for determination of coenzyme A, in *Methods of Biochemical Analysis,* Vol. II, Glick, D., Ed., Interscience Publishers, New York, 1955, 194.
34. **Wright, L. D. and Wright, E. Q.,** Urinary excretion of pantothenic acid by normal individuals, *Proc. Soc. Exp. Biol. Med.,* 49, 80, 1942.
35. **Gershberg, H., Rubin, S. H., and Ralli, E. P.,** Urinary pantothenate, blood glucose and inorganic serum phosphate in patients with metabolic disorders treated with doses of pantothenate, *J. Nutr.,* 39, 107, 1949.

Biotin

Although biotin is an essential cofactor for numerous enzymes,[1] a deficiency of the nutrient in the human has been reported only rarely.[2-5] In these reports, biotin deficiency has been induced experimentally[2] or as the result of the ingestion of diets that have included large amounts of raw egg white.[3-5]

Experimentally induced biotin deficiency resulted in a marked reduction in the urinary excretion of biotin. Excretion fell from a level of 29 to 62 μg of biotin/day on a normal diet to a level of only 3.5 to 7.3 μg/day on the low biotin diet.[2] Children with seborrheic dermatitis have been observed to also have reduced urinary excretions of biotin.[6] A biotin saturation test suggested that a depletion of biotin existed in these children.[6]

More recently, Baugh et al.[5] reported on a case of human biotin deficiency induced by raw egg consumption. Clinical manifestations associated with the deficiency included anorexia, nausea, vomiting, glossitis, pallor, depression, lassitude, substernal pain, scaly dermatitis, and desquamation of the lips. All symptoms cleared or improved markedly after 2 to 5 days of parenteral vitamin therapy providing 200 μg of biotin daily.

The biotin-deficient patient had a whole blood biotin level of 0.25 ng/ml and excreted an average of 8.4 μg of biotin in the urine daily.[5] Normal subjects were found to have a mean whole blood biotin level of 1.47 ng/ml (range: 0.82 to 2.7) which was similar to the values reported by others.[7-9] The mean urinary excretion of biotin/ 24 hr for normal subjects was 42.4 μg (range: 24 to 81).[5] This value was comparable to the earlier results of other investigators.[10,11] Blood and urine biotin levels returned to normal in the biotin-deficient patient while receiving parenteral biotin injections.[5]

Biotin may be measured in biological samples by microbiological assays. The test organisms most commonly used are *Lactobacillus plantarum* ATCC 8014, *L. casei* ATCC 7469, and *Saccharomyces cerevisiae* ATCC 7754.[12] *Ochromonas danica* has also been used.[12-14] *L. plantarum* has probably been the most widely used organism for biotin assays. Bound biotin in whole blood is liberated by papain digestion prior to microbiological assay.[5,13]

These limited reports would suggest that measurement of the biotin level in blood or the urinary excretion of biotin may provide evidence as to the existence of a deficiency of the vitamin in the rare patient that may be encountered with a suspected biotin deficiency.

REFERENCES

1. **Langer, B. W., Jr. and György, P.,** Biotin IX. Biochemical systems, in *The Vitamins,* Vol. II, 2nd ed., Sebrell, W. H., Jr. and Harris, R. S., Eds., Academic Press, New York, 1968, 322.
2. **Sydenstricker, V. P., Singl, S. A., Briggs, A. P., DeVaughn, N. M., and Isbell, H.,** Observations on the 'egg white injury' in man and its cure with a biotin concentrate, *J.A.M.A.,* 118, 1199, 1942.
3. **Williams, R. H.,** Clinical biotin deficiency, *N. Engl. J. Med.,* 288, 247, 1943.
4. **György, P. and Langer, B. W., Jr.,** Biotin XI. Deficiency effects in and requirements of man, in *The Vitamins,* Vol. II, 2nd ed., Sebrell, W. H., Jr. and Harris, R. S., Eds., Academic Press, New York, 1968, 347.
5. **Baugh, C. M., Malone, J. H., and Butterworth, C. E., Jr.,** Human biotin deficiency: A case history of biotin deficiency induced by raw egg consumption in a cirrhotic patient, *Am. J. Clin. Nutr.,* 21, 173, 1968.
6. **Berger, H.,** Urinary excretion of biotin in children with and without pathological skin conditions, with special reference to the relations of seborrhoeic dermatitis and eczema, *Int. Z. Vitaminforsch.,* 22, 190, 1950.
7. **Denko, C. W., Grundy, W. E., Porter, J. W., Berryman, G. H., Friedemann, T. E., and Youmans, J. B.,** Excretion of B-complex vitamins in the urine and feces of seven normal adults, *Arch. Biochem.,* 10, 33, 1946.
8. **Gardner, J., Neal, A. L., Peterson, W. H., and Parsons, H. T.,** Biotin, pantothenic acid, and riboflavin balances of young women on a milk diet, *J. Am. Diet. Assoc.,* 19, 683, 1943.
9. **Jensen, T.,** The excretion of biotin in the urine of psoriasis patients, *Acta Derm. Venereol.,* 28, 468, 1948.
10. **Denko, C. W., Grundy, W. E., and Porter, J. W.,** Blood levels in normal adults on restricted dietary intakes of B-complex vitamins and tryptophan, *Arch. Biochem.,* 13, 481, 1947.
11. **Nisenson, A. and Sherwin, L.,** Normal serum biotin levels in infants and adults: A modified assay method, *J. Pediatr.,* 69, 134, 1966.
12. **György, P.,** Biotin, in *The Vitamins,* Vol. VII, 2nd ed., György, P. and Pearson, W. N., Eds., Academic Press, New York, 1967, 303.
13. **Baker, H., Frank, O., Matovitch, V. B., Pasher, I., Aaronson, S., Hunter, S. H., and Sobotka, H.,** A new assay method for biotin in blood, serum, urine and tissues, *Anal. Biochem.,* 3, 31, 1962.
14. **Leevy, C. M., Cardi, L., Frank, O., Gellene, R., and Baker, H.,** Incidence and significance of hypovitaminemia in a randomly selected municipal hospital population, *Am. J. Clin. Nutr.,* 17, 259, 1965.

III. PROTEIN-CALORIE MALNUTRITION

Protein and Calorie Malnutrition

Protein-calorie-deficiency diseases are generally considered to represent the most common nutritional problem of children in developing countries.[1-8,10,12,13,35,37,38,96,97,100] Consequently, this problem continues to be a major concern of the nutrition programs of WHO, FAO and UNICEF.[3-5,163] Some evidence of inadequate protein intake has also been noted for the United States.[9]

Various attempts have been made to classify protein-calorie malnutrition diseases (PCM).[16,160] Some have classified protein-calorie malnutrition into three major conditions:[10]

    1. Kwashiorkor — edema, wasted muscles

    2. Marasmus (inanition) — muscles and subcutaneous fat, both wasted

    3. Nutritional growth failure — no clinical signs, only low weight corresponding to age.

The FAO and WHO have utilized additional classifications as exemplified in Table 18.[3-5,16] Nevertheless, it is generally agreed that kwashiorkor usually results from consumption of foods deficient in protein relative to calories and that marasmus is the consequence of insufficient food.[5] Kwashiorkor has its main incidence in the second year of life but can occur in infancy or in later childhood and even, though rarely, in the adult years.[1,3-5,10]

With severe forms of protein-calorie malnutrition, a clinical diagnosis can usually be made without biochemical information. Milder forms of protein malnutrition are more difficult to clinically diagnose.[5,11] Anthropometric measurements have been useful for this purpose although their limitations in sensitivity and specificity are recognized. The usual measurements as conducted in field studies are weight, height, arm, head, and chest circumferences, and the triceps skin-fold

TABLE 18

Simplified Classification of Protein-Calorie Malnutrition[a]

Condition	Body weight as % of standard	Edema	Deficit in weight for height
Underweight child	80 to 60	0	Minimal
Nutritional dwarfing	< 60	0	Minimal
Kwashiorkor	80 to 60	+	++
Marasmus	< 60	0	++
Marasmic kwashiorkor	< 60	+	++

[a]From FAO and WHO report (1971).[3]

thickness.[5,11,15,19,33,86,95,98,99,118] Whole body counting measurements for ^{40}K would be of assistance in estimating lean body mass and indirectly protein nutrition; but for survey studies and usually with clinical cases, such measurements are seldom feasible.[79]

Changes in hair morphology have been also proposed as indices for assessing early protein-calorie malnutrition in children.[95,133–143] It has long been recognized that children suffering from protein-calorie malnutrition have change in the texture, color, and pluckability of their hair.[1,5,6,136] Similar changes have been produced in experimentally protein-deprived adults.[133,134] Earlier, Latham and Velez[135] suggested that the reduction in hair tensile strength observed in malnourished children might possibly serve as a means of identifying children with an early stage of protein-calorie malnutrition. Recently, rate of hair growth and hair-shaft diameter,[136–138] hair-root (bulb) diameters[139–141] and hair-root atrophy[140–141] have been investigated as possible indices for this purpose. These hair tissue tests appear promising for the field assessment of the incidence and severity of protein-calorie malnutrition.[140,141]

Unfortunately, at present, no satisfactory biochemical measurement has been found that can be singly used to evaluate protein nutriture.[6,8,11,14,17–20,34,100–103] Nevertheless, a number of biochemical procedures are available that can provide useful information concerning protein nutritional status.[6,8,11,14,17–19,31,34,48,55,100–103] Some of these biochemical procedures will be briefly considered in this section.

Serum Total Protein and Albumin

Although total serum protein levels are commonly measured in nutrition surveys, the results themselves appear to be of little value as a sensitive and specific index for estimating protein intake or protein nutritional status.[8,18–20,100,104] In general, changes in serum proteins have been difficult to evaluate despite the voluminous literature on the subject. Often total serum protein levels are elevated in population groups living in the tropical and subtropical areas even in the presence of inadequate protein intakes.[17,18,26–29,104] These elevated serum protein levels appear to be largely due to environmental effects rather than of ethnic origin.[21,22]

Elevated serum protein levels are usually the result of an increase in the a-globulin fraction, frequently in association with infections and worm infestations.[17,21,22,104] However, the serum albumin level is often lowered in these subjects. Serum albumin normally represents 50 to 65% of the total serum protein concentration.[8,30,39–43] In normal subjects, the albumin: globulin ratio is 1.0 or above, while in kwashiorkor it may fall markedly below 1.0. Serum albumin levels are considered by many as a more reliable and sensitive index of protein nutritional status than total protein levels.[8,23,31,34,94,104] In children with clinical signs of protein malnutrition, serum total protein and albumin levels are usually markedly lowered.[16,31,34,35,63,65] Children with severe kwashiorkor may have albumin levels below 2.0 g/100 ml of serum.[23,31,35,57] However, clinically severe cases of marasmus may have reasonably normal serum total protein and albumin levels.[31,34,35,37,38] In this type of malnutrition, severe body-wasting occurs and an abnormal anthropometry is the major feature which can be measured (Table 18).[3,11,31,34] Slow but progressive hypoalbuminemia, culminating in edema, can occur in children exhibiting quite adequate rates of growth.[31] Although there is no unanimous agreement, the level of serum albumin has been suggested as an index of protein depletion and protein nutriture in children.[21,23,24,31,100] Usually, persistent low serum total protein and albumin levels suggest an inadequate protein intake, although other factors, such as hookworm infestation, may contribute to the problem. In most clinical cases and commonly in nutrition surveys, serum electrophoretic patterns are determined as an additional aid in the evaluation of protein nutriture. Various manual as well as automated digitized analytical systems can rapidly provide information on serum total proteins,

albumin, globulins, albumin-globulin ratios, electrophoretic patterns, etc.[2,6,9,32,36-43,109] Serum protein levels are relatively uninfluenced by age (except under 5 years of age) and sex but are affected by pregnancy, infection, cirrhosis, and various other disease states.[6,8,25,30,39-43] Guidelines that have been used to interpret serum protein data are indicated in Table 19.[6,24,30,31,35] In general, serum albumin levels have been a useful index for the assessment of protein nutritional status in a population group.[104]

Serum Amino Acid Ratios

Earlier studies revealed low total free amino acid concentrations in the plasma of children with

TABLE 19

Tentative Suggested Guidelines for the Interpretation of Biochemical Indices Used in Evaluating Protein and Calorie Deficiencies

Measurement or index	Less than acceptable (at risk)			References
	Deficient (high risk)	Low (medium risk)	Acceptable (low risk)	
1. Serum protein (g/100 ml)				2, 6, 30, 35, 156
0 to 11 months		< 5.0	≥ 5.0	
1 to 5 years		< 5.5	≥ 5.5	
6 to 17 years		< 6.0	≥ 6.0	
Adults	< 6.0	6.0 to 6.4	≥ 6.5	
Pregnant, 2nd and 3rd trimester	< 5.5	5.5 to 5.9	≥ 6.0	
2. Serum albumin (g/100 ml)				2, 6, 30, 31, 35, 156, 157
0 to 11 months		< 2.5	≥ 2.5	
1 to 5 years	(< 2.8)[6]	< 3.0	≥ 3.0	
6 to 17 years	(< 2.8)[6]	< 3.5	≥ 3.5	
Adults	< 2.8	2.8 to 3.4	≥ 3.5	
Pregnant, 1st trimester	< 3.0	3.0 to 3.9	≥ 4.0	
Pregnant, 2nd and 3rd trimester	< 3.0	3.0 to 3.4	≥ 3.5	
3. Nonessential/essential amino acid ratio (NE/E)[a] (all ages)	> 3.0	2.0 to 3.0	< 2.0	5, 7, 34, 45, 48, 49, 55, 60, 100, 102, 140
4. Hydroxyproline index (3 months to 10 years of age)	< 1.0	1.0 to 2.0	> 2.0	5, 34, 55, 60, 87, 100, 101, 103, 104, 116, 159
5. Creatinine height index (3 months to 17 years)	< 0.5	0.5 to 0.9	> 0.9	77, 80-82, 101, 147
6. Urea/creatinine ratio[b]	< 6.0	6.0 to 12.0	> 12.0	8, 17, 35, 58, 100, 101, 122, 140

[a] Value depends upon the analytical method employed and the procedure used to calculate the ratio.
[b] These values are considered exceedingly tentative in view of the effect of age and the wide range of values reported in the literature.

protein-calorie malnutrition.[17,46-48,59] Moreover, the essential and non-essential amino acids were no longer in balance.[17,47-49,130] In general, children with protein malnutrition were observed to have reduced serum concentrations of the essential amino acids and of certain nonessential ones, particularly tyrosine and arginine, whereas the concentrations of most of the other nonessential amino acids remained normal or were elevated.[44,47-50,52,59,130] The essential amino acids, isoleucine, leucine, methionine, and valine, were most markedly reduced while lysine and phenylalanine were the least affected.[47,50,52,59,103,130] As a result of these observations, Whitehead and Dean introduced the use of the non-essential/essential serum amino acid ratio (NE:E) as a means of evaluating protein nutritional status.[44,45,49,103] The procedure involved the separation of the free amino acids present in 100 to 200 $\mu\ell$ of *fasting blood* by one-dimensional paper chromatography into groups of amino acids.[44,45,55,103,158] The separated amino acids were reacted with ninhydrin, measured and expressed by the following ratio:

$$\text{Amino acid ratio (NE:E)} = \frac{\text{glycine + serine + glutamine + taurine}}{\text{isoleucine + leucine + valine + methionine}}$$

Several promising variations of the procedure have been proposed.[14,35,53,54,62,65,70] In some reports, the essential to nonessential amino acid ratio (E/N) was employed.[53,65,66] The amino acid ratio test has been utilized on numerous occasions with varied success.[14,34,35,48-61,70,100,102-104] The nonessential-essential amino acid ratio (NE:E) is raised in children with kwashiorkor but, little if any, in marasmic children.[34,48,51,55,57,59] In normal children, the amino acid ratio is usually less than 2.0 while, in cases of kwashiorkor, ratios above 3.0 are generally observed[34,48,55] (Table 19). Although these findings have been supported by other studies,[7,48,58,60-63,65,100,102] inconsistencies have been noted.[48,50,51,57,64,71] These variances appear to be related in part to the influence of factors such as infections, diarrhea, caloric deficiency, and circadian rhythm on the effectiveness of the amino acid ratio measurement.[34,48,51,52,72,73,85,103,158,162] Nevertheless, additional investigations are needed to evaluate what dietary factors, including vitamin and mineral deficiencies, may influence serum amino acid ratios.[162] Serum amino acid levels appear to be of limited value as an indicator of protein nutritional status in the adult.[67-69,74] The present view is that elevated serum amino acid ratios (NE:E) are probably an indication of primary protein malnutrition in children, although a normal ratio does not necessarily mean that a child is nutritionally normal.[11,34,48,100,102-104] Thus, if a deficiency of calories as well as a shortage of protein or a general lack of total food exists, the test may be of little value.[11,34,48,103] Regardless, even in population groups where a primary protein deficiency is commonplace, the use of the amino acid ratio test as the sole index of subclinical protein malnutrition would not be recommended.[11,162] Perhaps with the development of rapid and reliable gas chromatographic procedures for measuring urinary amino acids,[132] various modifications of the amino acid ratio index may come into more general use.

Urinary Creatinine-Height Index

The relationship of milligrams of creatinine excreted/unit of time/cm of body height (CHI) has been used in evaluating protein nutritional status in children.[11,14,17,75-77,80,101,147] Urinary excretion of creatinine is determined principally by the lean body mass which is sacrificed during protein deprivation.[77,78,101,104] Hence, children suffering from protein-calorie malnutrition have a lowered creatinine-height index:[17,75-78,80,101,104,147]

$$\text{Creatinine-height index (CHI)} = \frac{\text{Creatinine excretion by subject (mg/24 hr)}}{\text{Creatinine excretion by normal child of same height (mg/24 hr)}}$$

Although 24-hr urine collections are preferred, shorter collection periods have been used at the expense of precision.[17,82,83] Expressing creatinine excretion in terms of height is preferred over that of per kilogram of body weight since variations in adipose tissues do not affect the former.[14,17,77,80,82,83] Moreover, knowledge as to the exact age of the child is not essential since the CHI norms are based only on the expected creatinine excretion of normal children of the height of the malnourished child.[14,80,82,83] The creatinine-height index agreed closely with the potassium-height index as an indirect measure of the relative mass and the degree of protein depletion and repletion in malnourished children.[79,80,82] Suggested norms for use in comparing creatinine excretion in children in reference to height have been published[80-82] (Figure 27 and Table 19). Limitations in the use of the urinary creatinine-height index have been reviewed.[11,81-84] Although the requirement for carefully timed urine collections limits its field use, the measurement, if proven sufficiently sensitive could be of value in assessing the recovery of malnourished children as well as in the detection of marginal protein-calorie malnutrition.[11,80,83] Regardless, further studies are required to establish the reliability and usefulness of the measurement. Creatinine itself can be measured very quickly and accurately by automated or manual chemical methods.[6-9,32]

Urinary Hydroxyproline Index

Hydroxyproline, a product of collagen metabolism, is excreted in reduced amounts by malnourished and protein-depleted children.[11,34,55,60,] [87-93,104,105,115,117] From these observations, the hydroxyproline index was proposed:[11,60,87,116]

Urinary hydroxyproline index

$$= \frac{\mu M \text{ hydroxyproline/ml urine}}{\mu M \text{ creatinine/ml urine/kg body wt.}}$$

$$\text{or} \quad \frac{\mu M \text{ hydroxyproline/ml urine} \times \text{kg body wt.}}{\mu M \text{ creatinine/ml urine}}$$

Most reliable results are obtained when 24-hr urine collections are employed, although random samples have been reasonably satisfactory particularly in community survey studies.[11,34,91-93] In studies with children, 24-hr urine collections are not practical. However, expressing the urinary hydroxyproline excretion values in terms of creatinine excretion has permitted the use of random urine samples.[87,92,93] To avoid falsely high hydroxyproline excretions due to dietary ingestion of the amino acid, fasting morning urine collections are recommended.[105] When the hydroxyproline excretions are expressed in terms of creatinine excretion, differences between adult males and females are eliminated.[105] The age of the subject is, however, a major factor in the interpretation of urinary hydroxyproline levels.[92,93,]

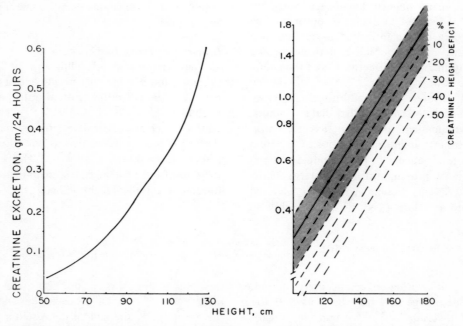

FIGURE 27. Relationship between creatinine excretion (g/24 hr) and height (cm) for children. (From Viteri et al.[80,82] and Mendez and Buskirk.[81])

[106,107,116,159] This is because the rate of hydroxyproline excretion in normal children decreases with increasing age, as the rate of growth drops,[106-108] while that of creatinine excretion increases.[78,92,103,116] Since in developing countries the exact age of the child is often unknown, a body weight factor was introduced by Whitehead into the urinary hydroxyproline index to avoid the need for an age control curve.[87,103,116,159] In normal children, the index is virtually constant over the age range of 6 months to 10 years[87,104,116,159] (Table 19). However, McLaren et al.[92] have incorporated an age adjustment into the hydroxyproline index as employed in their studies. This age adjustment allows for the increase in creatinine excretion with age that is not entirely offset by the increase in weight.[78] For older age groups, the index is probably not valid.[104,159] The highest absolute hydroxyproline excretion of any group of normal subjects is seen in the rapidly growing adolescent (11 to 16 years).[104,159] Between ages 16 and 24, there is a gradual reduction in hydroxyproline excretion.[159] The large variation in hydroxyproline excretion between normal individuals limits the use of the measurement to young children where the index appears to have virtue in the assessment of growth rate. For this age group, Whitehead and others[34,55,87,92,93,103,104] have found the urinary hydroxyproline index to be a useful biochemical test for evaluating nutritional status. However, the hydroxyproline index does not diagnose whether the growth retardation is due to protein and/or calorie malnutrition or to certain other disease conditions.[103-105] Perhaps of greater concern has been the observation that kwashiorkor patients infested with malaria, roundworm, or hookworm may have high rather than low excretions of hydroxyproline.[34,103] Consequently, until additional experience has been gained from studies by other investigators in various parts of the world, the reliability and value of the hydroxyproline excretion index to assess malnutrition in the field remains uncertain. Various methods have been employed to measure hydroxyproline in urine.[32,55,105,110-114]

Fasting Urinary Urea-Creatinine Ratio

Since urea is the principal end product of protein metabolism in the human, the use of nitrogen to creatinine ratios and urea to creatinine ratios have been proposed for evaluating dietary protein intakes.[2,8,11,14,17,18,119-123]

$$\text{Urea-creatinine ratio} = \frac{\text{mg urea nitrogen/ml urine}}{\text{mg creatinine/ml urine}}$$

Under laboratory conditions, an increase or a decrease in the level of protein intake is paralleled by marked changes in the urinary urea/creatinine ratio.[122,123,131] When the technique has been applied in the field, variable results have been reported.[2,8,14,35,58,94,100,120,122,124,125] Since 24-hr urine collections are difficult to obtain from children, especially in field nutrition studies, random urine samples have been commonly employed, recognizing their limitations.[119,122,124,125] The recommended procedure for collecting the fasting random urine sample is to discard the first urine void in the morning and collect the second.[11,122,127] Urea-creatinine ratio values must be interpreted with general caution as creatinine excretion is related to age, sex, diet, muscle mass, and other factors.[119,126] Clearly defined guidelines are not available[8,17,35,58,100] (Table 19). Nevertheless, the urea-creatinine ratio can be useful if it is recognized that it is primarily a measure of dietary rather than of nutritional status. The ratio is a reflection of the recent dietary intake and does not indicate the actual protein nutriture of an individual.[122,129] However, the ratio, when applied to population groups, may provide a general evaluation of the quantity of protein ingested. Automated procedures are available for measuring urinary urea.[32,167]

Miscellaneous Procedures

The urinary sulfur-creatinine ratio has also been proposed as an indicator of protein intake. This test could have the possible advantage of reflecting the dietary intake of high quality protein, in particular those with a high sulfur amino acid content.[11,166] The procedure has been seldom employed and, hence, the practical value of the test remains uncertain.[61,100,128,146,166]

Leucocyte pyruvic kinase activity has been observed to be reduced in protein-calorie malnutrition.[144] Various serum enzymes have likewise been studied in subjects suffering from protein-calorie malnutrition.[145,148,149] The enzyme changes observed held little promise of use as an index for evaluating protein malnutrition.[164] Serum transferrin (siderophilin) levels have recently been observed to be a good index of severity of kwashiorkor.[150-154,161] Patients with kwashiorkor have markedly depressed serum transferrin levels.[150,161] However, these reports did not suggest that serum transferrin measurements would be of any value in nutrition surveys or in diagnosing early stages of protein-calorie malnutrition. Most cases of marasmus had normal serum transferrin levels.[152] Moreover, under practical conditions, protein-calorie deficiency and iron deficiency may coexist and thereby further limit the usefulness of transferrin measurements as an indicator of protein malnutrition.

Recently, plasma and urine RNase activity levels and urine/plasma RNase activity ratios have been suggested as a means of diagnosing the severity of protein-calorie malnutrition in children suffering from this condition.[155] Plasma RNase was elevated in all malnourished children. Severely malnourished children had low urine/plasma RNase ratios, while less malnourished children had normal ratios. These interesting findings will require, however, additional investigations before the reliability and usefulness of the test can be established.

Summary

From the above considerations, it is apparent that no single biochemical procedure that can satisfactorily evaluate protein and calorie malnutrition in early or sub-clinical states is available. The severe forms of malnutrition, kwashiorkor and marasmus, are clinically recognizable. Anthropometric measurements such as weight, height, skinfold, arm circumference, and age, can be extremely useful in the diagnosis of these forms of malnutrition. However, even the available biochemical indices do not reliably distinguish between these two forms of malnutrition. Although Whitehead[34,103,165] has suggested that the use of the amino acid ratio, serum albumin and total serum protein levels, and hydroxyproline index might differentiate between calorie and protein malnutrition in children, this has not proven universally successful. Indices useful for evaluating protein nutritional status in the adult are even less certain. Nevertheless, the use of several biochemical measurements carefully interpreted can, when used in conjunction with clinical and anthropometric assessments, provide a reasonable evaluation of protein and calorie nutritional status.[11,165]

REFERENCES

1. **May, J. M.,** *Studies in Medical Geography. The Ecology of Malnutrition,* Vols. 1–11, Hafner Publishing Co., New York, 1961–1972.
2. Nutrition Survey Reports, Interdepartmental Committee on Nutrition for National Defense, Washington, D.C., 1957–1972.
3. Joint FAO/WHO Expert Committee on Nutrition, eighth report, FAO nutrition meetings report series No. 49, Food and Agriculture Organization, Rome, 1971.
4. Protein Requirements, Report of a Joint FAO/WHO Expert Group, FAO nutrition meetings report series No. 37, Food and Agriculture Organization, Rome, 1965.
5. **Jelliffe, D. B.,** The assessment of the nutritional status of the community, *W.H.O. Monogr.,* series No. 53, World Health Organization, Geneva, 1966.
6. *Manual for Nutrition Surveys,* 2nd ed., Interdepartmental Committee on Nutrition for National Defense, Superintendent of Documents, U.S. Government Printing Office, Washington, D.C. 20402, 1963.
7. Nutritional Evaluation of the Population of Central America and Panama: 1965–1967, Report of the Institute of Nutrition of Central America and Panama and of the Nutrition Program, Center for Disease Control, U.S. Dept. of Health, Education and Welfare Publication No. (HSM) 72–8120, 1972.
8. **Du Plessis, J. P.,** An Evaluation of Biochemical Criteria for Use in Nutrition Status Surveys, National Nutrition Research Institute, Council for Scientific and Industrial Research Report No. 261, Pretoria, S. Africa, 1967, 11.

9. Reports of the Ten-State Nutrition Survey: 1968–1970, U.S. Dept. of Health, Education and Welfare, Health Services and Mental Health Admin., Center for Disease Control, Atlanta, Georgia 30333, 1972.

10. **Brown, C. B.,** The incidence of protein-calorie malnutrition of early childhood, *Guy's Hosp. Rep.,* 120, 129, 1971.

11. Assessment of protein nutritional status. A committee report, *Am. J. Clin. Nutr.,* 23, 807, 1970.

12. *Progress in Meeting Protein Needs of Infants and Preschool Children,* National Academy of Sciences-National Research Council publication 843, Washington, D.C., 1961.

13. **Kevany, J.,** Nutritional problems in Latin America, *Proc. Western Hemisphere Nutrition Congress,* Nov. 1965, A.M.A., 535 N. Dearborn St., Chicago 60610, 50, 1966.

14. **Arroyave, G.,** Biochemical characteristics of malnourished infants and children, *Proc. Western Hemisphere Nutrition Congress,* Nov. 1965, A.M.A., 535 N. Dearborn St., Chicago 60610, 30, 1966.

15. **Rao, K., Visweswara and Singh, D.,** An evaluation of the relationship between nutritional status and anthropometric measurements, *Am. J. Clin. Nutr.,* 23, 83, 1970.

16. **Gomez, F., Galvan, R. R., Cravioto, J., and Frenk, S.,** Malnutrition in infancy and childhood with special reference to kwashiorkor, *Adv. Paediatr.,* 7, 131, 1955.

17. **Arroyave, G.,** The estimation of relative nutrient intake and nutritional status by biochemical methods: proteins, *Am. J. Clin. Nutr.,* 11, 447, 1962.

18. **Pearson, W. N.,** Assessment of nutritional status: biochemical methods, in *Nutrition: A Comprehensive Treatise,* Vol. III, Beaton, G. H. and McHenry, E. W., Eds., Academic Press, New York, 1966, 265.

19. Expert Committee on Medical Assessment of Nutritional Status, World Health Organization technical report series No. 258, World Health Organization, Geneva, 1963.

20. **Krehl, W. A. and Hodges, R. E.,** The interpretation of nutrition survey data, *Am. J. Clin. Nutr.,* 17, 191, 1965.

21. **Bronte-Stewart, B., Antonis, A., Rose-Innes, C., and Moodie, A. D.,** An interracial study on the serum protein pattern of adult men in Southern Africa, *Am. J. Clin. Nutr.,* 9, 596, 1961.

22. **Schofield, F. D.,** The serum protein pattern of West Africans in Britain, *Trans. R. Soc. Trop. Med. Hyg.,* 51, 332, 1957.

23. **Schendel, H. E., Hansen, J. D. L., and Brock, J. F.,** A comparative study of biochemical indices used in evaluating dietary protein in young children, *S. Afr. Med. J.,* 34, 791, 1960.

24. **Brock, J. F.,** Dietary proteins in relation to man's health, *Fed. Proc.,* Suppl. 7, 20, 61, 1961.

25. **Darby, W. J. et al.,** The Vanderbilt cooperative study of maternal and infant nutrition. IV. Dietary, laboratory and physical findings in 2,129 delivered pregnancies, *J. Nutr.,* 51, 565, 1953.

26. **Platt, B. S.,** Malnutrition and the pathogenesis of disease, *Trans. R. Soc. Trop. Med. Hyg.,* 52, 189, 1958.

27. **Bakker, A. W. I., Bliek, A., and Luyken, R.,** The serum proteins of malaria-free inhabitants of Central Netherlands, New Guinea, *Trop. Geogr. Med.,* 9, 1, 1957.

28. **Joubert, S. M., Hookins, K. W., and Hunter, W. G.,** A comparative study of serum protein moieties in European, African and Indian adult populations of Durban, *S. Afr. J. Lab. Clin. Med.,* 5, 1, 1959.

29. **Luyken, R.,** Specific nutritional and informational problems in tropical countries, *Voeding,* 24, 280, 1963.

30. **Oberman, J. W., Gregory, K. O., Burke, F. G., Ross, S., and Rice, E. C.,** Electrophoretic analysis of serum proteins in infants and children. I. Normal values from birth to adolescence, *N. Engl. J. Med.,* 255, 743, 1956.

31. **Whitehead, R. G., Frood, J. D. L., and Poskitt, E. M. E.,** Value of serum-albumin measurements in nutritional surveys: A reappraisal, *Lancet,* 2, 287, 1971.

32. **Coward, D. G., Sawyer, M. B., and Whitehead, R. G.,** Microtechniques for the automated analysis of serum total protein and albumin, urinary urea, creatinine, and hydroxyproline for nutrition surveys in developing countries, *Am. J. Clin. Nutr.,* 24, 940, 1971.

33. **Jelliffe, D. B. and Jelliffe, E. F.,** The arm circumference as a public health index of protein calorie malnutrition of early childhood, *J. Trop. Pediatr.,* 15, 253, 1969.

34. **Whitehead, R. G.,** Biochemical tests in differential diagnosis of protein and calories deficiencies, *Arch. Dis. Child.,* 42, 479, 1967.

35. **Bjørnesjφ, K. B., Belew, M., and Zaar, B.,** Biochemical study of advanced protein malnutrition in Ethiopia, *Scand. J. Clin. Lab. Invest.,* 18, 591, 1965.

36. **Chong, Y. H., Ho, G. S., and DeWitt, G. F.,** An evaluation of a simple refractometric method for determining plasma total proteins, *Med. J. Malaya,* 23, 115, 1968.

37. **McLaren, D. S. and Kanawat, A. A.,** The epidemiology of protein-calorie malnutrition in Jordan. Part I. Application of a simple scoring system, *Trans. R. Soc. Trop. Med. Hyg.,* 64, 754, 1970.

38. **Haddad, N. E. and Harfouche, J. K.,** Serum protein in Lebanese infants, *J. Trop. Pediatr.,* 17, 91, 1971.

39. **Bauer, S. and DeVino, T.,** Normal ranges of pediatric values determined by a survey model SAM 12/60, *Adv. in Automated Analyses,* 3, 31, 1969.

40. **Werner, M., Tolls, R. E., Hultin, J. V., and Melleker, J.,** Sex and age dependence of serum calcium, inorganic phosphorus, total protein, and albumin in a large ambulatory population, *Adv. in Automated Analyses,* 3, 59, 1969.

41. **Cutler, J. L., Collen, M. F., Siegelaub, A. B., and Feldman, R.,** Normal values for multiphasic screening blood chemistry tests, *Adv. in Automated Analyses,* 3, 67, 1969.

42. **Cunnick, W. R., Cromic, J. B., Beach, E. F., Seltzer, F., Tobin, J., and Culberson, S.,** Biochemical profiles in a healthy employee population: distribution of values classified by age and sex, *Adv. in Automated Analyses,* 3, 85, 1969.

43. **Craig, J. L. and Bartholomew, M. D.,** Blood profile ranges by age decades in 7,337 male employees, *Adv. in Automated Analyses,* 3, 105, 1969.

44. **Whitehead, R. G.,** Rapid determination of some plasma amino acids in subclinical kwashiorkor, *Lancet,* 1, 250, 1964.

45. **Whitehead, R. G. and Dean, R. F. A.,** Serum amino acids in kwashiorkor. II. An abbreviated method of estimation and its application, *Am. J. Clin. Nutr.,* 14, 320, 1964.

46. **Cravioto, J.,** Protein metabolism in chronic infantile malnutrition (kwashiorkor), *Am. J. Clin. Nutr.,* 6, 495, 1958.

47. **Arroyave, G., Wilson, D., DeFunes, C., and Béhar, M.,** The free amino acids in blood plasma of children with kwashiorkor and marasmus, *Am. J. Clin. Nutr.,* 11, 517, 1962.

48. **Simmons, W. K.,** The plasma amino acid ratio as an indicator of the protein nutrition status: A review of recent work, *Bull. W.H.O.,* 42, 480, 1970.

49. **Whitehead, R. G. and Dean, R. F. A.,** Serum amino acids in kwashiorkor. I. Relationship to clinical condition, *Am. J. Clin. Nutr.,* 14, 313, 1964.

50. **Migasena, P., Viseshakul, D., Changbumrung, S., and Harinasuta, C.,** Plasma amino acids in kwashiorkor and marasmus in Thailand, *South-East Asia J. Trop. Med. Public Health,* 2, 399, 1971.

51. **McLaren, D. S., Kamel, W. W., and Ayyoub, N.,** Plasma amino acids and the detection of protein-calorie malnutrition, *Am. J. Clin. Nutr.,* 17, 152, 1965.

52. **Saunders, S. J., Truswell, A. S., and Hansen, J. D. L.,** Plasma free amino acid pattern in protein-calorie malnutrition, *Lancet,* 2, 795, 1967.

53. **Arroyave, G.,** Comparative sensitivity of specific amino acid ratios versus "essential to nonessential" amino acid ratio, *Am. J. Clin. Nutr.,* 23, 703, 1970.

54. **Pereira, S. M., Begum, A., Sundararj, R., and Dumm, M. E.,** Effect of dietary protein on serum amino acids, *Am. J. Clin. Nutr.,* 21, 167, 1968.

55. **Katz, St. I.,** The amino acid ratio and hydroxyproline creatinine index in marginal protein-calorie malnutrition, *Trop. Geogr. Med.,* 22, 389, 1970.

56. **Grimble, R. F. and Whitehead, R. G.,** Fasting serum-amino acid patterns in kwashiorkor and after administration of different levels of protein, *Lancet,* 1, 918, 1970.

57. **Truswell, A. S., Wannenburg, P., Wittmann, W., and Hansen, J. D. L.,** Plasma-amino acids in kwashiorkor, *Lancet,* 1, 1162, 1966.

58. **Chong, Y. H., McKay, D. A., and Lim, R. K. H.,** Some results of recent nutrition surveys in West Malaysia, *Bull. Public Health Soc.,* 6, 55, 1972.

59. **Gürson, C. T., Neyzi, O., Uzman, Y., and Saner, G.,** An evaluation of the plasma amino acid ratio in marasmus, in *Nutrition and Health,* Vol. 1, Proc. Seventh International Congress of Nutrition, Hamburg 1966, Pergamon Press, New York, 1967, 112.

60. **Rutishauser, I. H. E. and Whitehead, R. G.,** Field evaluation of two biochemical tests which may reflect nutritional status in three areas of Uganda, *Br. J. Nutr.,* 23, 1, 1969.

61. **Bohdal, M., and Simmons, W. K.,** A comparison of the nutritional indices in healthy African, Asian and European children, *Bull. W.H.O.,* 40, 166, 1969.

62. **Ittyerah, T. R., Pereira, S. M., and Dumm, M. E.,** Serum amino acids of children on high and low protein intakes, *Am. J. Clin. Nutr.,* 17, 11, 1965.

63. **Hin, P. S., Rose, C. S., Muhilal, and Zuraida, S.,** Serum free amino acids in children with protein-calorie deficiency, *Am. J. Clin. Nutr.,* 20, 1295, 1967.

64. **Anasuya, A. and Rao, B. S. Narasinga,** Plasma amino acid pattern in kwashiorkor and marasmus, *Am. J. Clin. Nutr.,* 21, 723, 1968.

65. **Padilla, H., Sanchez, A., Powell, R. N., Umezawa, C., Swendseid, M. E., Prado, P. M., and Sigala, R.,** Plasma amino acids in children from Guadalajara with kwashiorkor, *Am. J. Clin. Nutr.,* 24, 353, 1971.

66. **Stegink, L. D. and Baker, G. L.,** Serum amino acid levels of Northern Alaska Eskimo infants and children, *Am. J. Clin. Nutr.,* 23, 1642, 1970.

67. **Swendseid, M. E., Tuttle, S. G., Figueroa, W. S., Mulcare, D., Clark, A. J., and Massey, F. J.,** Plasma amino acid levels of men fed diets differing in protein content. Some observations with valine-deficient diets, *J. Nutr.,* 88, 239, 1966.

68. **Swendseid, M. E., Yamada, C., Vinyard, E., and Figueroa, W. S.,** Plasma amino acid levels in young subjects receiving diets containing 14 or 3.5 g nitrogen per day, *Am. J. Clin. Nutr.,* 21, 1381, 1968.

69. **Young, V. R. and Scrimshaw, N. S.,** Endogenous nitrogen metabolism and plasma free amino acids in young adults given a 'protein-free' diet, *Br. J. Nutr.,* 22, 9, 1968.

70. **Snyderman, S. E., Holt, L. E., Jr., Norton, P. M., Roitman, E., and Phansalkar, S. V.,** The plasma aminogram. I. Influence of the level of protein intake and a comparison of whole protein and amino acid diets, *Pediatr. Res.,* 2, 131, 1968.

71. **Heard, C. R. C., Kriegsman, S. M., and Platt, B. S.,** The interpretation of plasma amino acid ratios in protein-calorie deficiency, *Br. J. Nutr.,* 23, 203, 1969.

72. **Feigin, R. D., Klainer, A. S., and Beisel, W. R.,** Circadian periodicity of blood amino acids in adult men, *Nature,* 215, 512, 1967.

73. **Wurtman, R. J., Rose, C. M., Chou, C., and Larin, F. F.,** Daily rhythms in the concentrations of various amino acids in human plasma, *N. Engl. J. Med.,* 279, 171, 1968.

74. **Crawford, M. A., Gale, M. M., Somers, K., and Hansen, I. L.,** Studies on plasma amino acids in East African adults in relation to endomyocardial fibrosis, *Br. J. Nutr.,* 24, 393, 1970.

75. **Arroyave, G., Sandstead, H., and Schumacher, R.,** Relation of urinary creatinine and vitamins to nutritional status in preschool children, *Fed. Proc.,* 17, 469, 1958.

76. **Standard, K. L., Wills, V. G., and Waterlow, J. C.,** Indirect indicators of muscle mass in malnourished infants, *Am. J. Clin. Nutr.,* 7, 271, 1959.

77. **Arroyave, G. and Wilson, D.,** Urinary excretion of creatinine of children under different nutritional conditions, *Am. J. Clin. Nutr.,* 9, 170, 1961.

78. **Stearns, G., Newman, K. J., McKinely, J. B., and Jeans, P. C.,** The protein requirements of children from one to ten years of age, *Ann. N. Y. Acad. Sci.,* 69, 857, 1958.

79. **Alleyne, G. A. O., Viteri, F., and Alvarado, J.,** Indices of body composition in infantile malnutrition: total body potassium and urinary creatinine, *Am. J. Clin. Nutr.,* 23, 875, 1970.

80. **Viteri, F. E. and Alvarado, J.,** The creatinine height index: its use in the estimation of the degree of protein depletion and repletion in protein calorie malnourished children, *Pediatrics,* 46, 696, 1970.

81. **Mendez, J. and Buskirk, E. R.,** Creatinine-height index, *Am. J. Clin. Nutr.,* 24, 385, 1971.

82. **Viteri, F. E., Alvarado, J., and Alleyne, G. A. O.,** Reply to Drs. Mendez and Buskirk, *Am. J. Clin. Nutr.,* 24, 386, 1971.

83. **Viteri, F. E.,** Creatinine-height index in malnourished children, *Nutr. Rev.,* 30, 24, 1972.

84. **Anon.,** Creatinine-height index in malnourished children, *Nutr. Rev.,* 29, 134, 1971.

85. **Feigin, R. E., Beisel, W. R., and Wannemacher, R. W.,** Rhythmicity of plasma amino acids and relation to dietary intake, *Am. J. Clin. Nutr.,* 25, 329, 1971.

86. **Davis, L. E.,** Epidemiology of famine in the Nigerian crisis: rapid evaluation of malnutrition by height and arm circumference in large populations, *Am. J. Clin. Nutr.,* 24, 358, 1971.

87. **Whitehead, R.,** Hydroxyproline creatinine ratio as an index of nutritional status and rate growth, *Lancet,* 2, 567, 1965.

88. **Picou, D., Alleyne, G. A. O., Waterlow, J. C., and Seakins, A.,** Hydroxyproline and creatinine excretion in protein-depleted infants, *Biochem. J.,* 95, 18P, 1965.

89. **Picou, D., Alleyne, G. A. O., and Seakins, A.,** Hydroxyproline and creatinine excretion in infantile protein malnutrition, *Clin. Sci.,* 29, 517, 1965.

90. **Anasuya, A. and Rao, B. S. Narasinga,** Urinary excretion of hydroxyproline in kwashiorkor, *Indian J. Med. Res.,* 54, 849, 1966.

91. **Prasad, L. S. and Rahman, A.,** Urinary excretion of hydroxpyroline and creatinine in malnutrition, *Indian Pediatrics,* 7, 54, 1970.

92. **McLaren, D. S., Loshkajian, H., and Kanawati, A. A.,** Urinary creatinine and hydroxyproline in relation to childhood malnutrition, *Br. J. Nutr.,* 24, 641, 1970.

93. **Howells, G. R., Wharton, B. A., and McCance, R. A.,** Value of hydroxypyroline indices in malnutrition, *Lancet,* 1, 1082, 1067.

94. **Du Plessis, J. P., De Lange, D. J., and Fellingham, S. A.,** Biochemical investigation of the nutrition status of urban school children aged 12-15 years: Protein status, *S. Afr. Med. J.,* 27, 509, 1966.

95. **Kanawati, A. A. and McLaren, D. S.,** Assessment of marginal malnutrition, *Nature,* 228, 573, 1970.

96. **Cravioto, J. and De Licardie, E. R.,** The long-term consequences of protein-calorie malnutrition, *Nutr. Rev.,* 29, 107, 1971.

97. **McLaren, D. S.,** A fresh look at protein-calorie malnutrition, *Lancet,* 2, 485, 1966.

98. **McKay, D. A., Lim, R. K. H., Notaney, K. H., and Dugdale, A. E.,** Nutritional assessment by comparative growth achievement in Malay children below school age, *Bull. WHO,* 45, 233, 1971.

99. **Seoane, N. and Latham, M. C.,** Nutritional anthropometry in the identification of malnutrition in childhood, *J. Trop. Pediatr.,* 17, 98, 1971.

100. **Simmons, W. K. and Bohdal, M.,** Assessment of some biochemical parameters related to protein-calorie nutrition in children, *Bull. WHO,* 42, 897, 1970.

101. **Arroyave, G.,** Proposed methodology for the biochemical evaluation of protein malnutrition in children, in *Protein-Calorie Malnutrition,* von Muralt, A., Ed., Springer-Verlag, Berlin and New York, 1969, 48.

102. **Prasanna, H. A., Desai, B. L. M., and Rao, M. Narayana,** Detection of early protein-calorie malnutrition (pre-kwashiorkor) in population groups, *Br. J. Nutr.,* 26, 71, 1971.

103. **Whitehead, R. G.,** The assessment of nutritional status in protein-malnourished children, *Proc. Nutr. Soc.,* 28, 1, 1969.

101

104. **Waterlow, J. C.,** The assessment of protein nutrition and metabolism in the whole animal, with special reference to man, in *Mammalian Protein Metabolism,* Vol. III, Munro, H. N., Ed., Academic Press, New York, 1969, 325.

105. **LeRoy, E. C.,** The technique and significance of hydroxyproline measurement in man, *Adv. Clin. Chem.,* 10, 213, 1967, Academic Press, New York.

106. **Jones, C. R., Bergman, M. W., Kittner, P. J., and Pigman, W. W.,** Urinary hydroxyproline excretion in normal children and adolescents, *Proc. Soc. Exp. Biol. Med.,* 115, 85, 1964.

107. **Smiley, J. D. and Ziff, M.,** Urinary hydroxyproline excretion and growth, *Physiol. Rev.,* 44, 30, 1964.

108. **Allison, D. J., Walker, A., and Smith, Q. T.,** Urinary hydroxyproline: creatinine ratio of normal humans at various ages, *Clin. Chim. Acta,* 14, 729, 1966.

109. **McPherson, I. G. and Everhard, D. W.,** Serum albumin estimation: modification of the bromcresol green method, *Clin. Chim. Acta,* 37, 117, 1972.

110. **Prockop, D. J. and Udenfriend, S.,** A specific method for the analysis of hydroxyproline in tissues and urine, *Anal. Biochem.,* 1, 228, 1960.

111. **Kivirikko, K. I., Laitinen, O., and Prockop, D. J.,** Modification of a specific assay for hydroxyproline in urine, *Anal. Biochem.,* 19, 249, 1967.

112. **Hosley, H. F., Olson, K. B., Horton, J., Michelsen, P., and Atkins, R.,** Automated analysis of urinary hydroxyproline for cancer research, *Adv. in Automated Analysis,* Vol. I, 105, 1969.

113. **Goverde, B. C. and Veenkamp, F. J. N.,** Routine assay of total urinary hydroxyproline based on resin-catalyzed hydrolysis, *Clin. Chim. Acta,* 41, 29, 1972.

114. **Ramamurthy, N. S., Zebrowski, E. J., and Golub, L. M.,** A modified procedure for determining hydroxyproline in normal and diabetic urine, *Biochem. Med.,* 5, 555, 1971.

115. **Anasuya, A. and Rao, B. S. Narasinga,** Urinary excretion of hydroxyproline in kwashiorkor, *Lancet,* 1, 94, 1966.

116. **Whitehead, R. G.,** Urinary excretion of hydroxyproline in kwashiorkor, *Lancet,* 1, 203, 1966.

117. **Cabacungan, N. B., Miles, C. W., Abernathy, R. P., and Ritchey, S. J.,** Hydroxyproline excretion and nutritional status of children, *Am. J. Clin. Nutr.,* 26, 173, 1973.

118. **Lowenstein, M. S. and Phillips, J. F.,** Evaluation of arm circumference measurement for determining nutritional status of children and its use in an acute epidemic of malnutrition: Owerri, Nigeria, following the Nigerian Civil War, *Am. J. Clin. Nutr.,* 26, 226, 1973.

119. **Powell, R. C., Plough, I. C., and Baker, E. M., III,** The use of nitrogen to creatinine ratios in random urine specimens to estimate dietary protein, *J. Nutr.,* 73, 47, 1961.

120. **Dubois, B., Leegwater, D. C., Pikaar, N. A., and Van Staveren, W.,** Correlation of protein intake and nitrogen and urea in urine, *Proc. Nutr. Soc.,* 29, 53A, 1970.

121. **Platt, B. S. and Heard, C. R. C.,** Biochemical evidences of protein malnutrition, *Proc. Nutr. Soc.,* 17, ii, 1958.

122. **Simmons, W. K.,** Urinary urea nitrogen/creatinine ratio as indicator of recent protein intake in field studies, *Am. J. Clin. Nutr.,* 25, 539, 1972.

123. **Albanese, A. A. and Oorto, L. A.,** Urinary excretion of amino acids, in *Newer Methods of Nutritional Biochemistry,* Vol. III, Albanese, A. A., Ed., Academic Press, New York, 1967, 1.

124. **Dugdale, A. E. and Edkins, E.,** Urinary urea/creatinine ratio in healthy and malnourished children, *Lancet,* 1, 1062, 1964.

125. **Fry, P. C., Fox, H. M., and Fry, E. I.,** Effect of diet on skin-fold measurements and creatinine and urea excretion of Hong Kong Chinese children, *Am. J. Clin. Nutr.,* 21, 1197, 1968.

126. **Pollack, H.,** Creatinine excretion as an index for estimating urinary excretion of micronutrients or their metabolic end products, *Am. J. Clin. Nutr.,* 23, 865, 1970.

127. **Arroyave, G. and Lee, M.,** Variation in urinary excretion of urea and N^1-methyl-nicotinamide during the day comparison with fasting levels, *Arch. Latinoam. Nutr.,* 16, 125, 1966.

128. **Bohdal, M., Gibbs, N. E., and Simmons, W. K.,** *Nutrition Survey and Campaign Against Malnutrition in Kenya, 1964-1968,* Ministry of Health, Nairobi, Kenya, 1968.

129. **Schendel, H. E. and Hansen, J. D. L.,** Daily urinary nitrogen partition and balance in infants with kwashiorkor, *Am. J. Clin. Nutr.,* 17, 36, 1965.

130. **Berry, H. K.,** Plasma amino acids, in *Newer Methods of Nutritional Biochemistry,* Vol. IV, Albanese, A. A., Ed., Academic Press, New York, 1970, 79.

131. **Kiriyama, S.,** Biological quality of dietary protein and urinary nitrogen metabolites, in *Newer Methods of Nutritional Biochemistry,* Vol. IV, Albanese, A. A., Ed., Academic Press, New York, 1970, 37.

132. **Coulter, J. R. and Hann, C. S.,** Gas chromatography of amino acids, in *New Techniques in Amino Acid, Peptide, and Protein Analysis,* Niederwieser, A. and Pataki, G., Eds., Ann Arbor Science Publishers, Inc., Ann Arbor, 48106, 1971, 75.

133. **Bradfield, R. B. and Margen, S.,** Morphological changes in human scalp hair during protein deprivation, *Science,* 157, 438, 1970.

134. **Bradfield, R. B.,** Protein deprivation: comparative response of hair roots, serum protein, and urinary nitrogen, *Am. J. Clin. Nutr.,* 24, 405, 1971.

135. **Latham, M. C. and Velez, H.,** The tensile strength of hair in protein-calorie malnutrition, in *Nutrition and Health,* Vol. 1, Proc. Seventh International Congress of Nutrition 1966, Hamburg, Pergamon Press, New York, 1967, 87.

136. **Sims, R. T.,** Hair growth in kwashiorkor, *Arch. Dis. Child.,* 42, 397, 1967.
137. **Bradfield, R. B., and Jelliffe, E. F. P.,** Early assessment of malnutrition, *Nature,* 225, 283, 1970.
138. **MacVandiviere, H., Dale, T. A., Driess, R. B., and Watson, K. A.,** Hair-shaft diameter as an index of protein-calorie malnutrition, *Arch. Environ. Health.,* 23, 61, 1971.
139. **Bradfield, R. B., Jelliffe, E. F. P., and Jelliffe, D. B.,** Assessment of marginal malnutrition, *Nature,* 235, 112, 1972.
140. **Nammacher, M. A., Bradfield, R. B., and Arroyave, G.,** Comparing nutritional status methods in a Guatemalan survey, *Am. J. Clin. Nutr.,* 25, 871, 1972.
141. **Bradfield, R. B.,** A rapid tissue technique for the field assessment of protein-calorie malnutrition, *Am. J. Clin. Nutr.,* 25, 720, 1972.
142. **Bradfield, R. B. and Cordano, A.,** Hair root changes in Andean Indian children during marasmic kwashiorkor, *Lancet,* 2, 1169, 1968.
143. **Bradfield, R. B., Cordano, A., and Graham, G. G.,** Hair root adaptation to marasmus in Andean Indian children, *Lancet,* 2, 1395, 1969.
144. **Yoshida, T., Metcoff, J., and Frenk, S.,** Reduced pyruvic kinase activity, altered growth patterns of ATP in leukocytes, and protein-calorie malnutrition, *Am. J. Clin. Nutr.,* 21, 162, 1968.
145. **Zaki, A. H., El Kammah, B., Fayand, L., Shehata, A. H., and Mahmoud, S.,** Serum enzymes in protein malnutrition, *Acta Biol. Med. Germ.,* 24, 137, 1970.
146. **Van Reen, R., Valyasevi, A., and Dhanamitta, S.,** Studies of bladder stone disease in Thailand. XII. The effect of methionine and pyridoxine supplements on urinary sulfate, *Am. J. Clin. Nutr.,* 23, 940, 1970.
147. **Alvarado, J. and Luthringer, D. G.,** Serum immunoglobulins in edematous protein-calorie malnourished children, *Clin. Pediatr.,* 10, 174, 1971.
148. **Reindorp, S. and Whitehead, R. G.,** Changes in serum creatinine kinase and other biological measurements associated with musculature in children recovering from kwashiorkor, *Br. J. Nutr.,* 25, 273, 1971.
149. **Waterlow, J. C. and Stephen, J. M. L.,** Enzymes and the assessment of protein nutrition, *Proc. Nutr. Soc.,* 28, 234, 1969.
150. **Antia, A. U., McFarlane, H., and Soothill, J. F.,** Serum siderophilin in kwashiorkor, *Arch. Dis. Child.,* 43, 459, 1968.
151. **McFarlane, H. and Udeozo, I. O. K.,** Immunochemical estimation of some proteins in Nigerian paired maternal and fetal blood, *Arch. Dis. Child.,* 43, 42, 1968.
152. **McFarlane, H., Ogbeide, M. I., Reddy, S., Adcock, K. J., Adeshina, H., Gurney, J. M., Cooke, A., Taylor, G. O., and Mordie, J. A.,** Biochemical assessment of protein-calorie malnutrition, *Lancet,* 1, 392, 1969.
153. **McFarlane, H., Reddy, S., Adcock, K. J., Adeshina, H., Cooke, A. R., and Akene, J.,** Immunity transferrin and survival in kwashiorkor, *Br. Med. J.,* 4, 268, 1970.
154. **Ismadi, S. D., Susheels, T. P., and Rao, B. S. Narasinga,** Usefulness of plasma ceruloplasmin and transferrin levels in the assessment of protein calorie malnutrition among pre-school children, *Indian J. Med. Res.,* 59, 1581, 1971.
155. **Brasel, J. A.,** Institute of Human Nutrition, Columbia University, College of Physicians and Surgeons, New York (personal communication). Presentation on "Newer enzymatic markers of malnutrition" at the Texas Medical Center's symposium on the Application of Nutrition in the Health Sciences, January 12-13, 1973, Houston, Texas.
156. **O'Neal, R. M., Johnson, O. C., and Schaefer, A. E.,** Guidelines for classification and interpretation of group blood and urine data collected as part of the National Nutrition Survey, *Pediatr. Res.,* 4, 103, 1970.
157. *Suggested Guidelines for Evaluation of the Nutritional Status of Preschool Children,* U.S. Dept. of Health, Education and Welfare, Social and Rehabilitation Service, Children's Bureau (Revised 1967), U.S. Govt. Printing Office Publ. No. 1967-0-275-984.
158. **Scriver, C. R., Chow, C. L., and Lamm, P.,** Plasma amino acids: screening, quantitation, and interpretation, *Am. J. Clin. Nutr.,* 24, 876, 1971.
159. **Crowne, R. S., Wharton, B. A., and McCance, R. A.,** Hydroxyproline indices and hydroxyproline/creatinine ratios in older children, *Lancet,* 1, 395, 1969.
160. **Whitehead, R. G. and Alleyne, G. A. O.,** Pathophysiological factors of importance in protein-calorie malnutrition, *Br. Med. Bull.,* 28, 72, 1972.
161. **Gabr, M., El-Hawary, M. F., and El-Dali, M.,** Serum transferrin in kwashiorkor, *J. Trop. Med. Hyg.,* 74, 216, 1971.
162. **Young, V. and Scrimshaw, N. S.,** The nutritional significance of plasma and urinary amino acids, in *Protein and Amino Acid Functions,* Vol. 11, Bigwood, E. J., Ed., Pergamon Press, Elmsford, N.Y., 1972, 541.
163. **Bengoa, J. M.,** Outline of WHO and PAG participation in research on protein-calorie malnutrition, in *Protein-Calorie Malnutrition,* von Muralt, A., Ed., Springer-Verlag, Berlin and New York, 1969, 10.
164. **Aebi, H.,** Enzymes and nutrition, in *Protein-Calorie Malnutrition,* von Muralt, A., Ed., Springer-Verlag, Berlin and New York, 1969, 19.
165. **von Muralt, A.,** The discussion. 1. Biochemical tests, in *Protein-Calorie Malnutrition,* von Muralt, A., Ed., Springer-Verlag, Berlin and New York, 1969, 111.
166. **Simmons, W. K.,** Use of sulfate sulfur/creatinine ratio in field studies, *Am. J. Clin. Nutr.,* 26, 72, 1973.
167. Technicon Laboratory Method File No. N-lc I/II. Urea nitrogen, Technicon Corporation, Tarrytown, N.Y., 1967.

Mineral Nutrition

In this section, consideration will be given to some of the laboratory tests which are routinely used for determining levels of either macro or micro elements and how the data from these tests may be interpreted on a nutritional basis. While no attempt will be made to cover all of the tests which can be used for determining the concentration of a particular element, an attempt will be made to present at least one method which is commonly used and has been found to be reliable to the satisfaction of many investigators. Also discussed will be some of the problems that may be inherent in the assay method. More than one procedure for determining the element in question will be presented when such methods appear to be equally reliable and feasible. Additionally, no attempt will be made to cover all of the elements in the periodic table, but only those for which the laboratory tests can give data which may be meaningful from a nutritional point of view. For the most part, emphasis will be placed on those elements which are considered essential for the human and with attention given to some of the elements which are considered important from either an environmental, toxicological, or pollutant aspect. Iron and iodine will be covered in a separate section.

Sodium and Potassium

Sodium and potassium can now be considered together on an analytical basis since the most widely used assay method for each is flame photometry. This method can be used to determine sodium and potassium in plasma and urine, usually in a matter of minutes and without the necessity of chemical separations which are required in many of the wet chemical techniques. Additional advantages to the flame photometric method include: (a) the ability to determine both sodium and potassium on a very small sample; (b) the two elements may be determined without the supervision of an experienced chemist; (c) it is highly specific; and (d) accuracy and sensitivity are usually equal, and frequently exceed, those of the chemical techniques.

There are limitations to flame photometry. The equipment is more expensive than the equipment required in the chemical methods. This limitation becomes much less important if the number of samples to be processed is large as would be obtained in a large-scale survey for determining nutritional status. Another limitation of flame photometry is that the method gives an answer which is not absolute, but relative, to a standard solution; and herein lies the limitation. In order to truly compare the sample with the standard, the standard should be in the same matrix (similar in composition) as the sample. This is necessary to compensate for any spectrophotometric interferences or enhancements which might occur. The preparation of such standards may be quite time consuming. However, this limitation, too, becomes of minor importance if a large number of samples are to be assayed. For a more complete review of flame photometry, the reader is referred to the article by Meloche.[7]

Another advantage of flame photometry for measuring sodium and potassium is that they can be determined simultaneously on one sample.[8] Furthermore, many of the scientific equipment companies now have available automated flame photometers which simultaneously assay for sodium and potassium which improves the feasibility of performing large nutritional status surveys. One such automated method for the simultaneous determination of sodium and potassium is the Technicon AutoAnalyzer system.[9] For information concerning some of the older, wet-chemistry methods for sodium and potassium determinations, the reader is referred to the review by Kallmann.[10]

"Normal" serum levels of sodium are similar for adult males and females, being reported as 143 ± 3 meq/l and 144 ± 2 meq/l, respectively.[11] A survey of the data from many authors suggests that a "normal range" for plasma sodium concentration might be 130 to 155 meq/l. The infant probably has a slightly lower level of plasma sodium than the adult[12] but still within the normal range mentioned above. "Normal" serum potassium for adults has been reported as 4.4 ± 0.3 meq/l[11] with a possible normal range (from many reports) of 4.0 to 5.5 meq/l. Since potassium is the principal cation of intracellular fluids, care must be taken in collecting the blood samples as any hemolysis would markedly increase the serum potassium concentration. Hemolysis would not be a particular problem in serum sodium determinations since sodium is primarily an extracellular fluid cation.

Attaching nutritional significance to fluctuations in serum sodium and potassium levels is difficult and probably inconclusive due to variations resulting from certain pathological states. However, a deficiency might be anticipated in specific cases in which excessive loss of sodium and potassium have occurred, such as in prolonged use of diuretics, diarrhea, chronic renal failure, vomiting, profuse sweating, etc. The ubiquity of sodium and potassium in nature probably renders meaningless their consideration from a conventional nutritional point of view. Conversely, their nutritional importance is increased under the conditions mentioned above where a deficiency may be induced, or, in cases in which salt tablets have been ingested to maintain osmotic equilibrium.

Chloride

On a nutritional basis, chloride should be considered along with sodium and potassium since nearly all dietary chloride occurs as sodium chloride. Additionally, the homeostatic control of chloride is closely related to potassium homeostasis. Thus, conditions that may lead to sodium and/or potassium deficiency would very likely result in a chloride deficiency as well. Chloride is also ubiquitous in nature and not easily considered along conventional nutritional lines.

Literature concerning analytical methodology for chloride is voluminous, perhaps because of the difficulty involved in obtaining accurate and precise measurements. The older gravimetric technique of precipitation as silver chloride has many limitations when considered on a biological sample basis, including differences in organic matter content, possible loss of chloride during ashing procedures, and lack of completeness of extraction. An automated technique[13] is currently being used in the authors' laboratory which is a photometric technique modified from Zall et al.[14] The technique results in the indirect determination of chloride through a coupled reaction. Mercuric thiocyanate is reacted with chloride to release thiocyanate which is subsequently reacted with ferric iron to form a red complex which is measured photometrically. Despite the indirectness of the assay, it has been used quite successfully. Using this procedure, chloride can be determined in plasma, serum, and urine.

The average serum chloride concentration in a group of "normal" subjects has been reported[11] as 103 ± 3.0 meq/l. A normal range for serum chloride based on numerous literature reports would appear to be 99 to 110 meq/l.

For a more comprehensive review of many of the techniques that have been tried for the determination of chloride, the reader is referred to the article by Armstrong et al.[15]

Sulfur

Sulfur is perhaps unique among the elements in that it functions predominantly (maybe exclusively) as a constitutive part of an organic molecule. It has been generally accepted that higher animals require only three of these organic sulfur compounds in the diet: thiamin, biotin, and methionine. Thus, tests for nutritional adequacy of sulfur should perhaps be concerned with measures of vitamin and protein nutriture, and these items are covered in other sections of this article. This is not to say that other important forms of biological sulfur do not exist. For instance, sulfomucopolysaccharides are of great biological importance but are synthesized from other forms of dietary sulfur, usually cysteine. If the investigator is merely interested in total sulfur in biological fluids or tissues, then one could use the gravimetric technique of precipitating the sulfate with barium and weighing.

Within the last decade, atomic absorption spectrophotometry (AAS) has been thoroughly developed and now enjoys widespread acceptance as an analytical method. This technique has made possible the determination of trace elements on a broad scale with a minimum of sample manipulation. The importance of AAS as a laboratory method for determining nutritional status will become increasingly evident as we discuss trace element nutrition later. The method is mentioned here because sulfur can also be determined by indirect AAS. To measure sulfur by this method, the gravimetric technique has been modified. Initially, Roe et al.[16] oxidized the sample, precipitated the sulfate with barium, repeatedly washed the precipitate, dissolved the precipitate in disodium ethylenediaminetetraacetic acid, and measured the barium by AAS. By calculation, or by comparison to a prepared sulfate standard curve, sulfur was determined. Subsequently, to avoid the washing step, an alternate technique was developed[17] which added a known amount of barium to precipitate the sulfate and then measured the residual barium in solution. Both procedures give excellent sulfur recovery data and can be applied to many types of biological samples including urine and blood. Other methods for sulfur determination may be found in the review by Heinrich et al.[18]

To the authors' knowledge, there are no well-defined "standard values" for total sulfur in biological samples (see section on Protein-calorie malnutrition).

Phosphorus

From a metabolic point of view, phosphorus is probably the central most element, being involved in both hard and soft tissue structure and essential at many steps in intermediary metabolism. Consequently, it is important to be able to determine phosphorus nutriture.

Perhaps one of the most widely used and accepted methods for determining phosphorus is some modification of the molybdenum blue procedure of Fiske and Subbarow.[19] This is a colorimetric technique which depends upon the development of a blue color following the reduction of the heteropoly acid formed between phosphate and molybdate. Some of the disadvantages of this method of phosphorus determination include spontaneous color development in the absence of phosphate and a progressive increase in the intensity of the color.[20] Many modifications of the molybdenum blue procedure have appeared in the literature since its original publication. Several of the modifications were concerned with the reducing agent used (originally aminonaphtholsulfonic acid was used) although none seems to greatly improve the procedure. The procedure currently in use in the authors' laboratory is, again, an automated method[21] which is a slight modification of the original molybdenum blue assay.[19] The sample (either plasma, serum or properly diluted urine) is dialyzed, acidic ammonium molybdate added (to form the phosphomolybdic acid) and then immediately reduced with aminonaphtholsulfonic acid. The mixture is then heated to enhance the development of the blue color and then assayed colorimetrically. The procedure is rapid and has been used quite successfully. Many other phosphorus assays may be found in the review article of Reiman and Beukenkamp.[22]

Certain precautions are necessary in order that plasma or serum phosphorus determinations are meaningful. For example, if blood is allowed to stand after drawing, hemolysis of the red blood cells readily occurs. Such hemolysis, even if it is slight, will invalidate plasma or serum phosphorus values since the red blood cell contains some 17 times the phosphorus of plasma.[23] The average normal range for serum phosphorus in the adult human appears to be 2.5 to 4.0 mg/100 ml, while in infants, serum phosphorus is somewhat higher at 5.0 to 6.5 mg/100 ml.

The number of factors that have been reported to alter plasma or serum phosphorus is too great to be within the scope of this review concerning methodology. However, it would be germane to the discussion here to mention a few of the more prominent factors which affect serum or plasma phosphorus since they might be suspect should the assay produce data which are outside the normal range. These factors have been summarized.[24] Blood inorganic phosphorus in rickets of children is markedly reduced. Vitamin D treatment of the disease will normalize the blood phosphorus picture. In persons with healing fractures, plasma phosphorus may be increased. In children, there appears to be a seasonal variation in plasma phosphorus; it rises during the summer and declines during the winter. This phenomenon is perhaps related, through the action of vitamin D, to solar ultraviolet radiation. In the diabetic, plasma phosphate levels may be quite variable since insulin injections tend to decrease the phosphorus in the plasma. For a more complete review of phosphorus alterations in biological systems, the reader is referred to the review of Bartter.[25] The information presented here is merely to show that the interpretation of laboratory test data from a nutritional point of view may be extremely difficult.

Calcium

Calcium is the major inorganic element of the body; thus, its nutritional importance is obvious. Unlike phosphorus, which is found in both hard and soft tissue structure, it is generally accepted that 99+% of the body content of calcium is present in bones and teeth. Calcium in the blood appears to be almost entirely in the plasma fraction. Consequently, hemolysis of the red blood cells does not create the analytical problem for calcium that it does for phosphorus. Normally, calcium should be determined on serum rather than plasma since most of the anticoagulants function by reacting with calcium.

Perhaps the most widely accepted method for the determination of serum calcium is that of Clark and Collip[26] wherein calcium is precipitated as the oxalate, the precipitate dissolved in acid, and the resultant solution titrated with permanganate. One of the chief disadvantages of this procedure is insuring complete precipitation of the calcium without excess oxalate, since it is the latter which is titrated.[27] Another disadvantage is that titration procedures, especially the manual ones, are quite time consuming. MacIntyre[28] presented a flame photometric technique which reportedly had good sensitivity in biological solutions. Flame photometry has the advantage, as indicated for sodium and potassium, that sample manipulation is minimal. In an effort to increase sample handling capacity, Kessler and Wolfman[29] developed an automated procedure for the simultaneous determination of calcium and phosphorus. Their calcium procedure is currently being used in the authors' laboratory and has been detailed.[30] This procedure can be used on either serum or urine and requires no preliminary sample treatment. Atomic absorption spectrophotometry has also been applied to serum calcium determinations[31] where direct dilution and aspiration of the sample have given results comparable to the calcium oxalate method. The presence of phosphate in diluted serum causes a slight depression of the AAS calcium signal which can be overcome by using a diluent containing a small amount of either strontium or lanthanum. Other procedures for calcium determination have been summarized.[32]

Compared with most other elements, the "normal" range for human serum calcium is quite narrow, probably about 9 to 11 mg/100 ml. Values for children seem to be slightly higher but not outside the normal range when compared with those of adults.[24] Another general factor which may slightly affect serum calcium levels is pregnancy, in which case a depression is sometimes observed in the late stages. Nutritional interpretation of sera calcium data, like that of phosphorus, is extremely difficult due to the highly developed homeostatic control system. In fact, blood calcium is controlled so closely that, should it vary outside the normal range, one might suspect pathological problems before nutritional aspects.

Magnesium

Magnesium is of great nutritional importance since it, like phosphorus, is a constituent of both bone and soft tissue. Additionally, magnesium is an activator of many enzymatic processes, especially reactions involving oxidative phosphorylation. The first description of magnesium deficiency as a specific entity in man[33] demonstrated that it was indistinguishable from hypocalcemic tetany except by chemical analysis. In magnesium deficiency, serum magnesium was markedly reduced, whereas serum calcium remained normal. Contrary to the above finding, Shils[34] reported that both serum calcium and serum potassium were reduced as hypomagnesemia persisted in experimental human magnesium deficiency.

Many procedures have been described for the determination of magnesium, and these have been reviewed.[35,36] Perhaps one of the oldest procedures is the gravimetric technique of McCrudden[37] which precipitates magnesium as magnesium ammonium phosphate. This procedure, or some modification, is still often used. One of the major modifications measures magnesium indirectly through a colorimetric determination of the precipitated phosphate.[38] Flame spectrometry has been used to determine magnesium in serum and urine.[39] Atomic absorption spectroscopy (AAS) is currently being used in the authors' laboratory for the determination of magnesium in serum and urine. For serum, magnesium can be determined on as little as one drop since the sensitivity will permit up to a 50-fold dilution.[40] The only interference in the determination of serum magnesium by AAS seems to be a small enhancement of the reading by protein. This can be corrected by adding a small amount of strontium to the diluent. Stewart et al.[41] precipitated the serum protein with 10% trichloroacetic acid to overcome the protein effect on sera magnesium assays. Magnesium in urine can be determined by AAS by simply diluting with water.[42]

A survey of many literature reports indicates that a "normal" value for serum magnesium would be approximately 1.7 meq/l with a "normal range" of about 1.3 to 2.0 meq/l. Many pathological states have been reported to alter serum magnesium, and these have been well reviewed.[36]

Zinc

Up to this point, only elements which are supplied in the diet in "macro" quantities have been discussed. With zinc, we begin consideration of a group of nutrients which are commonly termed "trace elements" (or micronutrients) because they are supplied in the diet in micro quantities. Zinc deficiency in man was first reported in 1961.[43] The symptoms were growth retardation and hypogonadism. Laboratory tests revealed that these zinc-deficient patients had reduced plasma and red blood cell zinc concentrations and that urinary zinc excretion was decreased compared to control subjects.[44]

The number of methods available for the determination of zinc are many.[45] Until recently, perhaps one of the most popular was the dithizone colorimetric procedure[46] or some modification of it. The procedure, while relatively precise, required a large degree of sample handling and was time-consuming. With the satisfactory development of atomic absorption spectrophotometry (AAS), many of the trace elements, including zinc, are now routinely determined by this method. Two procedures for determining zinc in serum by AAS seem to be well accepted. Sprague and Slavin[47] reported a method which required only a 1:1 dilution of the serum with water. The major disadvantage of this method was that the burner head of the AAS would frequently become clogged because of the high protein content of the diluted sample. Subsequently, it was reported that treating the serum with trichloroacetic acid (TCA), centrifuging, and assaying the supernatant solution for zinc would remove the burner clogging problem.[48] However, these workers found it necessary to purify (decontaminate) their TCA which was a laborious task. More recently, Olson and Hamlin[49] found that "reagent grade" commercial TCA was essentially free of contaminants and used the TCA precipitation method effectively for serum zinc determinations. Urinary zinc can normally be determined by AAS on either diluted or undiluted urine.[48]

"Normal" zinc values in the various blood components are not well established. There are many disease states which alter the blood zinc picture, and these have been summarized.[50,51] Some of these conditions include malignancy, anemias, atherosclerosis, infections, and pregnancies. Recently, the estrogenic containing oral contraceptives have been reported to decrease plasma zinc.[52] But perhaps an even more important factor in the lack of agreement concerning "normal" plasma or serum zinc values stems from the partition of zinc in the various blood fractions.

Red blood cells contain approximately 75% of whole blood fractions. Red blood cells contain approximately 75% of whole blood zinc, whereas plasma contains only 22%.[53] Thus, any hemolysis would cause marked variations in serum and plasma zinc concentrations. Platelets also contain significant amounts of zinc and, along with a volume difference, contribute to the difference between serum and plasma zinc levels.[54] Consequently, until procedures are standardized and "normal' values are determined, it will be extremely difficult to attach real nutritional significance to variations in blood zinc concentrations.

Copper

It goes without question that copper is an essential nutrient for all mammals.[55] However, frank copper deficiency in man is a debatable question[56] although there have been some suggestions of its existence,[57,58] especially in infants. Important symptoms of the reported deficiency were anemia, neutropenia, and skeletal lesions similar to those seen in scurvy.

Methodology for the determination of copper by wet chemistry has been adequately summarized.[59] One of these, which was widely used, was a colorimetric procedure using sodium diethyldithiocarbamate as a complexing agent.[60] However, as with many of the other tedious procedures, this colorimetric determination of copper has given way in recent years to atomic absorption spectroscopy (AAS). Copper, like zinc, has been measured by AAS in serum by simple dilution[47] or following trichloroacetic acid treatment.[48,49] Parker et al.[48] reported that urinary copper was so low that it had to be chelated and organically extracted in order to assay by AAS. Subsequently, Dawson et al.[61] reported that urinary copper could be determined directly by AAS if the urine was properly acidified. They reported a signal suppression due to the inorganic urinary components but corrected this bias by adding inorganic salts to the standards.

"Normal" values for serum copper have been reported as 95 μg/100 ml and 122 μg/100 ml for adult men and women, respectively.[61] A "normal range" would, from many reports, appear to be 75 to 150 μg/100 ml. Serum copper is somewhat reduced in newborn infants with values as low as 49 μg/100 ml being reported.[56] Serum copper variations associated with pathological states have been summarized.[51] Estrogenic oral contraceptives significantly increased serum copper whereas a progestogen type had no effect.[62] Factors such as these are certainly of extreme importance in determining nutritional status from concentrations of particular elements in body fluids.

Other Trace Elements

There are a number of trace elements not yet discussed which are regarded as essential to man: cobalt, because of its function in vitamin B_{12};[63] manganese, because of its function in bone structure and enzymatic reactions;[64] molybdenum, because of its role in the xanthine oxidase system;[65] fluoride, because of its involvement in teeth;[66] and chromium, because of its relation to glucose tolerance.[67] However, since frank deficiencies for these elements are either ill-defined or not defined at all, it is not within the scope of this article that they be discussed here. To be sure, these elements have been determined under various biological conditions, but "normal values" have not been adequately established. Consequently, a statement concerning nutritional status based upon the concentration of one of these elements in biological material would certainly be less than definitive.

There are also some trace elements that are of biological significance from a toxicological point of view but are not presently considered essential for man. Included in this group of elements would be lead, cadmium, and mercury. All three of these elements can be determined quite adequately by atomic absorption spectrophotometry.[68] Frequently, cadmium can be determined directly on urine and after nitric acid treatment on blood with no further sample preparation.[69] Since the concentration of lead and mercury is normally quite low in biological samples, they are usually concentrated by extracting into an organic solvent following chelation. Cadmium can also be determined by organic extraction as can many of the other elements previously mentioned.[70] One of the most popular of these organic solvent extraction techniques is to chelate the metal with ammonium pyrrolidine dithiocarbamate and extract into methyl isobutyl ketone. Not only can one concentrate the element by this procedure, but there is also an enhanced absorption signal with the organic matrix. To the interested reader, a complete coverage of atomic absorption spectroscopy has been published.[71] More recently, flameless atomic absorption spectrometry has been used for the determination of lead[72] and mercury.[73] Although it has not been mentioned with the discussions of atomic absorption spectrophotometry, it is extremely important that care be taken to avoid trace element contamination in glassware, water, reagents, and equipment if accurate and reliable results are to be obtained.

Underwood[51] has summarized the literature concerning our understanding of "normal" (or natural) amounts of cadmium, lead, and mercury in human biological fluids. For cadmium, a range of 0.3 to 5.4 µg/100 ml of blood appears normal; urinary cadmium concentrations appear to be in the range of from less than 7 to 22 µg/l. Normal blood lead was reported as 0.17 µg/ml with a range of 0.15 to 0.40 µg/ml, while "natural" urinary lead was 35 µg/l. Whole blood mercury for a normal population was reported as 0.005 µg/ml with red blood cells containing about twice the concentration of plasma. The reported normal urinary mercury was 0.023 µg/ml. All of these values reported by Underwood were from relatively small populations and should be verified by larger surveys. Also, all the urinary values suffer from the limitations outlined in the Introduction section.

General Comments

It was the original intent of this review to critically examine some of the more recent literature concerning laboratory testing procedures for the determination of nutritional status. In the area of inorganic elemental nutrition, such an intent was not always easily followed. This was especially true of the macro elements examined wherein the analytical methodology was developed many years ago and has undergone very little change since. To be sure, many of the techniques have been adapted to automated procedures, yet the test itself remains essentially the same. Thus, an attempt was made to present the "age-old" procedure and discuss some of its advantages and disadvantages. Similarly, it was not easy, in many instances, to attach a great deal of nutritional significance to deviations from the "normal ranges" of elemental concentration in either blood or urine. The reason for this is that an inorganic element can rarely stand alone in the nutritional sense. Even a superficial examination of the literature will reveal these complexities. For example, briefly consider the calcium-magnesium-phosphate interaction in biological systems. It was reported[74] that an increase of one gram of dietary magnesium at constant calcium intake resulted in sustained increases in serum calcium and urinary calcium and a decrease in urinary phosphorus. It has recently been emphasized[75] in the rat that serum calcium is more dependent upon the dietary calcium:phosphorus ratio than on the absolute amount of dietary calcium; and, when dietary phosphate is high, urinary calcium is reduced. In man, oral or intravenous administration of phosphate reduced urinary excretion of calcium and magnesium.[76] Further complicating the picture is a recent report that glucose ingestion increases urinary calcium and magnesium excretion rates.[77] These complexities are not presented to confuse the reader but rather to indicate the inconclusiveness of attempting to measure the concentration of one inorganic element in urine or blood and then attaching some nutritional significance to the data. While there may be nutritional implications, the "abnormal" data may be a result of some factor other than that resulting from the element under question. Nor are these biological interactions limited to the macro elements. Anemia immediately associated with iron deficiency can, in fact, result from low dietary copper.[78] High levels of dietary zinc significantly reduced serum copper.[79] Thus, inorganic element interactions in biological systems are numerous, and one must exercise caution in interpreting data based upon analysis of a single element.

This discussion of methods for determining nutritional status would not be complete without a brief consideration of some of the procedures which are currently "on the horizon." One such procedure which has shown great potential, at least for the determination of micro-element nutriture, but which has not yet been subjected to exhaustive study is the use of hair as the biological sample (rather than urine or blood). One of the advantages of using hair as a biopsy material, should it prove successful, is the ease with which such a sample could be obtained. Perhaps an even more important advantage would be that hair, by the very nature of the sample, should reflect a rather long-term nutritional state rather than recent (i.e., previous meal or day) dietary intake.

Growth rate, morphology, and color of hair reportedly respond to inadequate protein levels in the diet.[80-82] Low dietary levels of some of the essential micro-elements have been reported to result in corresponding decreases in hair concentra-

tion of the element.[83,84] Conversely, when the dietary level of lead (a toxic element) was high, the element accumulated in the hair.[85] Two studies have been reported in the literature in which the specific purpose was determining the value of hair as an effective biopsy sample, one for determining zinc nutriture,[4-6,86] and one for determining copper nutriture.[4-6,87] The general conclusions from the zinc study were that hair zinc varied with age (decreased during the first 10 years of life and increased during the second 10 years), did not vary with sex (but was somewhat reduced in either pregnant or lactating females), and should be used to compare nutriture of individuals or groups only on an age-matched basis. From the copper study, it was concluded that hair copper varied both with sex and with age, was correlated with plasma copper, and should be used as a nutriture comparator only on a sex- and age-matched basis.

One of the questions raised concerning the use of hair as a biopsy sample was whether or not some of the elements might not be adsorbed on the hair filament from environmental contamination such as sweat.[88] If such were the case, then the data obtained might be so biased as to not represent realistic nutritional status. However, Bate's contention[88] was based on work wherein radioisotopes were adsorbed onto previously washed hair which did not contain the natural oils, the latter presumably protects hair from contamination. This shortcoming (possible contamination) of hair as a biopsy sample has been effectively rebutted,[89] but no data were presented to contradict the original question.

Perhaps the most widely used method of determining trace elements in hair is by atomic absorption spectrophotometry.[90] Recovery data suggested that the method was certainly acceptable, whereas comparison with literature data was somewhat less definitive. This latter problem of differences with literature reports was attributed somewhat to variations in sample preparation, a procedure which has not been generally standardized. X-ray fluorescence has also been used for determining zinc and calcium in hair and has the advantage of being a nondestructive method.[91]

Since the use of hair as a biopsy material for determining nutritional status is still in the exploratory stage, "normal" values for the particular nutrients are not well defined. Based upon the work of Strain et al.,[84] it was suggested that, when hair zinc is less than 70 parts per million, other features of zinc deficiency may be observed.[92] Hair has also been used as a biological sample for the determination of chromium status[1-3,93,94] with the result that hair chromium was reduced in diabetic children and in parous women. The idea of using hair analyses for determining nutritional status is not without controversy. One group of workers[84] conclude that "hair analysis appears to be a reliable, simple and atraumatic method for assessing body zinc stores," while other investigators[95] report that their data "do not support the suggestion that the zinc content of hair is a reliable indicator of body zinc stores in prepubescent children." Perhaps age differences are responsible for this dichotomy of literature reports. Nevertheless, it appears that much more work will be required before hair can be accepted as biopsy material for nutriture determinations and before "normal ranges" can be set, although it does appear promising at the present time.

Fingernails may also serve as an effective biopsy material for determining nutritional status with respect to certain elements, but very little data are in the literature concerning "normal values." Atomic absorption has been used to assay fingernails for several elements,[96] and at least two studies were concerned with "normal" individuals.[97,98]

Other methods of analyses of biological samples, such as emission spectroscopy[99] and neutron activation,[100] are in the literature. However, these techniques are not yet widely used and are only mentioned here so that the interested reader may have a point of reference. A brief review[101] of some of the methodological problems inherent in nutritional studies discusses emission spectroscopy, atomic absorption spectroscopy, wet-chemical analyses, radioisotopic analysis, and contamination problems.

In summary, one can say that many methods are available for measuring the concentration of a particular inorganic element in biological samples. Some of these procedures have gained widespread acceptance, and an attempt has been made to evaluate them in this review. One facet which we feel has been inadequately explained in this particular section concerns the nutritional significance of deviations from "normal" elemental concentrations in biological fluids. In a few instances, definite nutritional aspects have been evident but, in most cases there is, sadly, not enough information available to conclude nutritional implications or even define "normal" status. No attempt has been made to consider the many pathological and clinical factors which may influence biological elemental concentrations since the intent of the article was to discuss methodology concerning nutritional status. Many new approaches are being made to better define "normal" nutrition by measuring the right parameters. When this is accomplished one can, hopefully, attach nutritional significance to the deviations from "normal values."

REFERENCES

1. **Hambidge, K. M. and Baum, J. D.,** Hair chromium concentration of human newborn and changes during infancy, *Am. J. Clin. Nutr.,* 25, 376, 1972.
2. **Hambidge, K. M., Franklin, M., and Jacobs, M. A.,** Changes in hair chromium concentrations with increasing distances from hair roots, *Am. J. Clin. Nutr.,* 25, 380, 1972.
3. **Hambidge, K. M., Franklin, M. L., and Jacobs, M. A.,** Hair chromium concentration: effects of sample washing and external environment *Am. J. Clin. Nutr.,* 25, 384, 1972.
4. **Klevay, L. M.,** Hair as a biopsy material, *Am. J. Clin. Nutr.,* 25, 263, 1972.
5. **Schroeder, H. A. and Nason, A. P.,** Trace metals in human hair, *J. Invest. Dermatol.,* 53, 71, 1969.
6. **Petering, H. G., Yeager, D. W., and Witherup, S. O.,** Trace metal content of hair. I. Zinc and copper content of human hair in relation to age and sex, *Arch. Environ. Health,* 23, 202, 1971.
7. **Meloche, V. W.,** Flame photometry, *Anal. Chem.,* 28, 1844, 1956.
8. **Ramsay, J. A., Brown, R. H. J., and Falloon, S. W. H. W.,** Simultaneous determination of sodium and potassium in small volumes of fluid by flame photometry, *J. Exptl. Biol.,* 30, 1, 1953.
9. Technicon laboratory method file N-20a, Technicon Corp., Ardsley, N.Y., 1963.
10. **Kallmann, S.,** The alkali metals, in *Treatise on Analytical Chemistry, Part II, Analytical Chemistry of the Elements,* Vol. 1, Kolthoff, I. M. and Elving, P. J., Eds., Interscience Publishers, New York, 1961, 301.

11. **Frank, H. A. and Carr, M. H.,** "Normal" serum electrolytes with a note on seasonal and menstrual variation, *J. Lab. Clin. Med.,* 49, 246, 1957.

12. **Overman, R. R., Etteldorf, J. N., Bass, A. C., and Horn, G. B.,** Plasma and erythrocyte chemistry of the normal infant from birth to two years of age, *Pediatrics,* 7, 565, 1951.

13. Technicon laboratory method file N-5b, Technicon Corp., Ardsley, N.Y., 1965.

14. **Zall, D. M., Fisher, D., and Garner, M. Q.,** Photometric determination of chlorides in water, *Anal. Chem.,* 28, 1665, 1956.

15. **Armstrong, G. W., Gill, H. H., and Rolf, R. F.,** The halogens, in *Treatise on Analytical Chemistry, Part II, Analytical Chemistry of the Elements,* Vol. 7, Kolthoff, I. M. and Elving, P. J., Eds., Interscience Publishers, New York, 1961, 335.

16. **Roe, D. A., Miller, P. S., and Lutwak, L.,** Estimation of sulfur in biological materials by atomic absorption spectrometry, *Anal. Biochem.,* 15, 313, 1966.

17. **Dunk, R., Mostyn, R. A., and Hoare, H. C.,** The determination of sulfate by indirect atomic absorption spectroscopy, *Atomic Absorption Newsletter,* 8, 79, 1969.

18. **Heinrich, B. J., Grimes, M. D., and Puckett, J. E.,** Sulfur, in *Treatise on Analytical Chemistry, Part II, Analytical Chemistry of the Elements,* Vol. 7, Kolthoff, I. M. and Elving, P. J., Eds., Interscience Publishers, New York, 1961, 1.

19. **Fiske, C. H. and Subbarow, Y.,** The colorimetric determination of phosphorus, *J. Biol. Chem.,* 66, 375, 1925.

20. **Lowry, O. H. and Lopez, J. A.,** The determination of inorganic phosphate in the presence of labile phosphate esters, *J. Biol. Chem.,* 162, 421, 1946.

21. Technicon laboratory method file N-4b, Technicon Corp., Ardsley, N.Y., 1965.

22. **Reiman, III, W. and Beukenkamp, J.,** Phosphorus, in *Treatise on Analytical Chemistry, Part II, Analytical Chemistry of the Elements,* Vol. 5, Kolthoff, I. M. and Elving, P. J., Eds., Interscience Publishers, New York, 1961, 317.

23. **Kay, H. D.,** The distribution of phosphorus compounds in the blood of certain mammals, *J. Physiol. (London),* 65, 374, 1928.

24. **Oser, B. L.,** *Hawk's Physiological Chemistry,* 14th ed., McGraw-Hill, New York, 1965, 1114.

25. **Bartter, F. C.,** Disturbances of phosphorus metabolism, in *Mineral Metabolism,* Vol. 2, Part A, Comar, C. L. and Bronner, F., Eds., Academic Press, New York, 1964, 315.

26. **Clark, E. P. and Collip, J. B.,** Determination of blood serum calcium, *J. Biol. Chem.,* 63, 462, 1925.

27. **Sendroy, J., Jr.,** Determination of serum calcium by precipitation with oxalate. A comparative study of factors affecting the results of several procedures. Note on gasometric determination of oxalic acid and calcium, *J. Biol. Chem.,* 152, 539, 1944.

28. **MacIntyre, I.,** The flame-spectrophotometric determination of calcium in biological fluids and an isotopic analysis of the errors in the Kramer-Tisdall procedure, *Biochem. J.,* 67, 164, 1957.

29. **Kessler, G. and Wolfman, M.,** An automated procedure for the simultaneous determination of calcium and phosphorus, *Clin. Chem.,* 10, 686, 1964.

30. Technicon laboratory method file N-3a, Technicon Crop., Ardsley, N.Y., 1965.

31. **Zettner, A. and Seligson, D.,** Application of atomic absorption spectrophotometry in the determination of calcium in serum, *Clin. Chem.,* 10, 869, 1964.

32. **Bronner, F.,** Dynamics and function of calcium, in *Mineral Metabolism,* Vol. 2, Part A, Comar, C. L. and Bronner, F., Eds., Academic Press, New York, 1964, 341.

33. **Vallee, B. L., Wacker, W. E. C., and Ulmer, D. D.,** The magnesium-deficiency tetany syndrome in man, *N. Engl. J. Med.,* 262, 155, 1960.

34. **Shils, M. E.,** Experimental human magnesium depletion. I. Clinical observations and blood chemistry alterations, *Am. J. Clin. Nutr.,* 15, 133, 1964.

35. **Wengert, G. B., Reigler, P. F., and Carlson, A. M.,** Magnesium, in *Treatise on Analytical Chemistry, Part II, Analytical Chemistry of the Elements,* Vol. 3, Kolthoff, I. M. and Elving, P. J., Eds., Interscience Publishers, New York, 1961, 43.

36. **Wacker, W. E. C. and Vallee, B. L.,** Magnesium, in *Mineral Metabolism,* Vol. 2, Part A, Comar, C. L. and Bronner, F., Eds., Academic Press, New York, 1964, 483.

37. **McCrudden, F. H.,** Magnesium ammonium phosphate method for magnesium in food, urine, and feces, *J. Biol. Chem.,* 7, 83, 1909.

38. **Simonsen, D. G., Westover, L. M., and Wertman, M.,** The determination of serum magnesium by the molybdivanidate method for phosphate, *J. Biol. Chem.,* 169, 39, 1947.

39. **Wacker, W. E. C. and Vallee, B. L.,** A study of magnesium metabolism in acute renal failure employing a multichannel flame spectrometer, *N. Engl. J. Med.,* 257, 1254, 1957.

40. **Willis, J. B.,** The analysis of biological materials by atomic-absorption spectroscopy, *Clin. Chem.,* 11, 251, 1965.

41. **Stewart, W. K., Hutchinson, F., and Fleming, L. W.,** The estimation of magnesium in serum and urine by atomic absorption spectrophotometry, *J. Lab. Clin. Med.,* 61, 858, 1963.

42. **Gimblet, E. G., Marney, A. F., and Bonsnes, R. W.,** Determination of calcium and magnesium in serum, urine, diet, and stool by atomic absorption spectrophotometry, *Clin. Chem.,* 13, 204, 1967.

43. **Prasad, A. S., Halsted, J. A., and Nadimi, M.,** Syndrome of iron deficiency anemia, hepatosplenomegaly, hypogonadism, dwarfism and geophagia, *Am. J. Med.,* 31, 532, 1961.

44. **Prasad, A. S., Miale, A., Jr., Farid, Z., Sandstead, H. H., and Schulert, A. R.,** Zinc metabolism in patients with the syndrome of iron deficiency anemia, hepatosplenomegaly, dwarfism, and hypogonadism, *J. Lab. Clin. Med.,* 61, 537, 1963.

45. **Kanzelmeyer, J. H.,** Zinc, in *Treatise on Analytical Chemistry, Part II, Analytical Chemistry of the Elements,* Vol. 3, Kolthoff, I. M. and Elving, P. J., Eds., Interscience Publishers, New York, 1961, 95.

46. **Hoch, F. L. and Vallee, B. L.,** Precipitation by trichloroacetic acid as a simplification in the determination of zinc in blood and its components, *J. Biol. Chem.,* 181, 295, 1949.

47. **Sprague, S. and Slavin, W.,** Determination of iron, copper and zinc in blood serum by an atomic absorption method requiring only dilution, *Atomic Absorption Newsletter,* 4, 228, 1965.

48. **Parker, M. M., Humoller, F. L., and Mahler, D. L.,** Determination of copper and zinc in biological material, *Clin. Chem.,* 13, 40, 1967.

49. **Olson, A. D. and Hamlin, W. B.,** Serum copper and zinc by atomic absorption spectrophotometry, *Atomic Absorption Newsletter,* 7, 69, 1968.

50. **Vallee, B. L.,** Biochemistry, physiology and pathology of zinc, *Physiol. Rev.,* 39, 443, 1959.

51. **Underwood, E. J.,** *Trace Elements in Human and Animal Nutrition,* 3rd ed., Academic Press, New York, 1971, 208.

52. **Briggs, M. H., Briggs, M., and Austin, J.,** Effects of steroid pharmaceuticals on plasma zinc, *Nature,* 232, 480, 1971.

53. **Vallee, B. L. and Gibson, J. G., 2nd,** The zinc content of normal human whole blood, plasma, leucocytes, and erythrocytes, *J. Biol. Chem.,* 176, 445, 1948.

54. **Foley, B., Johnson, S. A., Hackley, B., Smith, J. C., Jr., and Halsted, J. A.,** Zinc content of human platelets, *Proc. Soc. Exp. Biol. Med.,* 128, 265, 1968.

55. **Elvehjem, C. A.,** The biological significance of copper and its relation to iron metabolism, *Physiol. Rev.,* 15, 471, 1935.

56. **Cartwright, G. E. and Wintrobe, M. M.,** The question of copper deficiency in man, *Am. J. Clin. Nutr.,* 15, 94, 1964.

57. **Cordano, A., Baertl, J. M., and Graham, G. G.,** Copper deficiency in infancy, *Pediatrics,* 34, 324, 1964.

58. **Graham, G. G. and Cordano, A.,** Copper depletion and deficiency in the malnourished infant, *Johns Hopkins Med. J.,* 124, 139, 1969.

59. **Cooper, W. C.,** Copper, in *Treatise on Analytical Chemistry, Part II, Analytical Chemistry of the Elements,* Vol. 3, Kolthoff, I. M. and Elving, P. J., Eds., Interscience Publishers, New York, 1961, 1.

60. **Sandell, E. B., Colorimetric Determination of Traces of Metals,** 2nd ed., Interscience, New York, 1950, 300.

61. **Dawson, J. B., Ellis, D. J., and Newton-John, H.,** Direct estimation of copper in serum and urine by atomic absorption spectroscopy, *Clin. Chim. Acta,* 21, 33, 1968.

62. **Briggs, M., Austin, J., and Staniford, M.,** Oral contraceptives and copper metabolism, *Nature,* 225, 81, 1970.

63. **Stokstad, E. L. R.,** The biochemistry of the water soluble vitamins, *Ann. Rev. Biochem.,* 31, 472, 1962.

64. **North, B. B., Leichsenring, J. M., and Norris, L. M.,** Manganese metabolism in college women, *J. Nutr.,* 72, 217, 1960.

65. **Richert, D. A. and Westerfeld, W. W.,** Isolation and identification of the xanthine oxidase factor as molybdenum, *J. Biol. Chem.,* 203, 915, 1953.

66. **Sognnaes, R. F.,** Fluoride protection of bones and teeth, *Science,* 150, 989, 1965.

67. **Mertz, W.,** Biological role of chromium, *Fed. Proc.,* 26, 186, 1967.

68. **Willis, J. B.,** Determination of lead and other heavy metals in urine by atomic absorption spectroscopy, *Anal. Chem.,* 34, 612, 1962.

69. **Slavin, W., Sprague, S., Rieders, F., and Cordova, V.,** The determination of certain toxicological trace metals by atomic absorption spectrophotometry, *Atomic Absorption Newsletter,* 4, 7, 1964.

70. **Mulford, C. E.,** Solvent extraction techniques for atomic absorption spectroscopy, *Atomic Absorption Newsletter,* 5, 88, 1966.

71. **Slavin, W.,** *Atomic Absorption Spectroscopy,* Interscience Publishers, New York, 1968.

72. **Hwang, J. Y., Ullucci, P. A., Smith, S. B., Jr., and Malenfant, A. L.,** Microdetermination of lead in blood by flameless atomic absorption spectrometry, *Anal. Chem.,* 43, 1319, 1971.

73. **Manning, D. C.,** Non-flame methods for mercury determination by atomic absorption: A review, *Atomic Absorption Newsletter,* 9, 97, 1970.

74. **Briscoe, A. M. and Ragan, C.,** Effect of magnesium on calcium metabolism in man, *Am. J. Clin. Nutr.,* 19, 296, 1966.

75. **Clark, I.,** Importance of dietary Ca:PO_4 ratios on skeletal, Ca, Mg, and PO_4 metabolism, *Am. J. Physiol.,* 217, 865, 1969.

76. **Heaton, F. W., Hodgkinson, A., and Rose, G. A.,** Observations on the relation between calcium and magnesium metabolism in man, *Clin. Sci.,* 27, 31, 1964.

77. **Lemann, J., Jr., Lennon, E. J., Piering, W. R., Prien, E. L., Jr., and Ricanati, E. S.,** Evidence that glucose ingestion inhibits net renal tubular reabsorption of calcium and magnesium in man, *J. Lab. Clin. Med.,* 75, 578, 1970.

78. **Hart, E. B., Steenbock, H., Waddell, J., and Elvehjem, C. A.,** Iron in nutrition. VII. Copper as a supplement to iron for hemoglobin building in the rat, *J. Biol. Chem.,* 77, 792, 1928.

79. **Lee, D., Jr. and Matrone, G.,** Iron and copper effects on serum ceruloplasmin activity of rats with zinc-induced copper deficiency, *Proc. Soc. Exp. Biol. Med.,* 130, 1190, 1969.
80. **Bradfield, R. B., Bailey, M. A., and Margen, S.,** Morphological changes in human scalp hair roots during deprivation of protein, *Science,* 157, 438, 1968.
81. **Rook, A.,** Hair color in clinical diagnosis, *Ir. J. Med. Sci.,* 8, 415, 1969.
82. **Vandiviere, H. M., Dale, T. A., Driess, R. B., and Watson, K. A.,** Hairshaft diameter as an index of protein-calorie malnutrition, *Arch. Environ. Health,* 23, 61, 1971.
83. **Reinhold, J. G., Kfoury, G. A., Ghalambor, M. A., and Jean, C.,** Zinc and copper concentrations in hair of Iranian villagers, *Am. J. Clin. Nutr.,* 18, 294, 1966.
84. **Strain, W. H., Steadman, L. T., Lankau, C. A., Berliner, W. P., and Pories, W. J.,** Analysis of zinc levels in hair for the diagnosis of zinc deficiency in man, *J. Lab. Clin. Med.,* 68, 244, 1966.
85. **Kopito, L., Byers, R. K., and Schwachman, H.,** Lead in hair of children with chronic lead poisoning, *N. Engl. J. Med.,* 276, 949, 1967.
86. **Klevay, L. M.,** Hair as a biopsy material. I. Assessment of zinc nutriture, *Am. J. Clin. Nutr.,* 23, 284, 1970.
87. **Klevay, L. M.,** Hair as a biopsy material. II. Assessment of copper nutriture, *Am. J. Clin. Nutr.,* 23, 1194, 1970.
88. **Bate, L. C.,** Adsorption and elution of trace elements on human hair, *Intern. J. Appl. Radiat. Isot.,* 17, 417, 1966.
89. **Klevay, L. M.,** Hair as a biopsy material, *Am. J. Clin. Nutr.,* 23, 377, 1970.
90. **Harrison, W. W., Yurachek, J. P., and Benson, C. A.,** The determination of trace elements in human hair by atomic absorption spectroscopy, *Clin. Chim. Acta,* 23, 83, 1969.
91. **Zeitz, L., Lee, R., and Rothschild, E. O.,** Element analysis in hair by X-ray fluorescence, *Anal. Biochem.,* 31, 123, 1969.
92. **Hambidge, K. M., Hambidge, C., Franklin, M. F., and Baum, D.,** Zinc deficiency in children manifested by poor appetite and growth, impaired taste acuity, and low hair zinc levels, *Am. J. Clin. Nutr.,* 25, 453, 1972 (abstract).
93. **Hambidge, K. M., Rodgerson, D. O., and O'Brien, D.,** Concentration of chromium in the hair of normal children and children with juvenile diabetes mellitus, *Diabetes,* 17, 517, 1968.
94. **Hambidge, K. M. and Rodgerson, D.,** Comparison of hair chromium levels of nulliparous and parous women, *Am. J. Obstet. Gynecol.,* 103, 320, 1969.
95. **McBean, L. D., Mahloudji, M., Reinhold, J. G., and Halstead, J. A.,** Correlation of zinc concentrations in human plasma and hair, *Am. J. Clin. Nutr.,* 24, 506, 1971.
96. **Harrison, W. W. and Tyree, A. B.,** The determination of trace elements in human fingernails by atomic absorption spectroscopy, *Clin. Chim. Acta,* 31, 63, 1971.
97. **Vellar, O. D.,** Composition of human nail substance, *Am. J. Clin. Nutr.,* 23. 1272, 1970.
98. **Martin, G. M.,** Copper content of hair and nails of normal individuals and of patients with hepatolenticular degeneration, *Nature,* 202, 903, 1964.
99. **Vallee, B. L.,** Zinc and metalloenzymes, *Adv. Protein Chem.,* 10, 317, 1955.
100. **Coleman, R. F., Cripps, F. H., Stimson, A., and Scott, H. D.,** The determination of trace elements in human hair by neutron activation and the application to forensic science, *Atomic Weapons Res.,* Establishment Report No. 0-86/66, 1967.
101. **Livingston, D. M. and Wacker, W. E. C.,** Trace metal methods for nutritional studies, *Am. J. Clin. Nutr.,* 24, 1082, 1971.

V. IRON DEFICIENCY

Iron-Deficiency Anemia

The packed cell volume of whole blood (hematocrit)[1,2,35] is often used as a diagnostic for nutritional iron deficiency. The hematocrit is lowered due to insufficient hemoglobin formation resulting in microcytic hypochromic red blood cells. This measurement alone is not entirely conclusive in detection of iron deficiency although useful in the overall diagnosis.

Measurement of hemoglobin itself is a more direct means of estimating iron insufficiency because of the ultimate role of the element in this molecule; however, hemoglobin levels fall also in nutritional megaloblastic anemia. In whole blood, hemoglobin concentration has been determined by a variety of methods including gasometric measurement of oxygen capacity and carbon monoxide capacity and colorimetric determination of chemically induced derivatives of hemoglobin including oxyhemoglobin, carboxyhemoglobin, acid hematin, and cyanmethemoglobin. Automated instruments have been developed by differ-ent manufacturers which are based on some of these methods. The preferred method or basis is that which involves the conversion of all hemoglobin derivatives, except sulfhemoglobin, to cyanmethemoglobin[3],[4] using alkaline potassium ferricyanide and potassium cyanide.

Iron may be determined colorimetrically in whole blood also as an estimation of hemoglobin content. The direct measurement of iron in serum or plasma, together with the estimation of the degree of saturation of the iron transport protein transferrin, is extremely useful in detecting iron-deficiency states. The relative saturation of transferrin or iron-binding capacity of the serum may be approached by determining either total, unsaturated or latent iron-binding capacity, involving the addition of excess iron to the serum followed by either measurement of the excess unbound iron or direct determination of the bound iron after removal of the excess iron by either adsorption on magnesium carbonate or removal with an ion-exchange resin. The iron-binding capacity estimate permits distinction of nutritional deficiency from iron deficits due to infectious, inflammatory, or neoplastic diseases.

Principal emphasis in the area of colorimetric determination of serum iron has centered on the development of iron-specific chromogenic reagents which form iron complexes with increasingly higher molar absorptivities. Among the principal reagents used for serum iron are thiocyanate, ferrocyanide, 2,2'-bipyridyl, o-tolidine, dimethylglyoxime, bromoxime, haematoxylin, o-phenanthroline (1,10-phenanthroline), metamizol (sodium 1-phenyl-2,3-dimethyl-3-pyrazalone-5-1-4-methylaminomethane sulphonate), bathophenanthroline (4,7-diphenyl-1,10-phenanthroline), bathophenanthroline sulfonate, TPTZ (2,4,6-tripyridyl-5-triazine), ferrozine (3-(2-pyridyl)-5,6-bis(4-phenylsulfonic acid)-1,2,4-triazine) and 7-bromo-1,3-dihydro-1-(3-dimethylaminopropyl-5-(2-pyridyl)-2,H-1,4-benzodiazepin-2-1 dihydrochloride. Most modern colorimetric procedures involve the liberation of iron from protein by either acidification or detergent action and reduction of iron to the ferrous state for reaction with the chromogenic ligand. Protein precipitation or dialysis is usually interjected after iron liberation unless a blank unknown is also run. Turbid plasma or serum is a serious problem in the latter case.

Choice of methods for serum iron and iron-binding capacity will depend on equipment and amount of specimen available. Acceptable methods for manual determinations are available using the more sensitive color reagents bathophenanthroline,[5-7] bathophenanthroline sulfonate,[8],[9],[32] TPTZ,[10-12] and ferrozine.[13],[14] Bathophenanthroline sulfonate methods may be more preferable than those using bathophenanthroline because of the water solubility of the disodium salt of the sulfonic acid derivative. Ferrozine is also quite water soluble, as is TPTZ in the presence of acid. Methods for automated determination of serum iron and iron-binding capacity as well as semi-automated determination of iron-binding capacity using these reagents have been developed,[15-22],[31] all employing Technicon AutoAnalyzer* equipment. In the authors' laboratory, automated serum iron and semi-automated total iron-binding capacity are determined using bathophenanthroline sulfonate.[23] Using TPTZ, we have encountered the same difficulty that Bide[17] reports, i.e., the precipitation of the chromogen in the system. We have done some preliminary evaluation of the new reagent ferrozine, and it shows promise of being useful. We prefer to isolate the iron by dialysis from the serum or plasma background and determine total iron-binding capacity on another aliquot of the specimen. This increases the requirement for a sensitive chromogen but eliminates the problem encountered in blank correction for turbid specimens.

Iron and iron-binding capacity may also be determined satisfactorily using atomic absorption spectrophotometry[24],[25] and using radioactive iron[26] if necessary facilities and equipment are available.

Sideropenia

Iron deficiency may exist without manifest signs of anemia, although a low level of transferrin saturation may be observed and often protoporphyrins are elevated.[27],[45],[46] A recently published method[28] for routine estimation of porphyrins in whole blood is being evaluated in our laboratory as a more sensitive diagnostic for iron deficiency, as suggested by these authors, on nutrition survey specimens in which the other iron-deficiency parameters are also being determined. Blood porphyrin levels above 100 μg/100 ml of red blood cells have been considered abnormal and indicate an iron deficiency.[28],[46]

Interpretation of the results of analyses for hematocrit, hemoglobin, and serum iron para-

*Technicon and AutoAnalyzer are registered names used by Technicon Corp., Tarrytown, N.Y.

meters of iron deficiency require consideration of several characteristics of the subject, e.g., age, sex, physiological state, and altitude as shown in Tables 20 to 29. Certain criteria that have been proposed or utilized for the diagnosis of anemia are summarized in these tables. Problems associated with criteria of normality for hemoglobin concentration, for example, have been reviewed by Waters.[37] Table 20 provides information on mean hemoglobin and hematocrit values by age and sex as influenced by altitude. Table 21 summarizes suggested guidelines for the interpretation of blood data obtained in United States nutrition surveys.[30,39] Criteria for the diagnosis of anemia as suggested by the World Health Organization[36,37] are presented in Table 22. Somewhat different criteria were used in the Norwegian survey[40,41] (Table 23). Anemia was considered to exist in adult men with hemoglobin levels less than 14 g/100 ml or hematocrit values under 40%. For adult women, hemoglobin levels less than 12.5 g/100 ml or hematocrit values under 36% were designated as anemic. For both sexes, MCHC values below 30.5% were considered pathological. Recently, Viteri et al.[38] conducted a study to determine normal hematological values in the Central American population. The normal mean hemoglobin and hematocrit values for various age groups obtained are presented in Table 24. Degrees of risk are indicated as an aid in evaluating the prevalence of anemia in various population groups. Guidelines that have been suggested for interpretation of the influence of altitude on blood hemoglobin and hematocrit values are summarized in Tables 25 to 27. Hematological data obtained from the extensive nutrition survey conducted during 1965 to 1967 on populations of Central America and Panama[43,44] were evaluated with the use of the criteria presented in Tables 26 to 29. Although some differences do exist, the various criteria and guidelines employed to evaluate hematological data are in general agreement.

TABLE 20

Mean Blood Hemoglobin and Hematocrit Values at Various Ages

		Altitude			
		Sea level to 200 meters[a]		1750 meters (Denver, Colorado)[b]	
Age	Sex	Hemoglobin (g/100 ml)	Hematocrit (%)	Hemoglobin (g/100 ml)	Hematocrit (%)
2 months	M-F	13.3	38.9	11.4	33.4
6 months	M-F	12.3	36.2	12.5	36.9
1 year	M-F	11.6	35.2	12.6	37.8
2 years	M-F	11.7	35.5	12.9	38.2
4 years	M-F	12.6	37.1	13.1	39.0
6 years	M-F	12.7	37.9	13.3	39.6
8 years	M-F	12.9	38.9	13.4	40.3
10 years	M-F	13.0	39.0	13.6	40.8
12 years	M-F	13.4	39.6	13.9	41.6
14 years	M	—	—	14.6	44.1
	F	—	—	14.2	42.3
≥ 14 years	M	15.8	47.0	—	—
	F	13.9	42.0	—	—
16 years	M	—	—	15.5	46.2
	F	—	—	14.1	43.0
20 to 40 years	M	15.8	47.9	16.8	49.4
	F	14.1	42.9	14.6	43.2
> 40 years	M	15.6	46.3	—	—
	F	13.9	44.3	—	—

[a]From Diem and Lentner.[33]
[b]From McCammon.[34]

116

TABLE 21

Guidelines Used for the Interpretation of Blood Data[a]

Determination

Age (years)	Sex	Hemoglobin (g/100 ml)			Hematocrit (%)			Serum iron (μg/100 ml)		Transferrin saturation (%)	
		Deficient	Low	Acceptable	Deficient	Low	Acceptable	Deficient	Acceptable	Deficient	Acceptable
< 2	M-F	< 9.0	9.0 to 9.9	≥ 10.0	< 28	28 to 30	≥ 31	< 30	≥ 30	< 15	≥ 15
2 to 5	M-F	< 10.0	10.0 to 10.9	≥ 11.0	< 30	30 to 33	≥ 34	< 40	≥ 40	< 20	≥ 20
6 to 12	M-F	< 10.0	10.0 to 11.4	≥ 11.5	< 30	30 to 35	≥ 36	< 50	≥ 50	< 20	≥ 20
13 to 16	M	< 12.0	12.0 to 12.9	≥ 13.0	< 37	37 to 39	≥ 40	< 60	≥ 60	< 20	≥ 20
	F	< 10.0	10.0 to 11.4	≥ 11.5	< 31	31 to 35	≥ 36	< 40	≥ 40	< 15	≥ 15
> 16	M	< 12.0	12.0 to 13.9	≥ 14.0	< 37	37 to 43	≥ 44	< 60	≥ 60	< 20	≥ 20
	F	< 10.0	10.0 to 11.9	≥ 12.0	< 31	31 to 37	≥ 38	< 40	≥ 40	< 15	≥ 15
Pregnant											
2nd trimester		< 9.5	9.5 to 10.9	≥ 11.0	< 30	30 to 34	≥ 35	—	—	—	—
3rd trimester		< 9.0	9.0 to 10.4	≥ 10.5	< 30	30 to 32	≥ 33	—	—	—	—

M = males   F = females

[a]Adapted from the reports of O'Neal et al.[30] and of the Ten-State Nutrition Survey.[39]

TABLE 22

WHO Criteria for the Diagnosis of Anemia[a]

Determination	Levels considered anemic or iron-deficient
Hemoglobin (g/100 ml venous blood)	
Children aged 6 months to 6 years	< 11
Children aged 6 to 14 years	< 12
Adult males	< 13
Adult females; nonpregnant	< 12
Adult females; pregnant	< 11
Serum Iron (μg/100 ml)	
Adults	< 50
Transferrin Saturation (%)	
Adults	< 15%

[a]Adapted from World Health Organization Technical Report.[36,37]

TABLE 23

Norwegian Survey: Normal Values and Criteria for Anemia[a]

Age (years)	Sex	Hemoglobin (g/100 ml) Normal[b]	Anemia	Hematocrit (%) Normal[b]	Anemia	MCHC (%) Normal[b]	Anemia
7 to 9	M-F	12.7 ± 1.6	< 11.0	39 ± 5	34	33 ± 4	29
10 to 13	M-F	13.2 ± 1.6	< 11.5	40 ± 5	35	33 ± 4	29
14 to 16	M	15.0 ± 2.0	< 13.0	43 ± 6	37	34 ± 4	30
	F	14.2 ± 2.0	< 12.0	41 ± 6	35	34 ± 4	30
17 to 20	M	15.5 ± 2.0	< 13.5	45 ± 6	39	34 ± 4	30
	F	14.2 ± 2.0	< 12.0	42 ± 6	36	34 ± 4	30
> 20	M	15.7 ± 1.8	< 14.0	46 ± 6	40	33.6 ± 4	30.5
	F	14.3 ± 1.8	< 12.5	42 ± 6	36	33.6 ± 4	30.5

M = males   F = females

[a]Adapted from Natvig et al.[37,40,41]
[b]Mean ±2SD (= 95% of the population).

TABLE 24

Normal Hematological Values in the Central American Population[a]
(Altitude of 0 to 750 m)

Age (years)	Sex	Hemoglobin (g/100 ml) Risk Normal Mean	20% (−1 Sd)	75% (−1½ SD)	Hematocrit (%) Risk Normal Mean	20% (−1 SD)	75% (−1½ SD)
1 to 4	M-F	12.9	11.8	11.3	37.8	34.3	32.6
5 to 8	M-F	12.7	11.5	10.9	37.8	34.6	33.0
9 to 12	M-F	13.3	12.3	11.8	39.2	36.6	35.3
13 to 16	M	13.9	12.9	12.4	40.9	38.2	36.9
	F	13.6	13.0	12.7	41.0	39.0	38.0
17 to 20	M	14.7	13.8	13.4	44.1	41.9	40.8
	F	14.5	13.4	12.9	41.9	39.6	38.5
21 to 49	M	15.4	14.0	13.3	46.0	42.1	40.2
	F	13.6	12.4	11.8	40.3	36.9	35.2
≥ 50	M	14.6	13.0	12.2	43.1	37.7	35.0
	F	13.9	12.7	12.1	41.6	38.2	36.5

M = males   F = females

[a]From report of Viteri et al.[38]

TABLE 25

Suggested Guide to Interpretation of Blood Data Obtained from Various Altitudes[a]

	Deficient			Low			Acceptable		
	Sea Level	1500M	3700M	Sea Level	1500M	3700M	Sea Level	1500M	3700M
Hemoglobin (g/100 ml)									
6 to 23 months	< 9.0	< 9.3	< 10.3	9.0 to 9.9	9.3 to 10.2	10.3 to 11.2	≥ 10.0	≥ 10.3	≥ 11.3
2 to 5 years	< 10	< 10.3	< 11.3	10.0 to 10.9	10.3 to 11.2	11.3 to 12.2	≥ 11.0	≥ 11.3	≥ 12.3
6 to 12 years	< 10	< 10.3	< 11.3	10.0 to 11.4	10.3 to 11.7	11.3 to 12.9	≥ 11.5	≥ 11.8	≥ 13.0
13 to 16 years: male	< 12	< 12.3	< 13.3	12.0 to 12.9	12.3 to 13.2	13.3 to 14.4	≥ 13.0	≥ 13.3	≥ 14.5
13 to 16 years: female	< 10	< 10.3	< 11.3	10.0 to 11.4	10.3 to 11.7	11.3 to 12.9	≥ 11.5	≥ 11.8	≥ 13.0
> 16 years: male	< 12	< 12.3	< 13.3	12.0 to 13.9	12.3 to 14.2	13.3 to 15.4	≥ 14.0	≥ 14.3	≥ 15.5
> 16 years: female	< 10	< 10.3	< 11.3	10.0 to 11.9	10.3 to 12.2	11.3 to 13.4	≥ 12.0	≥ 12.3	≥ 13.5
Pregnant, 2nd trimester	< 9.5	< 9.8	< 10.8	9.5 to 10.9	9.8 to 11.2	10.8 to 12.4	≥ 11.0	≥ 11.3	≥ 12.5
Pregnant, 3rd trimester	< 9.0	< 9.3	< 10.3	9.0 to 10.4	9.3 to 10.7	10.3 to 11.9	≥ 10.5	≥ 10.8	≥ 12.0
Hematocrit (%)									
6 to 23 months	< 28	< 30	< 33	28 to 30	30 to 32	32 to 35	≥ 31	≥ 33	≥ 36
2 to 5 years	< 30	< 32	< 35	30 to 33	32 to 35	35 to 37	≥ 34	≥ 36	≥ 38
6 to 12 years	< 30	< 32	< 36	30 to 35	32 to 36	36 to 38	≥ 36	≥ 37	≥ 39
13 to 16 years: male	< 37	< 39	< 43	37 to 39	39 to 42	42 to 46	≥ 40	≥ 43	≥ 47
13 to 16 years: female	< 31	< 33	< 37	31 to 35	33 to 37	37 to 41	≥ 36	≥ 38	≥ 42
> 16 years: male	< 37	< 39	< 43	37 to 43	39 to 44	44 to 49	≥ 44	≥ 45	≥ 50
> 16 years: female	< 31	< 33	< 37	31 to 37	33 to 39	39 to 44	≥ 38	≥ 40	≥ 45
Pregnant, 2nd Trimester	< 30	< 32	< 36	30 to 34	32 to 36	36 to 40	≥ 35	≥ 37	≥ 41
Pregnant, 3rd Trimester	< 30	< 32	< 36	30 to 32	32 to 34	35 to 38	≥ 33	≥ 35	≥ 39

[a]Adapted from the reports of O'Neal et al.[30] and others.[29,33,34,42]

TABLE 26

Guide to Interpretation of Hemoglobin According to Altitude, Age, Sex, and Term of Pregnancy[a]

Altitude (feet)

Age	Sex	0 to 2499			2500 to 4999			5000 to 7499			7500+		
		Deficient	Low	Acceptable	Deficient	Low	Acceptable	Deficient	Low	Acceptable	Deficient	Low	Acceptable
3 to 11 months	M-F	< 9.0	9.0 to 9.5	≥ 9.6	< 9.2	9.2 to 9.7	≥ 9.8	< 9.4	9.4 to 9.9	≥ 10.0	< 9.5	9.6 to 10.1	≥ 10.2
12 to 35 months	M-F	< 9.5	9.5 to 10.2	≥ 10.3	< 9.7	9.7 to 10.4	≥ 10.5	< 9.9	9.9 to 10.6	≥ 10.7	< 10.1	10.1 to 10.8	≥ 10.9
3 to 11 years	M-F	< 10.1	10.1 to 11.0	≥ 11.1	< 10.3	10.3 to 11.2	≥ 11.3	< 10.5	10.5 to 11.4	≥ 11.5	< 10.7	10.7 to 11.6	≥ 11.7
12 to 17 years	M	< 11.9	11.9 to 13.8	≥ 13.9	< 12.1	12.1 to 14.0	≥ 14.1	< 12.3	12.3 to 14.2	≥ 14.3	< 12.5	12.5 to 14.4	≥ 14.5
12 to 17 years	F	< 10.8	10.8 to 11.7	≥ 11.8	< 11.0	11.0 to 11.9	≥ 12.0	< 11.2	11.2 to 12.1	≥ 12.2	< 11.4	11.4 to 12.3	≥ 12.4
18 to 44 years	M	< 12.1	12.1 to 14.0	≥ 14.1	< 12.3	12.3 to 14.2	≥ 14.3	< 12.5	12.5 to 14.4	≥ 14.5	< 12.7	12.7 to 14.6	≥ 14.7
18 to 44 years	F	< 10.1	10.1 to 11.0	≥ 11.1	< 10.3	10.3 to 11.2	≥ 11.3	< 10.5	10.5 to 11.4	≥ 11.5	< 10.7	10.7 to 11.6	≥ 11.7
45 to 64 years	M-F	< 11.1	11.1 to 12.5	≥ 12.6	< 11.3	11.3 to 12.7	≥ 12.8	< 11.5	11.5 to 12.9	≥ 13.0	< 11.7	11.7 to 13.1	≥ 13.2
≥ 65+ years	M-F	< 10.9	10.9 to 12.3	≥ 12.4	< 11.1	11.1 to 12.5	≥ 12.6	< 11.3	11.3 to 12.7	≥ 12.8	< 11.5	11.5 to 12.9	≥ 13.0
Pregnant Women													
1st Trimester		< 10.1	10.1 to 11.0	≥ 11.1	< 10.3	10.3 to 11.2	≥ 11.3	< 10.5	10.5 to 11.4	≥ 11.5	< .10.7	10.7 to 11.6	≥ 11.7
2nd Trimester		< 9.6	9.6 to 10.5	≥ 10.6	< 9.8	9.8 to 10.7	≥ 10.8	< 10.0	10.0 to 10.9	≥ 11.0	< 10.2	10.2 to 11.1	≥ 11.1
3rd Trimester		< 9.1	9.1 to 10.5	≥ 10.6	< 9.3	9.3 to 10.7	≥ 10.8	< 9.5	9.5 to 10.9	≥ 11.0	< 9.7	9.7 to 11.1	≥ 11.1

M = males   F = females

[a]From Central America and Panama Nutrition Survey.[43,44]

TABLE 27

Guide to Interpretation of Hematocrit According to Altitude, Age, Sex, and Term of Pregnancy[a]

Altitude (feet)

Age	Sex	0 to 2499			2500 to 4999			5000 to 7499			7500+		
		Deficient	Low	Acceptable	Deficient	Low	Acceptable	Deficient	Low	Acceptable	Deficient	Low	Acceptable
3 to 11 months	M-F	< 26.5	26.5 to 27.9	≥ 28.0	< 27.0	27.0 to 28.5	≥ 28.6	< 27.6	27.6 to 29.1	≥ 29.2	< 28.2	28.2 to 29.7	≥ 29.8
12 to 35 months	M-F	< 28.8	28.8 to 30.9	≥ 31.0	< 29.4	29.4 to 31.5	≥ 31.6	< 30.0	30.0 to 32.1	≥ 32.2	< 30.6	30.6 to 32.7	≥ 32.8
3 to 11 years	M-F	< 30.1	30.1 to 32.8	≥ 32.9	< 30.7	30.7 to 33.4	≥ 33.5	< 31.3	31.3 to 34.0	≥ 34.1	< 31.9	31.9 to 34.6	≥ 34.7
12 to 17 years	M	< 34.9	34.9 to 40.5	≥ 40.6	< 35.5	35.5 to 41.0	≥ 41.1	< 36.1	36.1 to 41.6	≥ 41.7	< 36.6	36.6 to 42.2	≥ 42.3
12 to 17 years	F	< 31.7	31.7 to 34.3	≥ 34.4	< 32.2	32.2 to 34.9	≥ 35.0	< 32.8	32.8 to 35.5	≥ 35.6	< 33.4	33.4 to 36.1	≥ 36.2
18 to 44 years	M	< 35.5	35.5 to 41.0	≥ 41.1	< 36.1	36.1 to 41.6	≥ 41.7	< 36.6	36.6 to 42.2	≥ 42.3	< 37.2	37.2 to 42.8	≥ 42.9
18 to 44 years	F	< 29.6	29.6 to 32.2	≥ 32.3	< 30.2	30.2 to 32.8	≥ 32.9	< 30.8	30.8 to 33.4	≥ 33.5	< 31.4	31.4 to 34.0	≥ 34.1
45 to 64 years	M-F	< 32.6	32.6 to 36.6	≥ 36.7	< 33.1	33.1 to 37.2	≥ 37.3	< 33.7	33.7 to 37.8	≥ 37.9	< 34.3	34.3 to 38.4	≥ 38.5
≥ 65 years	M-F	< 32.0	32.0 to 36.1	≥ 36.2	< 32.6	32.6 to 36.6	≥ 36.7	< 33.1	33.1 to 37.2	≥ 37.3	< 33.7	33.7 to 37.8	≥ 37.9
Pregnant Women													
1st Trimester		< 29.6	29.6 to 32.2	≥ 32.3	< 30.2	30.2 to 32.9	≥ 33.0	< 30.9	30.9 to 33.5	≥ 33.6	< 31.5	31.5 to 34.1	≥ 34.2
2nd Trimester		< 28.2	28.2 to 30.9	≥ 31.0	< 28.8	28.8 to 31.5	≥ 31.6	< 29.4	29.4 to 32.0	≥ 32.1	< 30.0	30.0 to 32.6	≥ 32.7
3rd Trimester		< 26.7	26.7 to 30.8	≥ 30.9	< 27.4	27.4 to 31.5	≥ 31.6	< 27.9	27.9 to 32.0	≥ 32.1	< 28.5	28.5 to 32.6	≥ 32.7

M = males   F = females

[a]From Central America and Panama Nutrition Survey.[43,44]

121

TABLE 28

Guide to Interpretation of Serum Iron According to Age, Sex, and Physiological State (All Altitudes)[a] (μg/100 ml)

		Classification category		
Age	Sex	Deficient	Low	Acceptable
3 to 11 months	M and F	< 18.0	18.0 to 29.9	⩾ 30.0
12 to 35 months	M and F	< 30.0	30.0 to 49.9	⩾ 50.0
3 to 11 years	M and F	< 30.0	30.0 to 49.9	⩾ 50.0
12 to 17 years	M	< 30.0	30.0 to 59.9	⩾ 60.0
12 to 17 years	F	< 30.0	30.0 to 59.9	⩾ 60.0
18 to 44 years	M	< 30.0	30.0 to 59.9	⩾ 60.0
18 to 44 years	F	< 30.0	30.0 to 59.9	⩾ 60.0
45 to 64 years	M and F	< 30.0	30.0 to 49.9	⩾ 50.0
⩾ 65	M and F	< 30.0	30.0 to 49.9	⩾ 50.0
Pregnant women				
1st Trimester		< 30.0	30.0 to 59.9	⩾ 60.0
2nd Trimester		< 30.0	30.0 to 59.9	⩾ 60.0
3rd Trimester		< 45.0	45.0 to 59.9	⩾ 60.0
Lactating women		< 30.0	30.0 to 59.9	⩾ 60.0

M = males   F = females
[a]From Central America and Panama Nutrition Survey (43,44)

TABLE 29

Guide to Interpretation of Percent Saturation of Transferrin According to Age, Sex, and Physiological State (All Altitudes)[a]

		Classification category		
Age	Sex	Deficient	Low	Acceptable
3 to 11 months	M and F	< 10.0	10.0 to 12.9	⩾ 13.0
12 to 35 months	M and F	< 15.0	15.0 to 19.9	⩾ 20.0
3 to 11 years	M and F	< 15.0	15.0 to 19.9	⩾ 20.0
12 to 17 years	M	< 15.0	15.0 to 19.9	⩾ 20.0
12 to 17 years	F	< 15.0	15.0 to 19.9	⩾ 20.0
18 to 44 years	M	< 15.0	15.0 to 19.9	⩾ 20.0
18 to 44 years	F	< 15.0	15.0 to 19.9	⩾ 20.0
45 to 64 years	M and F	< 15.0	15.0 to 19.9	⩾ 20.0
⩾ 65	M and F	< 15.0	15.0 to 19.9	⩾ 20.0
Pregnant Women				
1st Trimester		< 15.0	15.0 to 19.9	⩾ 20.0
2nd Trimester		< 15.0	15.0 to 19.9	⩾ 20.0
3rd Trimester		< 15.0	15.0 to 19.9	⩾ 20.0
Lactating Women		< 15.0	15.0 to 19.9	⩾ 20.0

M = males   F = females
[a]From Central America and Panama Nutrition Survey (43,44)

REFERENCES

1. **Wintrobe, M. M. and Landsberg, J. W.,** A standardized technique for the blood sedimentation test, *Am. J. Med. Sci.,* 189, 102, 1935.
2. **Strumia, M. M., Sample, A. B., and Hart, E. D.,** An improved micro hematocrit method, *Am. J. Clin. Pathol.,* 24, 1016, 1954.
3. **Wu, H.,** Studies on hemoglobin, *J. Biochem.,* 2, 173, 1922.
4. **Drabkin, D. L.,** The standardization of hemoglobin measurement, *Am. J. Med. Sci.,* 217, 710, 1949.
5. **Peterson, R. E.,** Improved spectrophotometric procedure for determination of serum iron, *Anal. Chem.,* 25, 1337, 1953.
6. **Peters, T., Giovanniello, J., Apt, L., and Ross, J. R.,** A simple improved method for the determination of serum iron, *J. Lab. Clin. Med.,* 48, 280, 1956.
7. **Forman, D. T.,** Determination of iron in serum using solvent extraction, *Am. J. Clin. Pathol.,* 42, 103, 1964.
8. **Trinder, P.,** The improved determination of iron in serum, *J. Clin. Pathol.,* 9, 170, 1956.
9. **Callahan, R.,** An improved serum iron measurement with sulfonated bathophenanthroline, *Clin. Chem.,* 9, 487, 1963.
10. **Caraway, W. T.,** Macro and micro methods for the determination of serum iron and iron-binding capacity, *Clin. Chem.,* 9, 188, 1963.
11. **Williams, H. L. and Conrad, M. E.,** A one-tube method for measuring the serum iron concentration and unsaturated iron-binding capacity, *J. Lab. Clin. Med.,* 67, 171, 1966.
12. **O'Malley, J. A., Hassan, A., Shiley, J., and Traynor, H.,** Simplified determination of serum iron and total iron-binding capacity, *Clin. Chem.,* 16, 92, 1970.
13. **Persijn, T., Van Der Slik, W., and Riethorst, A.,** Determination of serum iron and latent iron-binding capacity (LIBC), *Clin. Chim. Acta,* 35, 91, 1971.
14. **Carter, P.,** Spectrophotometric determination of serum iron at the submicrogram level with a new reagent (ferrozine), *Anal. Biochem.,* 40, 450, 1971.
15. **Zak, B. and Epstein, E.,** Automated determination of serum iron, *Clin. Chem.,* 11, 6, 1965.
16. **Kauppinen, V. and Gref, C. G.,** Automated determination of serum iron, *Scand. J. Clin. Lab. Invest.,* 20, 24, 1967.
17. **Bide, R. W.,** Some notes on the automated estimation of low levels of iron in biological fluids, *Anal. Biochem.,* 30, 271, 1969.
18. **Kunesh, J. P. and Small, L. L.,** Adaption of the Zak-Epstein automated micromethod for serum iron to determine iron-binding capacity and urinary iron, *Clin. Chem.,* 16, 148, 1970.
19. **Friedman, H. S. and Cheek, C. S.,** Simultaneous and completely automated methods for serum iron and iron-binding capacity determinations, *Clin. Chim. Acta,* 31, 315, 1971.
20. **Young, D. S. and Hicks, J. M.,** Method for the automatic determination of serum iron, *J. Clin. Pathol.,* 18, 98, 1965.
21. **Clarke, D. D. and Nicklas, R.,** A micro modification of the automatic determination of serum iron, *Technicon Symposia,* 181, 1967.
22. **Yee, H. Y. and Zin, Z.,** An autoanalyzer procedure for serum iron and total iron-binding capacity with use of ferrozine, *Clin Chem.,* 17, 950, 1971.
23. **Wise, W. R., Skala, J. H., and Sauberlich, H. E.,** Semiautomated determination of serum iron and total iron-binding capacity, *U.S. Army Med. Res. and Nutr. Lab. Rep.,* June 1972.
24. **Zettner, M. D., Sylvia, L. C., and Capacho-Delgado, L.,** The determination of serum iron and iron-binding capacity by atomic absorption spectroscopy, *Am. J. Clin. Pathol.,* 45, 533, 1966.
25. **Olson, A. D. and Hamlin, W. B.,** A new method for serum iron and total iron-binding capacity by atomic absorption spectrophotometry, *Clin. Chem.,* 15, 438, 1969.
26. **Brozovich, B. and Copestake, J.,** Semi-automated micromethod for estimating the unsaturated iron-binding capacity of serum using radioactive iron, *J. Clin. Pathol.,* 22, 605, 1969.
27. **Dagg, J. H., Goldberg, A., and Lochhead, A.,** Value of erythrocyte protoporphyrin in the diagnosis of latent iron deficiency (sideropenia), *Br. J. Haematol.,* 12, 326, 1966.
28. **Heller, S. R., Labbe, R. F., and Nutter, J.,** A simplified assay for porphyrins in whole blood, *Clin. Chem.,* 17, 525, 1971.
29. *Manual for Nutrition Surveys,* Interdepartmental Committee on Nutrition for National Defense, U.S. Govt. Printing Office, Washington, D. C., May 1947, 121.
30. **O'Neal, R. M., Johnson, O. C., and Schaefer, A. E.,** Guidelines for classification and interpretation of group blood and urine data collected as part of the National Nutrition Survey, *Pediatr. Res.,* 4, 103, 1970.
31. **Hünteler, L. A., Van Der Slik, W., and Persijn, T. P.,** Automated determination of serum iron and latent iron-binding capacity by continuous flow analysis without dialysis, *Clin. Chim. Acta,* 37, 391, 1972.
32. **Williams, H. L. and Conrad, M. E.,** Problems in the measurement of iron binding capacity in serum, *Clin. Chim. Acta,* 37, 131, 1972.
33. *Scientific Tables,* 7th ed., Diem, K. and Lentner, C., Eds., Ciba-Geigy Limited, Basle, Switzerland, and Ardsley, N.Y. 10502, 1970, 617.

34. **McCammon, R. W.,** *Human Growth and Development,* Charles C Thomas, Springfield, Ill., 1970, 224.

35. **England, J. M., Walford, D. M., and Waters, D. A. W.,** Re-assessment of the reliability of the haematocrit, *Br. J. Haematol.,* 23, 247, 1972.

36. *Nutritional Anaemias,* World Health Organization Technical Report Series No. 405, World Health Organization, Geneva, Switzerland, 1968.

37. **Waters, A. H.,** Anemia and normality, in *Metabolic Adaptation and Nutrition,* PAHO Scientific Publication No. 222, Pan American Health Organization, 525 Twenty-third Street, N. W., Washington, D. C. 20037, 1971, 105.

38. **Viteri, F. E., De Tuna, V., and Guzman, M. A.,** Normal haematological values in the Central American population, *Br. J. Haematol.,* 23, 189, 1972.

39. *Ten-State Nutrition Survey Reports, I-V,* Center for Disease Control, Atlanta, Georgia 30330, 1972.

40. **Natvig, H., Vellar, O. D., and Andersen, J.,** Studies on hemoglobin values in Norway. 7. Hemoglobin, hematocrit and MCHC values among boys and girls aged 7–20 years in elementary and grammar schools, *Acta Med. Scand.,* 182, 183, 1967.

41. **Natvig, H. and Vellar, O. D.,** Studies on hemoglobin values in adult men and women, *Acta Med. Scand.,* 182, 193, 1967.

42. *Manual for Nutrition Surveys,* 2nd ed., Interdepartmental Committee on Nutrition for National Defense, U.S. Govt. Printing Office, Washington, D.C. 20402, 1963.

43. *Nutritional Evaluation of the Population of Central America and Panama,* Institute of Nutrition of Central America and Panama and Nutrition Program, Center for Disease Control, DHEW Publication No. (HSM) 72–8120, Center for Disease Control, Atlanta, Georgia, 1972.

44. Evaluación Nutricional de la Población de Centro América y Panamá, Reports on Costa Rica, Guatemala, Honduras, Nicaragua, El Salvador, and Panama, Instituto de Nutrición de Centro América y Panamá (INCAP), Guatemala City, Guatemala, Central America, 1969.

45. **Smith, N. J., Labbe, R., and Cook, J.,** The use of erythrocyte porphyrin determination of iron deficiency, IX International Congress of Nutrition, Sept. 3-9, 1972, Mexico City, *Summaria* (abstracts), 123.

46. **McLaren, G., Carpenter, J., and Nino, H.,** RBC protoporphyrin in the detection of iron deficiency, IX International Congress of Nutrition, Sept. 3-9, 1972, Mexico City, *Summaria* (abstracts), 123.

VI. IODINE DEFICIENCY

Iodine Deficiency

The laboratory evaluation of thyroid status can be made by determination of hormonal iodine in blood as protein-bound iodine (PBI), urinary excretion of iodine and radioiodine uptake. In cases where there is a dietary insufficiency of iodine, the PBI and urinary iodine excretion are lowered and radioiodine uptake is increased. In either case, it is difficult to establish nutritional insufficiency as the cause solely on laboratory tests without supporting clinical and dietary history information because there are so many physiological states and drugs which produce similar trends in these parameters.[1,2]

Serum PBI, total serum iodine, and urinary iodine have been used extensively in nutrition work. The manual method of Zak et al.,[3] as modified by Benotti and Benotti,[4] was used by the Interdepartmental Committee on Nutrition for National Defense for all of these iodine measurements. The major interference in PBI determination is the presence of possible large amounts of nonhormonal iodine in serum; total iodine determination protects against potentially invalid conclusions. Other modifications of the Zak method have been made,[5,6] and automated procedures have been developed.[7-10] Approaches to the determination of PBI have varied primarily in the method of isolating the iodine normally associated with the hormone; the determination of iodine almost universally involves its catalytic action on the reduction of ceric salts by arsenious acid. Discussion of PBI determination principles and other thyroid parameters may be found in articles by Sunderman,[11] by Anido and Jarvis[12] and by Robbins and Rall.[13]

Serum PBI values for euthyroid individuals have generally been considered to fall in the range of 4.0 to 8.0 $\mu g/100$ ml;[14] however, Henry, in this reference, reviews the case for a lower limit to a range similar to that supported by values of 3.4 to 8.2 $\mu g/100$ ml reported by Nelson et al.[15] Urinary excretions of iodine of less than 50 $\mu g/g$ of creatinine are assumed to be indicative of deficiency.[16,17]

Radioiodine methods naturally require special equipment and technique. Rall[18] has published a review of isotope methods. Comparative studies between isotope techniques and PBI determinations have been made.[19,20] Urinary excretion of radioiodine has been used in nutrition survey work.[21]

REFERENCES

1. **Searcy, R. L.,** *Diagnostic Biochemistry,* McGraw-Hill, New York, 1969, chap. 58.
2. **Acland, J. D.,** The interpretation of the serum protein-bound iodine, *J. Clin. Pathol.,* 24, 187, 1971.
3. **Zak, B., Willard, H. H., Myers, G. B., and Boyle, A. J.,** Chloric acid method for determination of protein-bound iodine, *Anal. Chem.,* 24, 1345, 1952.
4. **Benotti, J. and Benotti, N.,** Protein-bound iodine and total iodine-Zak method modified, in *Manual for Nutrition Surveys,* 2nd ed., Interdepartmental Committee on Nutrition for National Defense, 1963, 155.
5. **Leffler, H. H.,** Determination of protein-bound iodine, *Am. J. Clin. Pathol.,* 24, 483, 1954.
6. **O'Neal, L. W. and Sims, E. S.,** Determination of protein-bound iodine in plasma or serum, *Am. J. Clin. Pathol.,* 23, 493, 1953.
7. **Stevens, C. O. and Levandoski, N.,** Automation of protein-bound iodine determinations, *Clin. Chem.,* 9, 400, 1963.
8. **Benotti, J. and Benotti, N.,** Protein-bound iodine, total iodine, and butanol-extractable iodine by partial automation, *Clin. Chem.,* 9, 408, 1963.
9. Technicon N-56 methodology, Protein-bound iodine, Copyright 1969, Technicon Corp., Tarrytown, New York.
10. **Stekelenburg, G. J. Van, Bree, P. K., and Stam, P. J.,** A micromodification of the flow diagram for the determination of protein-bound iodine with the Technicon AutoAnalyzer system, *Biochem. Med.,* 3, 431, 1970.
11. **Sunderman, F. W., Jr.,** Chemical measurements of serum hormonal iodine, *CRC Crit. Rev. Clin. Lab. Sci.,* 1, 551, 1970.
12. **Anido, G. and Jarvis, A.,** Thyroid function tests – the chemical thyroid profile, *Am. J. Med. Technol.,* 36, 317, 1970.
13. **Robbins, J. and Rall, J. E.,** The iodine containing hormones, in *Hormones in Blood,* Vol. 1, 2nd ed., Gray, C. H. and Bacharach, A. L., Academic Press, London, 1967, 383.
14. **Henry, R. J.,** *Clinical Chemistry,* Harper and Row, New York, 1964, Chap. 28.
15. **Nelson, J. C., Haynes, E., Willard, R., and Kuzma, J.,** The distribution of euthyroid serum protein-bound iodine levels, *J.A.M.A.,* 216, 1639, 1971.
16. **Follis, R. H., Jr., Vanprapa, K., and Damrongsakdi, D.,** Studies on iodine nutrition in Thailand, *J. Nutr.,* 76, 159, 1962.
17. **Stanbury, J. B.,** Iodine metabolism and physiological aspects of endemic goitre, *Bull. W.H.O.,* 18, 201, 1958.
18. **Rall, J. E.,** Recent advances in the diagnosis of the diseases of the thyroid, *Clin. Chim. Acta,* 25, 339, 1969.
19. **Webber, C. E., Johnstone, J. H., and Garnett, E. S.,** An improved automatic technic for the in vitro assessment of thyroid status, *Clin. Chem.,* 15, 219, 1969.
20. **Lucis, O. J., Cummings, G. T., Matthews, S., and Burry, C.,** Laboratory observations of assays of serum thyroxine and protein-bound iodine, *J. Nucl. Med.,* 10, 160, 1969.
21. **Delange, F. and Ermans, A. M.,** Role of a dietary goitrogen in the etiology of endemic goiter on Idjwi Island, *Am. J. Clin. Nutr.,* 24, 1354, 1971.

VII. ESSENTIAL FATTY ACID DEFICIENCY

Essential Fatty Acid Deficiency

Arachidonic acid or its precursor, linoleic acid, is essential for dermal integrity and growth in human infants.[1,2,4] The essential fatty acid requirement is quite low for infants with a recommendation that the level of linoleic acid in the infant formula should supply 3% of the calories.[2,3,5] Although a dietary deficiency of linoleic acid rarely occurs, essential fatty acid deficiency has been induced on several occasions in infants and in adults as a consequence of prolonged intravenous feeding with solutions that do not contain linoleic acid.[4,6-8]

Essential fatty acid deficiency can be diagnosed by determination of the level of certain unsaturated fatty acids in serum, plasma, or erythrocytes.[1,11] When linoleic acid is lacking in the diet, serum levels of linoleic and arachidonic acids decrease and the level of the trienoic acid, 5, 8, 11-eicosatrienoic, is increased.[1,4,6,8-11] Red blood cells show changes in fatty acid composition similar to those found in serum and plasma, but the changes become evident more slowly than in serum or plasma.[1,12,13] Moreover, the fatty acid composition of red cells of a-betalipoproteinemia patients may resemble that found with essential fatty acid deficiency.[14] Hence, a dietary deficiency of linoleic acid is most readily and reliably detected by the determination of 5, 8, 11-eicosatrienoic acid $(20:3\omega9)$ in serum or plasma lipids.[1,7,11]

The ratio of the endogenous eicosatrienoic acid

(20:3ω9) to the essential eicosatrienoic acid (20:4ω6) in serum lipids has been also used to assess the essential fatty acid status of the human.[1,5,6] In normal subjects, this ratio for serum is below 0.4, whereas ratios as high as 5.0 or higher have been observed in severely deficient infants.[4,6] Serum or plasma lipid classes are separated by column or thin-layer chromatography and the fatty acid composition of the separated lipids determined by gas chromatography.[6]

REFERENCES

1. **Wiese, H. F.,** Essential fatty acids. IX. Deficiency effects in human beings, in *The Vitamins,* Vol. III, 2nd ed., Sebrell, W. H., Jr. and Harris, R. S., Eds., Academic Press, New York, 1971, 327.

2. **Rahm, J. J. and Holman, R. T.,** Essential fatty acids. X. Requirements of animals and human beings, in *The Vitamins,* Vol. III, 2nd ed., Sebrell, W. H., Jr. and Harris, R. S., Eds., Academic Press, New York, 1971, 335.

3. *Recommended Dietary Allowances,* 7th revised ed., (publication 1964), National Academy of Sciences, Washington, D.C. 1968.

4. **Söderhjelm, L., Wiese, H. F., and Holman, R. T.,** The role of polyunsaturated acids in human nutrition and metabolism, in *Progress in the Chemistry of Fats and Other Lipids,* Vol. IX, Pergamon Press, Oxford, 1971, 555.

5. **Holman, R. T., Caster, W. O., and Wiese, H. F.,** The essential fatty acid requirement of infants and the assessment of their dietary intake of linoleate by serum fatty acid analysis, *Am. J. Clin. Nutr.,* 14, 70, 1964.

6. **Paulsrud, J. R., Pensler, L., Whitten, C. F., Stewart, S., and Holman, R. T.,** Essential fatty acid deficiency in infants induced by fat-free intravenous feeding, *Am. J. Clin. Nutr.,* 25, 897, 1972.

7. **Collins, F. D., Sinclair, A. J., Royle, J. P., Coats, D. A., Maynard, A. T., and Leonard, R. F.,** Plasma lipids in human linoleic acid deficiency, *Nutr. Metab.,* 13, 150, 1971.

8. **Caldwell, M. and Jonsson, H.,** Severe Essential Fatty Acid Deficiency (EFAD) in Man: Occurrence, Manifestations and Correction During Prolonged Total Parental Alimentation (TPA), IX International Congress of Nutrition, Mexico City, 1972, abstracts, 197.

9. **Woodruff, C. W., Bailey, M. C., Davis, J. T., Rogers, N., and Coniglio, J. C.,** Serum lipids in breast-fed infants and in infants fed evaporated milk, *Am. J. Clin. Nutr.,* 14, 83, 1964.

10. **Hanson, A. E., Wiese, H. F., Adam, D. J. D., Boelsche, A. N., Haggard, M. E., Davis, H., Newsom, W. T., and Pesut, L.,** Influence of diet on blood serum lipids in pregnant women and newborn infants, *Am. J. Clin. Nutr.,* 15, 11, 1964.

11. **Pikaar, N. A. and Fernandes, J.,** Influence of different types of dietary fat on the fatty acid composition of serum lipid fractions in infants and children, *Am. J. Clin. Nutr.,* 19, 194, 1966.

12. **Patil, V. S. and Hansen, A. E.,** Effect of diets with and without fat at low and high caloric levels on fatty acids in blood cells and plasma of dogs, *J. Nutr.,* 78, 167, 1962.

13. **Mohrhauer, H. and Holman, R. T.,** The effect of dietary essential fatty acids upon composition of polyunsaturated fatty acids in depot fat and erythrocytes of the rat, *J. Lipid Res.,* 4, 346, 1963.

14. **Bieri, J. G. and Poukka, R. K. H.,** Red cell content of vitamin E and fatty acids in normal subjects and patients with abnormal lipid metabolism, *Int. I. Vitam. Nutr.,* 40, 344, 1970.

ADDITIONAL REFERENCES

I. VITAMINS

Vitamin A (Retinol)

1. **Zaklama, M. S., Gabr, M. K., El Maraghy, S., and Patwardhan, V. N.,** Serum vitamin A in protein-calorie malnutrition, *Am. J. Clin. Nutr.,* 26, 1202, 1973.
2. **Glick, Z. and Reshef, A.,** Vitamin A status and related nutritional parameters of children in East Jerusalem, *Am. J. Clin. Nutr.,* 26, 1229, 1973.
3. **Smith, F. R., Goodman, D. S., Zaklama, M. S., Gabr, M. K., El Maraghy, S., and Patwardhan, V. N.,** Serum vitamin A, retinol-binding protein, and prealbumin concentrations in protein-calorie malnutrition. I. A functional defect in hepatic retinol release, *Am. J. Clin. Nutr.,* 26, 973, 1973.
4. **Smith, F. R., Goodman, D. S., Arroyave, G., and Viteri, F.,** Serum vitamin A, retinol-binding protein, and prealbumin concentrations in protein-calorie malnutrition. II. Treatment including supplemental vitamin A, *Am. J. Clin. Nutr.,* 26, 982, 1973.
5. **Mitchell, G. V., Young, M., and Seward, C. R.,** Vitamin A and carotene levels of a selected population in metropolitan Washington, D.C., *Am. J. Clin. Nutr.,* 26, 992, 1973.
6. **Bieri, J. G.,** Effects of excessive vitamins C and E on vitamin A status, *Am. J. Clin. Nutr.,* 26, 382, 1973.
7. **Russell, R. M., Multack, R., Smith, V., Krill, A., and Rosenberg, I. H.,** Subclinical vitamin A deficiency: the use of retinol function tests for diagnosis and evaluation of therapy, *Am. J. Clin. Nutr.,* 26, 463, 1973.
8. **Reddy, V. and Mohanram, M.,** Urinary excretion of lysosomal enzymes in hypovitaminosis and hypervitaminosis A in children, *Int. J. Vitam. Nutr. Res.,* 41, 321, 1971.
9. **Mohanram, M. and Reddy, V.,** Urinary excretion of acid mucopolysaccharides in kwashiorkor and vitamin A-deficient children, *Clin. Chim. Acta,* 34, 93, 1971.
10. **Kahan, J.,** Automated fluorometric assay of serum vitamin A, *Int. J. Vitam. Nutr. Res.,* 43, 127, 1973.
11. **De Luca, L. and Wolf, G.,** Vitamin A and mucus secretion, *Int. J. Vitam. Nutr. Res.,* 40, 284, 1970.
12. **Sundaresan, P. R.,** Recent advances in the metabolism of vitamin A, *J. Sci. Ind. Res.,* 31, 581, 1972.
13. **Hayes, K. C., McCombs, H. L., and Faherty, T. P.,** The fine structure of vitamin A deficiency. II. Arachnoid granulations and CSF pressure, *Brain,* 94, 213, 1971.
14. **Sinha, D. P. and Bang, F. B.,** Seasonal variation in signs of vitamin-A deficiency in rural West Bengal children, *Lancet,* 2, 228, 1973.
15. **Corey, J. E. and Hayes, K. C.,** Cerebrospinal fluid pressure, growth, and hematology in relation to retinol status of the rat in acute vitamin A deficiency, *J. Nutr.,* 102, 1585, 1972.
16. **Smith, J. C., Jr., McDaniel, E. G., Fan, F. F., and Halsted, J. A.,** Zinc: a trace element essential in vitamin A metabolism, *Science,* 181, 954, 1973.
17. **Olson, J. A.,** The biological role of vitamin A in maintaining epithelial tissues, *Isr. J. Med. Sci.,* 8, 1170, 1972.
18. **Olson, J. A.,** The prevention of childhood blindness by the administration of massive doses of vitamin A, *Isr. J. Med. Sci.,* 8, 1199, 1972.
19. **Varma, R. N. and Beaton, G. H.,** Quantitative aspects of the urinary and fecal excretion of radioactive metabolites of vitamin A in the rat, *Can. J. Physiol. Pharmacol.,* 50, 1026, 1972.
20. **Bashor, M. M., Toft, D. O., and Chytil, F.,** In vitro binding of retinol to rat-tissue components, *Proc. Natl. Acad. Sci. USA,* 70, 3483, 1973.
21. **Montes, L. F., Krumdieck, C., and Cornwell, P. E.,** Hypovitaminosis A in patients with mucocutaneous Candiasis, *J. Infect. Dis.,* 128, 227, 1973.
22. **Bubb, F. A. and Murphy, G. M.,** Determination of serum phytofluene and retinol, *Clin. Chim. Acta,* 48, 329, 1973.
23. **Pollack, J. D., Owen, G. M., Garry, P. J., and Clark, D.,** Plasma retinol assay by elution from silicic acid with cymene (p-isopropyl toluene), *Clin. Chem.,* 19, 977, 1973.
24. **Muto, Y., Smith, F. R., and Goodman, D. S.,** Comparative studies of retinol transport in plasma, *J. Lipid Res.,* 14, 525, 1973.
25. **Sundaresan, P. R. and Sundaresan, G. M.,** Studies on the urinary metabolites of retinoic acid in the rat, *Int. J. Vitam. Nutr. Res.,* 43, 61, 1973.
26. **Sundaresan, P. R. and Bhagavan, H. N.,** Metabolic studies on retinoic acid in the rat, *Biochem. J.,* 122, 1, 1971.
27. *The Prevention of Blindness,* report of a WHO Study Group, Geneva, Switzerland, November 6-10, 1972, WHO Tech. Rep. Ser. No. 518, Geneva, Switzerland, 1973.
28. *WHO Consultation on Prevention of Xerophthalmia in South-East Asia,* in Hyderabad, India, March 27-29, 1972, document no. NUTR/72.5, Nutrition, WHO, 1211 Geneva, Switzerland.
29. **Thompson, J. N., Erdody, P., and Maxwell, W. B.,** Simultaneous fluorometric determinations of vitamins A and E in human serum and plasma, *Biochem. Med.,* 8, 403, 1973.

Vitamin C (Ascorbic Acid)

1. McLeroy, V. J. and Schendel, H. E., Influence of oral contraceptives on ascorbic acid concentrations in healthy, sexually mature women, *Am. J. Clin. Nutr.,* 26, 191, 1973.
2. Goad, W. C., Skala, J. H., Harding, R. S., and Sauberlich, H. E., A semiautomated technique for the determination of vitamin C (ascorbic acid) in serum or plasma samples. Laboratory Report No. 337, September, 1973. U.S. Army Medical Research and Nutrition Laboratory, Fitzsimons Army Medical Center, Denver, CO, 80240.
3. Pelletier, O. and Brassard, R., A new automated method for serum vitamin C, *Advances in Automated Analysis,* 1972 Technicon Int. Cong. 9, 73, 1973, Mediad Inc., P.O. Box 417, Tarrytown, N.Y., 10591.
4. Croft, L. K., Davis, R. K., and Rose, M. E., Ascorbic acid status of the drug addict patient, *Am. J. Clin. Nutr.,* 26, 1042, 1973.
5. Yew, M. S. and Lo, Y., Levels of optimal vitamin C intake in individuals as estimated by the lingual tests, *Proc. Soc. Exp. Biol. Med.,* 144, 626, 1973.
6. Hankes, L. V., Leklem, J., Brown, R. R., Mekel, R. C., and Jansen, C. R., Abnormal tryptophan metabolism in patients with scurvy-type skin, *Biochem. Med.,* 7, 184, 1973.
7. Barnes, M. J. and Kodicek, E., Biological hydroxylations and ascorbic acid with special regard to collagen metabolism, *Vitam. Horm.,* 30, 1, 1972.
8. Schrauzer, G. N. and Rhead, W. J., Ascorbic acid abuse: effects of long term ingestion of excessive amounts on blood levels and urinary excretion, *Int. J. Vitam. Nutr. Res.,* 43, 201, 1973.
9. King, C. G., The biological synthesis of ascorbic acid, *World Rev. Nutr. Diet.,* 18, 47, 1973.
10. Lewin, S., Evaluation of potential effects of high intakes of ascorbic acid, *Comp. Biochem. Physiol.,* 46B, 427, 1973.
11. Ascorbic acid sulfate (AAS), A metabolite of ascorbic acid with antiscorbutic activity, *Nutr. Rev.,* 31, 251, 1973.

Thiamin (Vitamin B$_1$)

1. Cambier, J., Masson, M., Dairou, R., Delacoux, E., and Bournique, J., Evaluation biochimique de la carence en vitamine B$_1$. Etude de comparée de la pyruvicémie et de la transcétolase, *Ann. Med. Intern.,* 124, 189, 1973.
2. Bamji, M. S., Changes in hepatic and erythrocyte transketolase activity and thiamine concentration in liver in experimental deficiency of water soluble vitamins, *Int. J. Vitam. Nutr. Res.,* 42, 184, 1972.
3. Massod, M. F., McGuire, S. L., and Werner, K. R. Analysis of blood transketolase activity, *Am. J. Clin. Pathol.,* 55, 465, 1971.
4. Smeets, E. H. J., Muller, H., and De Wael, J., A NADH-dependent transketolase assay in erythrocyte hemolysates, *Clin. Chim. Acta,* 33, 379, 1971.
5. Hoffmann, I., Knapp, A., Rietz, K., and Milner, C., Die Bestimmung die Transketolase-Aktivitat im Blut, *Clin. Chim. Acta,* 33, 415, 1971.

Riboflavin

1. Rosenthal, W. S., Adham, N. F., Lopez, R., and Cooperman, J. M., Riboflavin deficiency in complicated chronic alcoholism, *Am. J. Clin. Nutr.,* 26, 858, 1973.
2. Sterner, R. T. and Price, W. R., Restricted riboflavin: within-subject behavioral effects in humans, *Am. J. Clin. Nutr.,* 26, 150, 1973.
3. Bamji, M. S., Sharada, D., and Naidu, A. N., A comparison of the fluorometric and microbiological assays for estimating riboflavin content of blood and liver, *Int. J. Vitam. Nutr. Res.,* 43, 351, 1973.
4. Mellor, N. P. and Maas, A. R., An automated fluorometric method for the determination of riboflavin in human urine, *Advances in Automated Analysis,* 1972 Technicon Int. Cong. 9 (Pharmaceutical Sciences), 67, 1973, Mediad Inc., P.O. Box 417, Tarrytown, N.Y., 10591.
5. Cooperman, J. M., Cole, H. S., Gordon, M., and Lopez, R., Erythrocyte glutathione reductase as a measure of riboflavin nutritional status of pregnant women and newborns, *Proc. Soc. Exp. Biol. Med.,* 143, 326, 1973.
6. Glatzle, D., Weiser, H., Weber, F., and Wiss, O., Correlations between riboflavin supply, glutathione reductase activities and flavin levels in rats, *Int. J. Vitam. Nutr. Res.,* 43, 187, 1973.
7. Shapiro, B. L., Smith, Q. T., and Warwick, W. J., Red cell glutathione and glutathione reductase in cystic fibrosis, *Proc. Soc. Exp. Biol. Med.,* 144, 181, 1973.
8. Frischer, H., Bowman, J. E., Carson, P. E., Rieckmann, K. H., Willerson, D., Jr., and Colwell, E. J., Erythrocytic glutathione reductase, glucose-6-phosphate dehydrogenase, and 6-phosphogluconic dehydrogenase deficiencies in populations of the United States, South Vietnam, Iran, and Ethiopia, *J. Lab. Clin. Med.,* 81, 603, 1973.
9. Benöhr, H. C., Lehmann, W., and Eriksson, A. W., Activation of red cell glutathione reductase by flavin-adenine-dinucleotide, *Klin. Wochenschr.,* 50, 462, 1972.

Vitamin B$_6$

1. Heller, S., Salkeld, R. M., and Körner, W. F., Vitamin B$_6$ status in pregnancy, *Am. J. Clin. Nutr.,* 26, 1339, 1973.
2. Salkeld, R. M., Knörr, K., and Körner, W. F., The effect of oral contraceptives on vitamin B$_6$ status, *Clin. Chim. Acta,* 49, 195, 1973.

3. **Luhby, A. L., Reyniak, J. V., Brin, M., Sambour, M., and Brin, H.,** Abnormal vitamin B_6 metabolism in menopausal women given estrogenic steroids and its correction by pyridoxine, *Am. J. Clin. Nutr.,* 26, 468, 1973.

4. **Gröbe, H.,** Homocystinurie, *Dtsch. Med. Wochenschr.,* 98, 1313, 1973.

5. **Pfeiffer, R., and Ebadi, M.,** On the mechanism of the nullification of CNS effects of L-DOPA by pyridoxine in Parkinsonian patients, *J. Neurochem.,* 19, 2175, 1972.

6. **Seashore, M. R., Durant, J. L., and Rosenberg, L. E.,** Studies of the mechanism of pyridoxine-responsive homocystinuria, *Pediatr. Res.,* 6, 187, 1972.

7. **Ebadi, M. S. and Costa, E., Ed.,** *Role of vitamin B_6 in neurobiology.* Advances in Biochemical Psychopharmacology. Vol. 4. Raven Press, New York, N.Y. 1972.

8. **Morrow, G., III and Barness, L. A.,** Combined vitamin responsiveness in homocystinuria, *J. Pediatr.,* 81, 946, 1972.

9. Vitamin B_6 deficiency in rats and the metabolism of O-phosphorylethanolamine, *Nutr. Rev.,* 31, 292, 1973.

10. **Gaull, G. E.,** Homocystinuria, vitamin B_6, and folate: metabolic interrelationships and clinical significance. *J. Pediatr.,* 81, 1014, 1972.

11. **Shelley, W. B., Rawnsley, H. M., and Morrow, G., III,** Pyridoxine-dependent hair pigmentation in association with homocystinuria, *Arch. Dermatol.,* 106, 228, 1972.

12. **Stoica, E., Meyer, J. S., Kawamura, Y., Hiromoto, H., Hashi, K., Aoyagi, M., and Pascu, I.,** Central neurogenic control of cerebral circulation. Effects of intravertebral injection of pyrithioxin on cerebral blood flow and metabolism, *Neurology,* 23, 687, 1973.

13. **Adams, P. W., Rose, D. P., Folkard, J., Wyn, V., Seed, M., and Strong, R.,** Effect of pyridoxine hydrochloride (vitamin B_6) upon depression associated with oral contraception, *Lancet,* 1, 898, 1973.

14. **Hall, C. D., Weiss, E. A., Morris, C. E., and Prange, A. J., Jr.,** Rapid deterioration in patients with Parkinsonism following tryptophan-pyridoxine administration, *Neurology,* 22, 231, 1972.

15. **Hsu, T. H., Bianchine, J. R., Preziosi, T. J., and Messiha, F. S.,** Effect of pyridoxine on Levodopa metabolism in normal and Parkinsonian subjects, *Proc. Soc. Exp. Biol. Med.,* 143, 578, 1973.

16. **Davis, R. E. and Smith, B. K.,** Pyridoxine and depression associated with oral contraception, *Lancet,* 1, 1245, (1973).

17. **Beaconsfield, P., Rainsbury, R., and Ginsburg, J.,** Correlation of experimental and clinical investigations of the pill, *Lancet,* 1, 1245, 1973.

18. **Horrigan, D. L.,** Pyridoxine-responsive anemia: Influence of tryptophan on pyridoxine responsiveness, *Blood,* 42, 187, (1973).

19. **Bremer, H. J. and Endres, W.,** Primary cystathioninuria: Methionine load tests and response to pyridoxine, *Helv. Paediatr. Acta,* 27, 525, 1972.

20. **Ury, A. G. and Chassy, J. R.** Increased activity of serum aspartate aminotransferase in the presence of added pyridoxal-5'-phosphate, *Clin. Chem.,* 19, 140, 1973.

21. **Morin, L. G. and Prox, J.,** Technical improvements in measurement of L-aspartate: 2-oxoglutarate aminotransferase activity in serum by diazonium salt coupling, *Clin. Chem.,* 19, 776, 1973.

Folacin (Folic Acid, Pteroylmonoglutamic Acid, Folate)

1. **Saraya, A. K., Choudhry, V. P., and Ghai, O. P.,** Interrelationships of vitamin B_{12}, folic acid, and iron in anemia of infancy and childhood: effect of vitamin B_{12} and iron therapy on folate metabolism, *Am. J. Clin. Nutr.,* 26, 640, 1973.

2. **Cowan, D. H. and Hines, J. D.,** Thrombokinetics in dietary-induced folate deficiency in human subjects, *J. Lab. Clin. Med.,* 81, 577, 1973.

3. **Kamen, B. A. and Caston, J. D.,** Direct radiochemical assay for serum folate: competition between ^{3}H-folic acid and 5-methyltetrahydrofolic acid for a folate binder, *J. Lab. Clin. Med.,* 83, 165, 1974.

4. **Skelley, D. S., Brown, L. P., and Besch, P. K.,** Radioimmunoassay, *Clin. Chem.,* 19, 146, 1973.

5. **O'Broin, J. D., Scott, J. M., and Temperley, I. J.,** A comparison of serum folate estimations using two different methods, *J. Clin. Pathol.,* 26, 80, 1973.

6. **Shaw, W.,** Radioassay of serum folate: some criticisms, *Clin. Chem.,* 19, 281, 1973.

7. **Rothenberg, S. P. and da Costa, M.,** Radioassay of folate, *Clin. Chem.,* 19, 785, 1973.

8. **Tajuddin, M. and Gardyna, H. A.,** Radioassay of serum folate, with use of a serum blank and nondialyzed milk as folate binder, *Clin. Chem.,* 19, 125, 1973.

9. **Eichner, E. R., Pierce, H. I., and Hillman, R. S.,** Folate balance in dietary-induced megaloblastic anemia, *N. Engl. J. Med.,* 284, 933, 1971.

10. **Eichner, E. R. and Hillman, R. S.,** Effect of alcohol on serum folate level, *J. Clin. Invest.,* 52, 584, 1973.

11. **Harrison, J. W., Sade, B. A., and Shaw, W.,** Relationships among urinary aminoimidozolecarboxamide in urine and folate, and vitamin B_{12} concentrations in serum, *Clin. Chem.,* 19, 1049, 1973.

12. **Rothenberg, S. P., da Costa, M., and Rosenberg, Z.,** A radioassay for serum folate: use of a two-phase sequential-incubation, ligand-binding system, *N. Engl. J. Med.,* 286, 1335, 1972.

13. **Dunn, R. T. and Foster, L. B.,** Radioassay of serum folate, *Clin. Chem.,* 19, 1101, 1973.

14. **Shojania, A. M. and Hornady, G. J.,** Oral contraceptives and folate absorption, *J. Lab. Clin. Med.,* 82, 869, 1973.

15. **Wilcken, B. and Turner, B.,** Homocystinuria. Reduced folate levels during pyridoxine treatment, *Arch. Dis. Child.,* 48, 58, 1973.

16. **Himes, R. H. and Harmony, J. A. K.,** Formyltetrahydrofolate synthetase, *CRC Crit. Rev. Biochem.,* 2, 501, 1973.

17. **Waxman, S. and Schreiber, C.,** Measurement of serum folate levels and serum folic acid-binding protein by ^{3}H-PGA radioassay, *Blood*, 42, 281, 1973.

18. **Waxman, S. and Schreiber, C.,** Characteristics of folic acid-binding protein in folate-deficient serum, *Blood,* 42, 291, 1973.

19. **Markkanen, T., Pajula, R.-L., Himanen, P., and Virtanen, S.,** Serum folic acid activity (*L. casei*) in Sephadex gel chromatography, *J. Clin. Pathol.,* 26, 486, 1973.

20. *Nutritional anaemias,* report of a WHO Group of experts, Geneva, Switzerland, October 11-15, 1971, WHO Tech. Rep. Ser. No. 503, Geneva, Switzerland, 1972.

21. **Da Costa, M. and Rothenberg, S. P.,** Appearance of a folate binder in leukocytes and serum of women who are pregnant or taking oral contraceptives, *J. Lab. Clin. Med.,* 83, 209, 1974.

Vitamin B$_{12}$ (Cyanocobalamin, Corrinoids)

1. **Alvarado, J., Vargas, W., Diaz, N., and Viteri, F. E.,** Vitamin B$_{12}$ absorption in protein-calorie malnourished children and during recovery: influence of protein depletion and of diarrhea, *Am. J. Clin. Nutr.,* 26, 595, 1973.

2. **Bernstein, L. and Herbert, V.,** The role of pancreatic exocrine secretions in the absorption of vitamin B$_{12}$ and iron, *Am. J. Clin. Nutr.,* 26, 341, 1973.

3. **Duran, M., Ketting, D., Wadman, S. K., Trijbels, J. M. F., Bakkeren, J. A. J. M., and Waelken, J. J. J.,** Propionic acid, an artefact which can leave methylmalonic acidemia undiscovered, *Clin. Chim. Acta,* 49, 177, 1973.

4. Procedures for the determination of vitamin B$_{12}$ levels in serum by competitive protein binding (1973), available from Schwarz/Mann, Mountain View Avenue, Orangeburg, N.Y. 10962.

5. **Frenkel, E. P., White, J. D., Reisch, J. S., and Sheehan, R. G.,** Comparison of two methods for radioassay of vitamin B$_{12}$ in serum, *Clin. Chem.,* 19, 1357, 1973.

6. **Gutcho, S., Johnson, J., and McCarter, H.,** Liquid-scintillation counting of (^{57}Co) − application to the radioassay of vitamin B$_{12}$, *Clin. Chem.,* 19, 998, 1973.

7. **Rothenberg, S. P.,** Application of competitive ligand binding for the radioassay of vitamin B$_{12}$ and folic acid, *Metabolism,* 22, 1075, 1973.

8. **Davis, R. E., Moulton, J., and Kelly, A.,** An automated microbiological method for the measurement of vitamin B$_{12}$, *J. Clin. Pathol.,* 26, 494, 1973.

9. **Desai, H. G. and Antia, F. P.,** Vitamin B$_{12}$ malabsorption due to intrinsic factor deficiency in Indian subjects, *Blood,* 40, 747, 1972.

10. **Van Der Weyden, M. B., Rother, M., and Firkin, B. G.,** The metabolic significance of reduced serum B$_{12}$ in folate deficiency, *Blood,* 40, 23, 1972.

11. *Nutritional anaemias,* report of a WHO Group of experts, Geneva, Switzerland, October 11-15, 1971, WHO Tech. Rep. Ser. No. 503, Geneva, Switzerland, 1972.

Vitamin E (Tocopherol)

1. **Thompson, J. N., Beare-Rogers, J. L., Erdody, P., and Smith, D. C.,** Appraisal of human vitamin E requirements based on examination of individual meals and a composite Canadian diet, *Am. J. Clin. Nutr.,* 26, 1349, 1973.

2. **Lewis, J. S., Pian, A. K., Baer, M. T., Acosta, P. B., and Emerson, G. A.,** Effect of long-term ingestion of polyunsaturated fat, age, plasma cholesterol, diabetes mellitus, and supplemental tocopherol upon plasma tocopherol, *Am. J. Clin. Nutr.,* 26, 136, 1973.

3. **Ramirez, I., Santini, R., Corcino, J., and Santiago, P. J.,** Serum vitamin E levels in children and adults with tropical sprue in Puerto Rico, *Am. J. Clin. Nutr.,* 26, 1045, 1973.

4. **Carpenter, M.,** Vitamin E and microsomal drug hydroxylations, *Ann. N.Y. Acad. Sci.,* 203, 81, 1972.

5. **Witting, L. A.,** The recommended dietary allowance for vitamin E, *Am. J. Clin. Nutr.,* 25, 257, 1972.

6. **Fujii, T. and Shimizu, H.,** Investigation on serum lipid components and serum vitamin E in iron deficiency anemia, *J. Nutr. Sci. Vitaminol.,* 19, 23, 1973.

7. **Kayden, H. J., Chow, C-K., and Bjornson, L. K.,** Spectrophotometric method for determination of tocopherol in red blood cells, *J. Lipid Res.,* 14, 533, 1973.

8. **Thompson, J. N., Erdody, P., and Maxwell, W. B.,** Simultaneous fluorometric determinations of vitamins A and E in human serum and plasma, *Biochem. Med.,* 8, 403, 1973.

Vitamin D

1. **Palmisano, P. A.,** Vitamin D: A reawakening, *J.A.M.A.,* 224, 1526, 1973.

2. **Avioli, L. V. and Haddad, J. G.,** Progress in endocrinology and metabolism. Vitamin D: Current concepts, *Metabolism,* 22, 507, 1973.

3. **Haddad, J. G., Jr., Chyu, K. J., Hahn, T. J., and Stamp, T. C. B.,** Serum concentration of 25-hydroxyvitamin D in sex-linked hypophosphatemic vitamin D-resistant rickets, *J. Lab. Clin. Med.,* 81, 23, 1973.

4. Haddad, J. G., Jr. and Hahn, T. J., Natural and synthetic sources of circulating 25-hydroxyvitamin D in man, *Nature,* 244, 515, 1973.
5. Belsey, R., De Luca, H. F., and Potts, J. T., Jr., Competitive binding assay for vitamin D and 25-OH vitamin D. *Calcium, Parathyroid Hormone and the Calcitonins,* Talmage, R. V., and Munson, P. L., Eds., Excerpta Medica, Amsterdam, 1972, p. 237.

Vitamin K
1. Burdick, C. O., Partial thromboplastin time in heparin therapy, *Am. J. Clin. Pathol.,* 55, 384, 1971.
2. Quick, A. J., Prothrombin time standardization, *Am. J. Clin. Pathol.,* 55, 385, 1971.
3. Morse, E. E., Panek, S., and Menga, R., Automated fibrinogen determination, *Am. J. Clin. Pathol.,* 55, 671, 1971.

Pantothenic Acid
1. Markkanen, T., The metabolic significance of pantothenic acid as assessed by its levels in serum in various clinical and experimental conditions, *Int. J. Vitam. Nutr. Res.,* 43, 302, 1973.

Miscellaneous: General
1. Guthrie, H. A., Owen, G. M., and Guthrie, G. M., Factor analysis of measures of nutritional status of preschool children, *Am. J. Clin. Nutr.,* 26, 497, 1973.
2. Chase, H. P., Larson, L. B., Massoth, D. M., Martin, D. L., and Niernberg, M. M., Effectiveness of nutrition aides in a migrant population, *Am. J. Clin. Nutr.,* 26, 849, 1973.
3. Silink, S. J., Nobile, S., and Woodhill, J. M., Nutrition in the elderly: Clinical and biochemical assessment of nutritional status, *J. Geriatr.,* 3, 27, 1972.
4. Woodhill, J. M. and Nobile, S., Nutrition in the elderly: Calories, protein and vitamin C, *J. Geriatr.,* 3, 35, 1972.
5. Eichner, E. R. and Hillman, R. S., The evolution of anemia in alcoholic patients, *Am. J. Med.,* 50, 218, 1971.
6. Eichner, E. R., Buchanan, B., Smith, J. W., and Hillman, R. S., Variations in the hematologic and medical status of alcoholics, *Am. J. Med. Sci.,* 263, 35, 1972.
7. Nutrition Canada: National Survey (1973), Catalogue No. H58-36/1973, Information Canada, 171 Slater Street, Ottawa, Canada.
8. Ryabinin, I. F., Study of the vitamin C, B_1, B_2, B_6, PP balance in men in the Mirny station in Antarctica, *Nahrung,* 16, 617, 1972.
9. Scriver, C. R., Progress in endocrinology and metabolism: Vitamin-responsive inborn errors of metabolism, *Metabolism,* 22, 1319, 1973.
10. Recommended Daily Dietary Allowances, Revised 1973, Food and Nutrition Board, National Academy of Sciences-National Research Council, Washington, D.C. 20418.
11. Greene, H. L., Vitamins in total parenteral nutrition, *Drug Intell. Clin. Pharm.,* 6, 355, 1972.
12. *Symposium on Total Parenteral Nutrition,* Nashville, TN, January 17-19, 1972, Council on Foods and Nutrition, American Medical Association, 535 North Dearborn Street, Chicago, Ill. 60610.
13. Harper, A. E., Recommended Dietary Allowances (Revised — 1973), *Nutr. Rev.,* 31, 393, 1973.

II. PROTEIN-CALORIE MALNUTRITION

1. Ratnakar, K. S., Emanuel, V., and Ramachandraiah, U., Nonspecific protective substances of serum in protein deficiency: an in vitro experimental study, *Am. J. Clin. Nutr.,* 26, 571, 1973.
2. Malcolm, L. A., Balasubramaniam, E., and Edwards, G., Effect of protein supplementation on the hair of chronically malnourished New Guinean schoolchildren, *Am. J. Clin. Nutr.,* 26, 479, 1973.
3. Singh, P. I., Sood, S. C., and Saini, A. S., Plasma nonessential to essential amino acid ratio in marasmus, *Am. J. Clin. Nutr.,* 26, 484, 1973.
4. Said, A., El-Hawary, M. F. S., Sakr, R., Aldel Khalek, M. K., and Ibrahim, A. M., Protein-calorie malnutrition in Egypt. I. Immunoelectrophoretic studies on urinary proteins, *Am. J. Clin. Nutr.,* 26, 1355, 1973.
5. Gurney, J. M. and Jelliffe, D. B., Arm anthropometry in nutritional assessment: nomogram for rapid calculation of muscle circumference and cross-sectional muscle and fat areas, *Am. J. Clin. Nutr.,* 26, 912, 1973.
6. Sigulem, D. M., Brasel, J. A., Velasco, E. G., Rosso, P., and Winick, M., Plasma and urine ribonuclease as a measure of nutritional status in children, *Am. J. Clin. Nutr.,* 26, 793, 1973.
7. Ritchey, S. J., Derise, N. L., Abernathy, R. P., and Korslund, M. K., Variability of creatinine excretion in preadolescent girls consuming a wide range of dietary nitrogen, *Am. J. Clin. Nutr.,* 26, 690, 1973.
8. Weller, L. A., Margen, S., Calloway, D. H., and Meissner, E. F., Serum amino acids in young men consuming diets differing in level and pattern of amino acids, *Am. J. Clin. Nutr.,* 26, 722, 1973.
9. Mikhail, M. M., Patwardhan, V. N., and Waslien, C. I., Plasma and red blood cell amino acids of Egyptian children suffering from protein-calorie malnutrition, *Am. J. Clin. Nutr.,* 26, 387, 1973.
10. Paolucci, A. M., Spadoni, M. A., and Pennetti, V., Modifications of serum-free amino acid patterns of Babinga adult pygmies after short-term feeding of a balanced diet, *Am. J. Clin. Nutr.,* 26, 429, 1973.

11. **Cabacungan, N. B., Miles, C. W., Abernathy, R. P., and Ritchey, S. J.,** Hydroxyproline excretion and nutritional status of children, *Am. J. Clin. Nutr.,* 26, 173, 1973.

12. **Hoeldtke, R. D. and Wurtman, R. J.,** Excretion of catecholamines and catecholamine metabolites in kwashiorkor, *Am. J. Clin. Nutr.,* 26, 205, 1973.

13. **Loewenstein, M. S. and Phillips, J. F.,** Evaluation of arm circumference measurement for determining nutritional status of children and its use in an acute epidemic of malnutrition: Owerri, Nigeria, following the Nigerian Civil War, *Am. J. Clin. Nutr.,* 26, 226, 1973.

14. **Golderg, M. and Sardi, A.,** Serum globulin assay, *Clin. Chem.,* 19, 292, 1973.

15. **Habicht, J. P., Schwedes, J. A., Arroyave, A., and Klein, R. E.,** Biochemical indices of nutrition reflecting ingestion of a high protein supplement in rural Guatemalan children, *Am. J. Clin. Nutr.,* 26, 1046, 1973.

16. **Simmons, W. K.,** Biochemical measurements in the assessment of the protein nutrition status, *Arch. Latinoamericanos Nutr.,* 22, 385, 1972.

17. **Korte, R., Wiersinga, A., and Simmons, W. K.,** The use of osmolarity in lieu of creatinine to express urinary rations in nutritional field studies, *Arch. Latinoamericanos Nutr.,* 21, 139, 1971.

18. **Kumar, V., Chase, H. P., Hammond, K., and O'Brien, D.,** Alterations in blood biochemical tests in progressive protein malnutrition, *Pediatrics,* 49, 736, 1972.

19. **McLaren, D. S. and Read, W. W. C.,** Classification of nutritional status in early childhood, *Lancet,* 2, 146, 1972.

20. **Swendseid, M. E. and Kopple, J. D.,** Nitrogen balance, plasma amino acid levels, and amino acid requirements, *Trans. N.Y. Acad. Sci.,* 35, 471, 1973.

21. **Yoshimura, H.,** Physiological effect of protein deficiency with special reference to evaluation of protein nutrition and protein requirement, *World Rev. Nutr. Diet.,* 14, 100, 1972.

22. Hormones, amino acids, and malnutrition, *Nutr. Rev.,* 31, 306, 1973.

23. Leukocyte and placental metabolism as indices of fetal malnutrition, *Nutr. Rev.,* 31, 315, 1973.

24. **Gold, R. J. M. and Scriver, C. R.,** The amino acid composition of hair from different racial origins, *Clin. Chim. Acta,* 33, 465, 1971.

25. **Kulkarni, M. and Kilgore, L.,** Diurnal variations of hydroxyproline and creatinine excretion in children, *Am. J. Clin. Nutr.,* 26, 1069, 1973.

26. **Kyaw, A. and Hla-Pe, U.,** A more efficient oxidizing system for hydroxyproline assay, *Clin. Chem.,* 19, 1415, 1973.

27. **Statland, B. E., Winkel, P., and Bokelund, H.,** Factors contributing to intra-individual variation of serum constituents: 2. Effects of exercise and diet on variation of serum constituents in healthy subjects, *Clin. Chem.,* 19, 1380, 1973.

28. **Harper, A. E., Payne, P. R., and Waterlow, J. C.,** Assessment of human protein needs, *Am. J. Clin. Nutr.,* 26, 1168, 1973.

29. **Armstrong, M. D. and Stave, U.,** A study of plasma free amino acid levels. I. Study of factors affecting validity of amino acid analysis, *Metabolism,* 22, 549, 1973.

30. **Armstrong, M. D. and Stave, U.,** A study of plasma free amino acid levels. II. Normal values for children and adults, *Metabolism,* 22, 561, 1973.

31. **Armstrong, M. D. and Stave, U.,** A study of plasma free amino acid levels. III. Variations during growth and aging, *Metabolism,* 22, 571, 1973.

32. **Armstrong, M. D. and Stave, U.,** A study of plasma free amino acid levels. IV. Characteristic individual levels of the amino acids, *Metabolism,* 22, 821, 1973.

33. **Armstrong, M. D. and Stave, U.,** A study of plasma free amino acid levels. V. Correlations among the amino acids and some other blood constituents, *Metabolism,* 22, 827, 1973.

34. **Knudsen, J. J., Skala, J. H., and Sauberlich, H. E.,** A semi-automated method for the determination of total nitrogen in urine, feces and diets, U.S. Army Medical Research and Nutrition Laboratory Report, September 1973, U.S. Army Medical Research and Nutrition Laboratory, Fitzsimons Army Medical Center, Denver, CO 80240.

III. MINERAL NUTRITION

1. **Caddell, J. L., Ratananon, N., and Trangratapit, P.,** Parenteral magnesium load tests in postpartum Thai women, *Am. J. Clin. Nutr.,* 26, 612, 1973.

2. **Irwin, M. I. and Kienholz, E. W.,** Monograph: A conspectus of research on calcium requirements of man, *J. Nutr.,* 103, 1019, 1973.

3. **Valyasevi, A., Dhanamitta, S., and Van Reen, R.,** Studies of bladder stone disease in Thailand. XVI. Effect of 4-hydroxy-L-proline and orthophosphate supplementations on urinary composition and crystalluria, *Am. J. Clin. Nutr.,* 26, 1207, 1973.

4. **Hambidge, K. M.,** Increase in hair copper concentration with increasing distance from the scalp, *Am. J. Clin. Nutr.,* 26, 1212, 1973.

5. **Sandstead, H. H.,** Zinc as an unrecognized limiting nutrient, *Am. J. Clin. Nutr.,* 26, 790, 1973.

6. **Butler, L. C. and Daniel, J. M.,** Copper metabolism in young women fed two levels of copper and two protein sources, *Am. J. Clin. Nutr.,* 26, 744, 1973.

7. **Nomoto, S., Decsy, M. I., Murphy, J. R., and Sunderman, F. W., Jr.,** Isolation of [63]Ni-labeled nickeloplasmin from rabbit serum, *Biochem. Med.,* 8, 171, 1973.

8. **Hadded, J. G., Jr., Chyu, K. J., Hahn, T. J., and Stamp, T. C. B.,** Serum concentration of 25-hydroxyvitamin D in sex-linked hypophosphatemic vitamin D-resistant rickets, *J. Lab. Clin. Med.,* 81, 23, 1973.
9. **Halsted, J. A. and Smith, J. C., Jr.,** Plasma zinc in health and disease, *Lancet,* 1, 322, 1970.
10. **Steele, T. H.,** Dissociation of zinc excretion from other cations in man, *J. Lab. Clin. Med.,* 81, 205, 1973.
11. **Sandstead, H. H.,** Zinc nutrition in the United States, *Am. J. Clin. Nutr.,* 26, 1251, 1971.
12. **Nielsen, F. H.,** "Newer" trace elements in human nutrition, *Food Technol.,* 28, 38, 1974.
13. **Reinhold, J. G., Lahimgarzadeh, A., Nasr, K., and Hedayati, H.,** Effect of purified phytate and phytate-rich bread upon metabolism of zinc, calcium, phosphorus, and nitrogen in man, *Lancet,* 1, 283, 1973.
14. **Fell, G. S., Cuthbertson, D. P., Morrison, C., Fleck, A., Queen, K., Bessent, R. G., and Husain, S. L.,** Urinary zinc levels as an indication of muscle catabolism, *Lancet,* 1, 280, 1973.
15. **Mazess, R. B., Cameron, J. R., and Miller, H.,** Direct readout of bone mineral content using radionuclide absorptiometry, *Int. J. Appl. Radiat. Isot.,* 23, 471, 1972.
16. **Fox, M. R. S.,** The status of zinc in human nutrition, *World Rev. Nutr. Diet.,* 12, 208, 1970.
17. **Betro, M. G. and Pain, R. W.,** Hypophosphataemia and hyperphosphataemia in a hospital population, *Br. Med. J.,* 1, 273, 1972.
18. **Hohnadel, D. C., Sunderman, F. W., Jr., Nechay, M. W., and McNeely, M. D.,** Atomic absorption spectrometry of nickel, copper, zinc, and lead in sweat collected from healthy subjects during sauna bathing, *Clin. Chem.,* 19, 1288, 1973.
19. **Statland, B. E., Winkel, P., and Bokelund, H.,** Factors contributing to intra-individual variation of serum constituents: 1. Within-day variation of serum constituents in healthy subjects, *Clin. Chem.,* 19, 1374, 1973.
20. **Epstein, S., Mieghem, W. V., Sagel, J., and Jackson, W. P. U.,** Effect of single large doses of oral calcium on serum calcium levels in the young and the elderly, *Metabolism,* 22, 1163, 1973.
21. *Zinc in Human Nutrition,* Summary of workshop proceedings, December 4-5, 1970, Food and Nutrition Board, National Research Council, Washington, D.C. 20418.
22. **Delves, H. T.,** The determination of trace elements and their significance in clinical chemistry, *At. Absorption Newsletter,* 12, 50, 1973.

IV. IRON DEFICIENCY

1. **Seelig, M. S.,** Proposed role of copper-molybdenum interaction in iron-deficiency and iron-storage diseases, *Am. J. Clin. Nutr.,* 26, 657, 1973.
2. **Basu, R. N., Sood, S. K., Ramachandran, K., Mathur, M., and Ramalingaswami, V.,** Etiopathogenesis of nutritional anemia in pregnancy: a therapeutic approach, *Am. J. Clin. Nutr.,* 26, 591, 1973.
3. **Bollet, A. J. and Owens, S.,** Evaluation of nutritional status of selected hospitalized patients, *Am. J. Clin. Nutr.,* 26, 931, 1973.
4. **Chang, L. L.,** Tissue storage iron in Singapore, *Am. J. Clin. Nutr.,* 26, 952, 1973.
5. **Elwood, P. C.,** Evaluation of the clinical importance of anemia, *Am. J. Clin. Nutr.,* 26, 958, 1973.
6. **Wise, W. R., Skala, J. H., and Sauberlich, H. E.,** Automated determination of iron in biological materials. Laboratory Report No. 341, September 1973, U.S. Army Medical Research and Nutrition Laboratory, Fitzsimons Army Medical Center, Denver, CO 80240.
7. **Piomelli, S.,** A Micromethod for free erythrocyte porphyrins: The FEP test, *J. Lab. Clin. Med.,* 81, 932, 1973.
8. **Porter, F. S.,** The effect of iron content on the behavior of human ferritin in an inhibition-type radioimmunoassay, *J. Lab. Clin. Med.,* 83, 147, 1974.
9. **Bainton, D. F. and Finch, C. A.,** The diagnosis of iron deficiency anemia, *Am. J. Med.,* 37, 62, 1964.
10. **White, J. W. and Flashka, H. A.,** An automated procedure, with use of ferrozine, for assay of serum iron and total iron-binding capacity, *Clin. Chem,* 19, 526, 1973.
11. **Olsen, E. D., Jatlow, P. I., Fernandez, F. J., and Kahn, H. L.,** Ultramicro method for determination of iron in serum with the graphite furnace, *Clin. Chem.,* 19, 326, 1973.
12. **Mayet, F. G. H., Adams, E. B., Moodley, T., Kleber, E. E., and Cooper, S. K.,** Dietary iron and anaemia in an Indian community in Natal, *S. Afr. Med. J.,* 46, 1427, 1972.
13. **Langer, E. E., Haining, R. G., Labbe, R. F., Jacobs, P., Crosby, E. F., and Finch, C. A.,** Erythrocyte protoporphyrin, *Blood,* 40, 112, 1972.
14. *Extent and Meanings of Iron Deficiency in the U.S.,* Summary of workshop proceedings, March 8-9, 1971, Food and Nutrition Board, National Research Council, Washington, D.C. 20418.
15. *Nutritional anaemias,* report of a WHO Group of experts, Geneva, Switzerland, October 11-15, 1971. WHO Tech. Rep. Ser. No. 503, Geneva, Switzerland, 1972.

V. IODINE DEFICIENCY

1. **Ingenbleek, Y. and Beckers, C.,** Evidence for intestinal malabsorption of iodine in protein-calorie malnutrition, *Am. J. Clin. Nutr.,* 26, 1323, 1973.

2. **Koutras, D. A., Christakis, G., Trichopoulos, D., Dakou-Voutetaki, A., Kyriakopoulos, V., Fontanares, P., Livadas, D. P., Gatsios, D., and Malamos, B.,** Endemic goiter in Greece: nutritional status, growth, and skeletal development of goitrous and nongoitrous populations, *Am. J. Clin. Nutr.,* 26, 1360, 1973.

3. **Trowbridge, F. L., Matovinovic, J., and Nichaman, M. Z.,** Goiter prevalence and iodine status of children, *Am. J. Clin. Nutr.,* 26, 461, 1973.

4. **Frey, H. M. M., Rosenlund, B., and Torgersen, T. P.,** Value of single urine specimens in estimation of 24 hour urine iodine excretion, *Acta Endocrinol.,* 72, 287, 1973.

5. **Mantel, M.,** Improved method for the determination of iodine in urine, *Clin. Chim. Acta,* 33, 39, 1971.

6. **Garry, P. J., Lashley, D. W., and Owen, G. M.,** Automated measurement of urinary iodine, *Clin. Chem.,* 19, 950, 1973.

7. *Iodine Nutriture in the United States,* Summary of workshop proceedings, October 31, 1970, Food and Nutrition Board, National Research Council, Washington, D.C. 20418.

VI. ESSENTIAL FATTY ACID DEFICIENCY

1. **Helmkamp, G. M., Wilmore, D. W., Johnson, A. A., and Pruitt, B. A.,** Essential fatty acid deficiency in red cells after thermal injury: correction with intravenous fat therapy, *Am. J. Clin. Nutr.,* **26, 1331, 1973.**

INDEX

erythrocyte glutathione reductase activity, relation to, 33–35
  determination of, 33, 34
  guideline for interpretation of, 34
urinary excretion of, 30–35
  determination of, 32
  guidelines for interpretatin of, 30–32
  load test, 31–33

T

Thiamin, 22–30
  body levels of, 26
  carbohydrate index in relation to, 26
  deficiency of, manifestations, 22
  erythrocyte transketolase activity, relation to, 25, 26
    determination of, 25, 26
    guidelines for interpretation of, 25
  urinary excretion of, 22–25
    determination of, 22
    guidelines for interpretation of, 23, 24
    load tests, 24, 25
Tocopherol, *see* Vitamin E

V

Vitamin A, 4–13
  deficiency of, clinical manifestations, 4, 6
  determination in serum (or plasma), 6, 7
  functions, 4
  guidelines for interpretation of biochemical data, 7, 8
  levels in serum (or plasma), 4–8
  metabolites of, in urine, 9
  retinal evaluation of deficiency of, 4, 6–8
  retinol binding protein, 9
  storage of, 4, 5
Vitamin B_1, *see* Thiamin
Vitamin B_6, 37–49
  blood levels of, 42, 43
    determination of, in serum (or plasma), 43
    guideline for interpretation of, tentative, 42
  blood transaminase activities, relation to, 41–43
    determination of, 43
    erythrocyte transaminase index, derived, 42, 43

metabolites of, in urire, 41, 42
  guideline for interpretation of excretion of 4-pyrodoxic acid in, tentative, 42
methionine load test, 43, 44
tryptophan load test, relation to, 38–40, 42
  determination of metabolites resulting from, 39
  guideline for interpretation of, tentative, 42
  method for, 38
urinary excretion of, 39–42
  determination of, 40, 41
  guideline for interpretation of, tentative, 41, 42
Vitamin B_{12}, 60–70
  deficiency of, clinical and hematological changes, 60, 61
  determination of, in serum, 61
  guidelines for interpretation of serum levels of, 61, 62
  levels in serum, 61, 62
  malabsorption of, 60, 64
    pernicious anemia, distinction from, 64
  methylmalonic acid excretion, relation to, 62–64
    determination of, 63, 64
Vitamin C, 13–22
  body pools of, 13
  determination of, in serum or plasma, 17, 18
  functions of, 13
  guidelines for interpretation of biochemical data, 15, 16
  leucocyte levels of, 15, 16
    determination of, 16
  lingual evaluation of (statas), 18
  metabolites of, 17
  saturation tests, 17
  serum of plasma levels of, 13–17
  tissue levels, 15
  urinary excretion of, 16, 17
  whole blood levels of, 15–17
Vitamin D, 80–83
  alkaline phosphatase in serum, relation to, 80, 81
  calcium in serum, relation to, 81, 82
  epiphyseal enlargement, due to, 82
  phosphorus in serum, relation to, 81, 82
Vitamin E, 74–80
  deficiency of, biochemical changes, 74, 75
  determination of, in blood, 76
  guidelines for interpretation of serum levels and hemolysis test for, 76, 77
  hemolysis test for deficiency of, 75, 76
  levels in blood and blood components, 76, 77
Vitamin K, 83–88
  diagnostic tests for deficiency of, 84–87
    clotting time, 86
    quick one-stage prothrombin time, 84